Neonatal and Pediatric Respiratory Medicine

Butterworths International Medical Reviews

Pediatrics

Published titles

1 Hematology and Oncology
Michael Willoughby and Stuart E. Siegel

2 Perinatal Medicine
Robert Boyd and Frederick C. Battaglia

Next title

Genetic and Metabolic Disease in Pediatrics
June K. Lloyd and Charles R. Scriver

Neonatal and Pediatric Respiratory Medicine

Edited by

Anthony D. Milner, MD, FRCP, DCH
Professor of Paediatric Respiratory Medicine, Department of Child Health,
Queen's Medical Centre, Nottingham, UK

and

Richard J. Martin, MB, FRACP
Associate Professor of Pediatrics, Department of Pediatrics, Rainbow Babies and
Children's Hospital, Case Western Reserve University, Cleveland, Ohio, USA

Butterworths
London Boston Durban Singapore Sydney Toronto Wellington

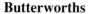

First published 1985

© Butterworth & Co. (Publishers) Ltd. 1985

British Library Cataloguing in Publication Data

Neonatal and pediatric respiratory medicine.–
(Butterworths international medical reviews/
Pediatrics, ISSN 0260-0161; 4)
1. Pediatric respiratory diseases
I. Milner, Anthony D.   II. Martin, Richard J.
618.9′22   RJ431

ISBN 0-407-02311-9

Photoset by Butterworths Litho Preparation Department
Printed and bound in England by Robert Hartnoll Ltd., Bodmin, Cornwall

Preface

In compiling this volume we invited experts from North America, the United Kingdom and Australia to write articles reviewing topics in paediatric respiratory medicine, encouraging them to provide clear personal statements with the clinician in mind. The subjects have been chosen on the grounds that they are either controversial or have changed rapidly in the last few years. This selection process obviously rests on the interests of the two editors to some extent but we hope that the ground covered, although far from comprehensive, will be of interest to neonatal, pulmonary and general paediatricians alike.

Finally, we would like to thank all the contributors for their support and time and hope that they are as pleased with the final result as we are.

A. Milner
R. Martin

Contributors

Eduardo Bancalari, MD
Professor of Pediatrics and Director, Division of Neonatology, University of Miami
School of Medicine, Miami, Florida, USA

Waldemar A. Carlo, MD
Assistant Professor of Pediatrics, Department of Pediatrics, Rainbow Babies and
Children's Hospital, Case Western Reserve University, Cleveland, Ohio, USA

Ivan D. Frantz III, MD
Associate Professor of Pediatrics, Tufts University School of Medicine; Director,
Tufts Affiliated Programs in Newborn Medicine, Boston, Massachusetts, USA

Joan E. Hodgman, MD
Professor of Pediatrics, University of Southern California; Director, Newborn
Service, Los Angeles County, University of Southern California Medical Center,
Los Angeles, California, USA

Richard J. Martin, MB, FRACP
Associate Professor of Pediatrics, Department of Pediatrics, Rainbow Babies and
Children's Hospital, Case Western Reserve University, Cleveland, Ohio, USA

Anthony D. Milner, MD, FRCP, DCH
Professor of Paediatric Respiratory Medicine, Department of Child Health,
Queen's Medical Centre, Nottingham UK

Jacqueline Y. Q. Mok, MD, MRCPE
Senior Registrar, Royal Hospital for Sick Children, Edinburgh, UK

Anthony Olinsky, MB, BCh, DipPaed, FCPSA, FRACP
Director, Professorial Department of Thoracic Medicine, Royal Children's
Hospital, Parkville, Victoria, Australia

Contributors

Peter D. Phelan, BSc, MD, FRACP
Professor of Paediatrics, Department of Paediatrics, University of Melbourne, Parkville, Victoria, Australia

Don M. Roberton, MD, FRACP
Immunologist and Senior Lecturer in Paediatrics, Royal Children's Hospital, Victoria, Australia

Michael Silverman, MD, FRCP
Senior Lecturer in Paediatrics, Department of Paediatrics and Neonatal Medicine, Royal Postgraduate Medical School, Hammersmith Hospital, London, UK

Hamish Simpson, RD, MD, FRCPE, DCH
Professor of Child Health, University of Leicester, Leicester Royal Infirmary, Leicester, UK

Harish Vyas, MRCP
MRC Research Fellow, Department of Child Health, Queen's Medical Centre, Nottingham, UK

Robert W. Wilmott, BSc, MD, MRCP
Director of Pulmonology, Children's Hospital of Philadelphia; Assistant Professor, Department of Pediatrics, University of Pennsylvania, Philadelphia, Pennsylvania, USA

Nicola Wilson, MB, BS, DCH
Clinical Lecturer in Paediatrics, Department of Paediatrics and Neonatal Medicine, Royal Postgraduate Medical School, Hammersmith Hospital, London, UK

Robert E. Wood,, PhD, MD
Associate Professor of Pediatrics and Chief, Pediatric Pulmonary Medicine, University of North Carolina, Chapel Hill, North Carolina, USA

Contents

1
Resuscitation of the newborn

A. D. Milner and H. Vyas

HISTORICAL BACKGROUND

The transition from a fluid environment to an air milieu makes birth the most perilous time in a human life. Clement Smith (1967) called this hazardous period 'The Valley of the Shadow of Birth'. Failure to adapt rapidly leads to birth asphyxia and its dire consequences. This high risk situation has been recognized for a long time. Our first report on sudden death from respiratory failure in newborn infants dates back to H Wang T (2698–2599 BC), an Emperor of China. References to increased respiratory problems were also made in *Eber's Papyrus* (Egypt, circa 1552 BC). The first description of active intervention, presumably an active form of mouth-to-mouth ventilation, is to be found in the Old Testament:

> 'And he went up, and lay upon the child, and put his mouth upon his mouth, and his eyes lay upon his eyes, and his hands upon his hands: He stretched himself upon the child; and the flesh of the child waxed warm. Then he returned, and walked in the home to and fro; and went up and stretched himself upon him; and the child sneezed seven times, and the child opened his eyes'.
>
> II Kings, Chapter 4, Verses 34–35

By the fifth century BC the Chinese were managing respiratory failure by 'counter irritation'. Soon after, Hippocrates (circa 400 BC) described experimental endotracheal intubation. The Babylonian Talmud expounded on the concepts of resuscitation for the newborn, later to be written up by Moses Maimonides. Although Vesalius (1514–1569 AD) used tracheotomy for ventilatory support in a sow, it was Robert Hook in 1667 who demonstrated that it was possible to keep animals alive with mechanical ventilation for a long period. Robert Boyle (1670) performed further studies on asphyxiated kittens, giving a clear account of both resuscitation ('pinching') and primary apnoea.

Chaussier gave the final detailed description of endotracheal intubation of asphyxiated infants in 1806 (Faulconer and Keys, 1965). By the early nineteenth century mouth-to-mouth breathing was a common way of resuscitation in adults, but in 1812 the Royal Humane Society put an end to this by publishing a health warning in their annual report. The authors of the report felt that a mouthful of air used was: 'chiefly carbonic, or what arises from burning charcoal and more likely to

1

destroy than to promote the action of the lungs'. This Society did, however, redeem itself to some extent by sponsoring the development of an intermittent positive pressure ventilator in 1845.

Although Billard's textbook of paediatrics (Billard, 1828) was retrogressive, recommending blood-letting and leeches, Evanson and Maunsell (1842) were still using mouth-to-mouth breathing in asphyxiated neonates. They describe a 'sthenic' type of asphyxia in which the infant had a good pulse and an 'asthenic' type in which the baby was virtually moribund. The description of the technique they used is a joy to read and they concluded: 'the disadvantages of using air already deteriorated by having been respired is more than counterbalanced by the other advantages of this plan'. However, their excellent advice went unheeded and there followed a whole variety of procedures recommended, including the use of slapping (still practised), tickling, applying hot and cold water and even tongue pulling!

As mentioned earlier, intermittent positive pressure ventilation had already been used in the second half of the nineteenth century. Truehead (1869) and O'Dwyer (1887) demonstrated that intubation and intermittent positive pressure ventilation could be successfully used to manage childhood respiratory failure. Egon Braun in Vienna (Doe, 1889) successfully demonstrated resuscitating asphyxiated newborns using intermittent positive pressure ventilation.

Flagg (1928), in America, published details of the apparatus and technique which he had devised for direct laryngoscopy, intubation and intermittent positive pressure insufflation with an oxygen and carbon dioxide mixture, for resuscitation of asphyxiated infants. Working independently, Blaikley and Gibberd (1935) were the first to publish details of tracheal intubation and treatment of 'asphyxia neonatorum' in the UK. They were the first individuals to recommend that an insufflation pressure of $30\,cm\,H_2O$ was necessary for lung expansion. Since their publication, endotracheal intubation and intermittent positive pressure ventilation was accepted as the standard method of resuscitation until 1950 when AKerren and Furstenberg introduced the idea that intragastric oxygen would be sufficient to support life. It took ten years before Coxon (1960) finally discredited their finding.

No further vogues have come into fashion and now intermittent positive pressure ventilation, either through a face mask or an endotracheal tube, is the accepted way of resuscitating asphyxiated neonates.

PHYSIOLOGICAL RESPONSES TO ASPHYXIA

Birth constitutes a severe physiological challenge. In 1964 Saling convincingly demonstrated a progressive fall in scalp blood Po_2, O_2 content and pH with a corresponding rise in Pco_2 during normal human labour, assuming that these changes were due to uterine contraction and resultant fall in placental blood flow (Saling, 1964). Dawes *et al.* (1963) in their rhesus monkey studies confirmed that there was a fall in intrauterine femoral arterial Po_2 at or after uterine contractions. Recently, catecholamine levels have been used to assess the degree of stress during labour. Fetal concentrations have been found to be increased 10-fold during normal vaginal delivery and even higher levels have been noted in complicated deliveries (Lagercrantz and Bistoletti, 1977; Eliot *et al.*, 1980; Lagercrantz, Bistoletti and Nylund, 1981).

However, whatever the cause, the principal effect of the stress of birth on the fetus is that of asphyxia with progressive hypoxia and acidosis. Extensive animal experimentations have shown that animals respond to this in a predictable way (Dawes, 1968; Hull, 1971). With the onset of acute total asphyxia, the fetal monkey starts making rhythmic respiratory effort, clonic movements and convulsions. This is followed by a profound bradycardia while the animal remains atonic and without any spontaneous movements. During this period (primary apnoea) the skin is initially cyanosed, but over a period of minutes becomes progressively paler due to intense vasoconstriction. The vasoconstriction is probably related to the outpouring of vast quantities of catecholamines. After the initial apnoeic phase the fetus starts to gasp at progressively increasing rates. By 5 min the gasping becomes weaker and around 8.5 min secondary or terminal apnoea sets in. If active resuscitation is not commenced at this stage, the animal dies. The time to the last gasp is very much dictated by the pH of the animal at delivery. If the fetus is grossly acidotic (pH <6.8), no gasps are observed at all. The course of events is very similar in the mature fetal lamb but the time to the last gasp is shorter, only 5.4 min (Dawes *et al.*, 1963).

The phenomenon of primary apnoea can be greatly extended by drugs such as morphine or even by general anaesthetic. Barbiturates have been also known to extend the period of primary apnoea (Cockburn, Daniel, Dawes *et al.*, 1969). Although often it is not possible to differentiate between primary and secondary apnoea, the former will nearly always respond to stimuli such as tactile stimulation or analeptics, with the onset of gasping. In the secondary apnoeic phase, active resuscitation with intermittent positive pressure ventilation is necessary to sustain life.

While it is often assumed that the human neonate responds in a similar manner, we should be wary of such assumptions. As stated by Hull (1971) 'it is not easy to evaluate the relevance of animal investigations to the clinical (human) situation', particularly as in the animal kingdom, labour and birth are rapid events. Only in the human is the process of labour and delivery a protracted one. This may modify the infant's responses. There is no conclusive evidence that primary and secondary apnoea occur in human infants. However, occasionally babies are delivered with acute total asphyxia who do not have any spontaneous gasping. These babies do not respond to tactile stimuli and probably would only survive if rapid resuscitatory measures were taken and might represent the terminal apnoeic phase. Much more frequently the babies respond rapidly to manual resuscitation, particularly seen after Caesarean section, in a manner similar to animals in primary apnoea. The duration of this period cannot, however, be assessed properly for obvious ethical reasons.

The respiratory behaviour of the asphyxiated infant cannot be discussed on its own without reference to the corresponding cardiovascular changes. In the fetal lamb and monkey, asphyxia results in a transient rise in blood pressure and a fall in the heart rate (Dawes, 1968). As the pH continues to drop there is a simultaneous decline in the heart rate and a steady fall in the cardiac output. The blood pressure falls to a very low level at the last gasp. Cassin, Swann and Cassin (1960) recorded pressures of 9/7 mmHg in their animal studies during anoxic death. The hypoxia and acidaemia result in intense pulmonary vasoconstriction only relieved by adequate ventilation of the lungs. Adamson *et al.* (1964) have shown the importance of improving acid–base balance as well as oxygenation in accelerating recovery following asphyxia.

FACTORS LEADING TO ONSET OF RESPIRATION AT BIRTH

We now know that the fetus makes intrauterine respiratory efforts before birth. It is thus appropriate to think of extrauterine respiration as an extension of breathing activity *in utero*. Thus, to understand the factors leading to onset of extrauterine breathing, the control of intrauterine activity is essential.

Ahfield (1888) was the first person to associate abdominal pulsation with intrauterine fetal breathing. However, it was not until 1971 that Boddy and Robinson (1971) made direct observations using A-scan ultrasound to assess the human fetus. The fetus initiates respiratory activity as early as 11 weeks' gestation: Initially the fetal breathing is irregular and infrequent but it becomes more frequent and organized with increasing gestation. Patrick *et al.* (Patrick *et al.*, 1978, 1980; Patrick, Natale and Richardson, 1978) have extensively investigated fetal breathing using real-time ultrasound in the last ten weeks of pregnancy. They observed fetal breathing for 31% of the time at both 30–31 weeks' and 38–39 weeks' gestation. However, fetal breathing is abolished during labour, possibly related to fetal hypoxia. Apart from labour, many other factors are known to affect fetal breathing *in utero* including hypoxia, hypoglycaemia, alcohol (all reducing fetal breathing) and smoking (enhancing the rate of fetal breathing).

Animal studies have shown that the fetal breathing movements occur predominantly in 'rapid eye movement sleep' (Dawes *et al.*, 1972; Ioffe *et al.*, 1980), a state in which the cortical activity heavily modifies the respiratory drive. Recent research indicates that respiration at birth is initiated by a variety of triggering factors. Some may be of primary importance whilst others serve as back-up systems. There are thus both intrinsic and extrinsic factors which are responsible for the initiation of respiration at birth.

Intrinsic factors

As mentioned earlier, the intrauterine breathing activity is inhibited towards the last stage. In sheep preparation this has been shown to be due to uterine contractions causing fetal asphyxia. The longer the contractions, the longer PaO_2 takes to return to normal levels after each contraction. Harned *et al.* (1966) observed fetal gasps following umbilical cord occlusion. Biscoe, Purves and Sampson (1969) showed that carotid body chemoreceptors are inactive and insensitive to chemical or drug stimulation. Jansen *et al.* (1981) studied the effect of *in utero* carotid chemoreceptor denervation on their fetal lamb preparations after birth. Four of their carotid sinus denervated fetuses were allowed to be delivered spontaneously and all established regular respiration after birth. Their experiment indicated that fetal carotid chemoreceptors are not essential for spontaneous intrauterine breathing activity during rapid eye movement sleep (REM sleep) nor for the establishment of effective breathing at birth. However, little is known about the function of central chemoreceptors in the fetus.

Extrinsic factors

Although birth asphyxia is probably the strongest stimulus for the newborn to breathe, other factors are responsible for maintaining respiration. Experimental evidence indicates that these factors can initiate breathing in the term fetus via sensory stimulation alone.

(*a*) *Temperature*. Cooling of the fetal snout can initiate respiration. Cooling of the skin can also induce breathing and, conversely, warming lambs can induce apnoea.
(*b*) *Pain*. Painful stimuli can induce respiratory responses in the fetus though these are not often sustained. This was the rationale for using varieties of 'torture' on the newborn who had failed to breathe.

Stimuli, such as touch, proprioception and audiovisual input, must play an important part in initiating and maintaining breathing but are obviously very difficult to quantify. Cordorelli and Carpelli (1975) suggested that these peripheral stimuli recruit central neurones and thus increase central arousal.

Recently, endorphins have been implicated in the pathogenesis of apnoea. These can be modified by naloxone (Chernick, Madansky and Lawson, 1980). However, the role of endogenous opiates in fetus still remains unclear.

The factors that lead to failure of respiration include:

(i) Severe birth asphyxia (usually pH <7.0)
(ii) Maternal analgesia/anaesthesia.

If the intrinsic factors fail to initiate respiration, extrinsic factors should be recruited. If these too fail, active resuscitation should be commenced.

INDICATIONS FOR RESUSCITATION

The newborn baby is more tolerant of asphyxia than the adult or older child, and there are well-recorded instances of babies who have not commenced respiratory efforts for 10–15 min and yet escaped neurologically intact (Scott, 1976). However, some infants who are slow to breathe have already suffered moderately severe hypoxia by the time of birth and such an additional delay would then almost inevitably lead to death or severe neurological damage. For this reason we follow the standard criteria for commencing active resuscitation, namely:

(1) Failure of regular respiration to occur by 2 min after delivery
(2) Apnoea and a heart rate of less than 80 per min before the age of 2 min.

Inevitably, using these indications many babies (probably in the region of 85%) would have started to breathe spontaneously within the next 1–2 min. However, irreversible damage would have affected the remaining 15%, more than justifying intervention at these levels.

The need for intubation seems to be falling in many units from a high in the region of 10% in the 1960s. In Nottingham the frequency of intubation has fallen from 3.3% in 1978 to 2.1% of all deliveries in 1982. We strongly suspect that this represents improvements in obstetric care.

The requirement for intubation is closely related to the type of delivery, so that less than 1% of babies born by normal spontaneous delivery require intubation, while 8% of breech deliveries and over 6% of babies born by Caesarean section will require active resuscitation (*Table 1.1*). Prematurity is also important and at least

Table 1.1 Effect of mode of delivery on need for intubation

Mode of delivery	Percentage needing intubation	Percentage of all intubated
Normal spontaneous	0.8	32
Forceps	2.5	19
Caesarean section	6.2	41
Breech	8.0	8

Table 1.2 High-risk deliveries requiring presence of a paediatric resident

Caesarean section
Breech delivery
Multiple pregnancy
Preterm delivery
Meconium staining with fetal distress
Rhesus incompatibility in moderately to severely affected fetus (as judged by antibodies)
Instrumentation: all Kielland's deliveries
                  Neville Barnes or Wrigleys liftout when associated with fetal distress
Prepartum haemorrhage if associated with fetal distress or bleeding

40% of babies born with a gestation of less than 32 weeks will require intubation. However, since the majority of deliveries are normal, at least one-third of all intubations are likely to be unexpected. Conversely, if the paediatric resident attends all of what are generally recognized as high risk deliveries (*Table 1.2*), there will be no delay proceeding with resuscitation in the remaining 60% at a cost of attending just over 20% of all deliveries.

PHYSIOLOGICAL EFFECTS OF RESUSCITATION

The pattern of resuscitation now generally accepted has evolved from very little information obtained from studies on stillborn babies and data collected by Karlberg and his colleagues on a small group of babies breathing spontaneously at birth (Karlberg *et al.*, 1962). We are now in a position where we can assess the babies' responses and evaluate efficacy by measuring tidal exchange with a pneumotachograph and inflation and intrathoracic pressures with suitable pressure transducers.

Babies' response to inflation

Measurements of intrathoracic pressure and tidal volume have shown that the baby may respond to the first few inflations in three ways: passive response, Head's paradoxical reflex and rejection response (Boon, Milner and Hopkin, 1979).

Passive response

In some situations the baby makes no active response. In this situation the oesophageal pressure trace mimics the change in tidal exchange to a degree which is determined by the compliance characteristics of the chest wall and respiratory muscles (*Figure 1.1*). There is an apparent 'opening pressure' due to the prolonged

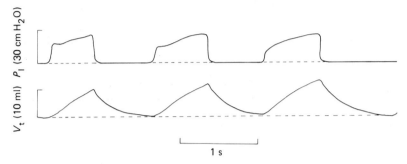

Figure 1.1 Inflation pressure (P_I) and tidal volume (V_t) at the onset of resuscitation showing a passive response. (Reproduced from Boon *et al.*, 1979, by courtesy of the Editors and Publishers, *Archives of Disease in Childhood*)

time constant of the fluid-filled lung, producing a slowly rising tidal volume in the presence of square wave inflation. This pattern was seen in 30% of the first three breaths in 20 full-term babies requiring resuscitation (Boon, Milner and Hopkin, 1979).

Head's paradoxical reflex

In a further 18% of these breaths the inflation pressure stimulated the babies to make a spontaneous inspiratory effort, often dramatically augmenting the inspiratory volume (*Figure 1.2*). As the babies tended to inspire at rates of greater than $31 \cdot \text{min}^{-1}$, the bias flow normally selected, the inflation pressure of 30 cm of water was often reversed, a situation which cannot be considered ideal (*Figure 1.3*).

Rejection response

The common pattern seen was for the baby to produce large positive intrathoracic pressures, often exceeding 90 cm of water, starting soon after the onset of the inflation. These pressures were almost always sufficient to squeeze air out of the lungs during the period of positive inflation (*Figure 1.4*). The nature of these rejection responses remains uncertain. Measurement of both intragastric and intrathoracic pressure with the dual pressure transducer system has shown that the positive pressures are generated below the diaphragm (*Figure 1.5*), presumably by the abdominal muscles. The relatively long time course suggests that these are not part of the cough reflex but represent a coordinated active expiration in response to the positive inflation.

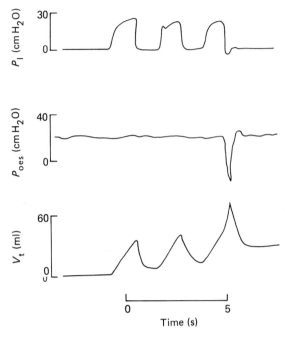

Figure 1.2 Inflation (P_I), oesophageal pressure (P_{oes}), and tidal volume (V_t) during resuscitation. On the third inflation the baby makes an inspiratory effort, increasing tidal exchange (Head's paradoxical reflex)

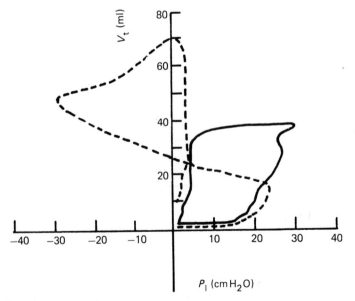

Figure 1.3 Pressure/volume loops at the onset of resuscitation. During the second inflation (dotted line) a Head's paradoxical reflex leads to reversal of the pressure within the airway. (Reproduced from Boon *et al.*, 1979, by courtesy of the Editors and Publishers, *Archives of Disease in Childhood*)

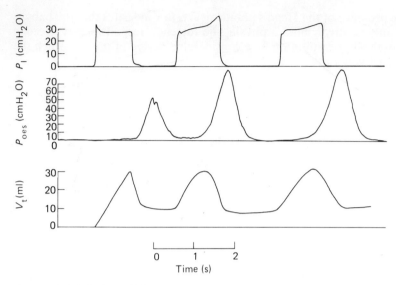

Figure 1.4 Inflation (P_I) and oesophageal pressure (P_{oes}) and tidal volume during resuscitation. The inflation pressures stimulate high intrathoracic rejection responses. (Reproduced from Boon *et al.*, 1979, by courtesy of the Editors and Publishers, *Archives of Disease in Childhood*)

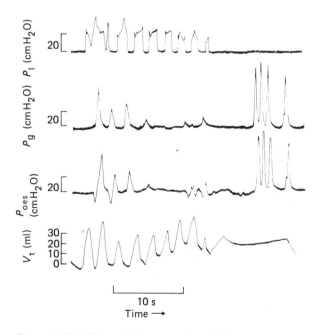

Figure 1.5 Inflation (P_I), intragastric (P_g), oesophageal pressure (P_{oes}), and tidal volume during resuscitation. The positive rejection responses are recorded by both the oesophageal and gastric pressure transducers

Although the presence of the Head's paradoxical reflex indicates that the baby is suffering from only relatively mild asphyxia, the rejection responses may precede the onset of spontaneous respiration by a considerable period of time in which the baby responds passively to the inflations.

Tidal exchange

The inflation volume resulting from an inflation pressure in the region of 30 cm of water maintained for approximately 1 s was measured in the first breath of the 20 full-term babies (Boon, Milner and Hopkin, 1979). The mean volume was only 15.2 ml (*Table 1.3*). This was only 50% of the mean inspiratory volume measured in 24 babies who breathed spontaneously at birth, and who had very similar intrathoracic pressure changes. This suggests that a negative pressure applied on the outside of the lung is more effective than a similar pressure applied down the trachea, a concept unacceptable to physiologists who claim that it is the differential pressure alone which determines volume changes (Milner and Vyas, 1982). The inflation volumes can, however, be increased to the levels achieved by the spontaneously breathing babies if the inflation pressure is maintained for up to 5 s (*Table 1.3*). Thus, the difference in inflation volume between the two situations

Table 1.3 Comparison of the pressure volume changes occurring during the first spontaneous breath and first resuscitative inflation in full-term babies

	Spontaneous	*1-s inflation*	*3–5-s inflation*
Inspiratory/inflation pressure (cmH$_2$O)	33 (6.1–103.0)	30	30
Tidal exchange (ml)	40.3 (2.7–90.0)	18.6 (0–62.5)	33.6 (16.9–70.0)
Functional residual capacity (ml)	18.7 (2.7–40.0)	7.5 (0–15.5)	15.9 (11.7–23.2)

The values are the mean with the range in parentheses.

appears to be secondary to the very long time constant which exists during resuscitation (Milner and Vyas, 1982). Why the baby should be able to expand his lungs so effectively in a tenth of this time when breathing by himself remains unclear. It may be that the baby's efforts alter the configuration of the chest and lung structures, reducing viscous resistance. As resuscitation is continued there is a tendency for the tidal exchange to increase, i.e. for the 'dynamic compliance' to rise. A further increase occurs as soon as the baby makes his first inspiratory effort.

Formation of the functional residual capacity

Resuscitation after intubation rarely leads to the formation of a functional residual capacity (FRC) in the first few inflations. In only three of the 20 babies was there a measurable volume of air remaining in the lungs at the end of inflation, compared to 48 of 50 babies who breathed spontaneously and managed to achieve a mean FRC of 18.7 ml (Milner and Vyas, 1982). Thirty seconds after the onset of resuscitation the FRC in the 20 babies was 34.8 ml, very similar to the 36.4 ml found 30 s after the onset of respiration in the babies breathing spontaneously. Why there is a failure for the FRC to form after resuscitation requires further clarification. There was no close association between the initial inspiratory volume and whether or not an FRC was formed. Interestingly, after prolonged inflation, i.e. greater than 3 s, an FRC was formed in all nine babies (Vyas, Milner and Hopkin, 1981). Although some babies did form a small FRC during the initial phase of resuscitation, almost always the baby's first inspiratory effort led to the retention of significant volumes of air in the lung (Milner and Vyas, 1982). As already seen, this first respiratory effort produces changes in the dynamic compliance characteristics of the lung and is probably also associated with an increase in tone in the respiratory muscles. The size of the first inflation, often a Head's paradoxical reflex, may also create conditions which favour the retention of air in the lungs.

Whether the delay in the formation of an FRC is important is not currently nor ever likely to be known.

PHYSIOLOGICAL RESPONSE TO FACE MASK RESUSCITATION

Many units depend on face mask resuscitation devices with self-filling gas reservoirs as the first line of therapy for birth asphyxia. The pressures generated are limited either by a leak, in which case the pressure is flow dependent, or by a spring-loaded relief valve. Although the pressure generating characteristics of these devices have been well documented in the *in vitro* situation by manufacturers and investigators, there have been no previous studies of their efficacy at birth. For this reason we modified a commonly used system, the Laerdal manual resuscitator, by incorporating a pneumotachograph between the body of the device and the face mask and also measured inflation pressure within the face mask with a transducer. Data was then collected on nine babies requiring resuscitation at birth, using standard criteria. Inflation pressures were found to be very similar to those achieved by the intubation system, i.e. 28 cm of water. Inflation volume proved impossible to measure due to a leak around the face mask but expiratory volumes were very small, less than 25% of those found after intubation (*Table 1.4*). Even when the pressure relief valve was over-ridden and inflation pressures of up to

Table 1.4 Comparison of the pressure volume changes occurring during resuscitation by face mask and endotracheal systems

	Face mask	Endotracheal
Inflation pressure (cm H_2O)	28.3 (26.5–33.3)	31.4 (24.2–36.5)
Expiratory tidal volume (ml)	3.0 (0–11.1)	14.3 (3.3–43.7)

Values are the mean with the range in parentheses.

80 cm of water were generated, tidal exchange remained inadequate, often throughout the entire period of resuscitation. Thus, the system depended on stimulating the babies to make respiratory efforts, rather than on improving oxygenation in the babies to any significant extent, and so is unlikely to be of use in severely asphyxiated babies. Perhaps it is of value in selecting those who do not require intubation at birth. The reason for the small tidal exchange is that the devices have been designed so that rapid respiratory rates can be achieved. This limits the inspiratory time to less than 0.5 s, far too short a period to allow adequate inflation to occur. This pattern of inflation, however, does not lead to significant passage of air down the oesophagus, presumably again due to the short inspiratory time (Milner, Vyas and Hopkin, 1981).

RECOMMENDATIONS FOR RESUSCITATION

From the information now available it is possible to at least make provisional statements on the efficacy of current techniques and whether these need to be modified.

Face mask resuscitation

As has been demonstrated, current devices are unlikely to produce adequate respiratory exchange, at least until an FRC has formed and the viscous resistance has fallen. Use of higher inflation pressures may help but may well increase the risk of pneumothorax. More effective exchange is likely if the inflation pressure can be maintained for at least 1 s initially. This could be achieved by redesigning the devices, by using a larger gas reservoir in gadgets which have a spring-loaded relief valve rather than purely a leak, or by using an anaesthetic re-breathing bag with relatively high gas flows, i.e. in excess of $8 l \cdot min^{-1}$. With care, the operator can then maintain the inflation pressure sufficiently long for lung expansion to occur, assessing progress by observing movement of the chest wall and abdomen and by auscultation.

Resuscitation after intubation

Systems

The use of a water column to limit the inflation pressure is no longer acceptable. Occlusion of the T-piece leads to transient pressures of up to 60 or 70 cm of water, due to the inertial characteristics of the water column (Hey and Lenney, 1973). These alone are probably not dangerous, in view of their rapid decay. Of greater importance is the fact that the turbulence produced by the gas escaping into the water creates far higher pressures than are generally appreciated, so that with the end of the blow off tube 30 cm below the water surface, inflation pressures of greater than 60 cm of water are often produced. The alternatives are either to use an anaesthetic re-breathing bag or a hand-held self-filling resuscitator, or to replace the water column with an appropriate pressure-limiting valve.

Pressures to be selected

The pressure generally selected for resuscitation at birth is 30 cm of water. This was based initially on a small number of studies carried out on stillborn babies (Blaikley and Gibberd, 1935). A further study (Rosen and Laurence, 1965) claimed that inflation pressures in excess of 60 cm of water are likely to burst the lungs, but since this information was obtained on isolated lungs from stillborn babies, its relevance is limited as the chest wall and abdominal contents will have a protective effect on the lung at high volumes, limiting over-expansion in the same way as the outer tyre protects an inner tube at pressures which would surely burst the unprotected inner tube.

Our data (Milner and Vyas, 1982) and that of Hull (1969) indicate that the large majority of full-term babies can be successfully resuscitated with an inflation pressure of 30 cm of water, but that higher pressures will occasionally be required. We would recommend that the first inflation should be maintained for at least 2 s as this will expand the lungs more effectively and create an air reservoir. If the hand-held resuscitation devices are used, these will need to be modified to increase the inspiratory time. If the chest wall fails to move and no air entry is apparent on auscultation within two or three inflations, it is acceptable to increase the inflation pressure to either 40 or even 50 cm of water, dropping this pressure as soon as lung expansion has occurred. This should avoid the risk of pneumothorax, which may occur if the lung is overstretched.

Selection of gas

Most units use 100% oxygen for resuscitation at birth. Some authorities have recommended that 40% is entirely adequate and also preferable, as there is a risk that exposure of the very preterm baby to high oxygen concentrations for even a short period may increase the risk of retrolental fibroplasia. There is currently no evidence to suggest that the use of oxygen in this way does have a significant effect (Lucey and Dangman, 1984).

Surprisingly, breathing 80% oxygen for up to 20 min in the first six hours of life does not appear to produce the atelectasis which is seen later, possibly due to the formation of foam within the lungs. On balance, it would seem reasonable to use 40% if this can be provided without undue expense.

Preterm babies

We currently have very little information on the resuscitation of preterm babies. What information is available suggests that an inflation pressure of 30 cm of water is usually adequate but, as with larger babies, higher pressures will sometimes be required.

The more preterm the baby, the greater will be the need for intubation. Many centres now routinely intubate all babies with a gestation of less than 30 weeks, in the hope that active resuscitation will lead to more rapid lung expansion and reduce the incidence of respiratory distress syndrome (RDS). It is well documented that the incidence of respiratory distress is higher in babies who have been asphyxiated at birth and some information that the incidence of RDS has fallen following the introduction of more aggressive resuscitation policies (Robson and Hey, 1982). Whether elective intubation of all very preterm babies regardless of their condition is a good practice is unknown, as the procedure virtually always produces a period of hypoxia and this may, on occasions, be responsible for the formation of an intraventricular haemorrhage. Control studies are urgently needed to resolve this controversial point.

Position for resuscitation

It has been traditional for babies to be resuscitated in the head-down position, partly from convenience but also on the assumption that since the babies were asphyxiated the head-down position would improve venous return, increase cardiac output and thus improve cerebral perfusion. Recently, there has been a trend towards resuscitating babies flat, claiming that the head-down position impedes respiration since the abdominal contents will then lie on the diaphragm, and also that the increased venous pressure may exacerbate any tendency to cerebral oedema and even intraventricular haemorrhage in preterm babies. Measurements on full-term babies in the first six hours of life have shown that the mechanical characteristics of the lungs are identical in the head-down or supine position, and that the mean intrathoracic pressure changes by less than 1 cm of water, making it extremely unlikely that the baby's respiratory system is at a disadvantage when the baby is tilted (*Table 1.5*). The changes in intracranial pressure will also be very small, particularly when compared with the situation which exists after the delivery of the head, while the abdomen and chest are still compressed by pressures of up to 250 cm of water. Crying and even grunting will also produce increases in intracranial pressure which are many times higher than those produced by tilting.

Table 1.5 Effect of nursing babies flat or tilted head down on tidal volume rate (V_t), oesophageal pressure (P_{oes}), dynamic compliance (C_D) and total respiratory work per min (W_T)

	V_t (ml)	Rate (min^{-1})	P_{oes} (cm H_2O)	C_D (ml/cm H_2O)	W_T (g · cm · min^{-1})
Flat	19.2	44.5	7.15	4.0	4630
Tilted	19.1	47.5	7.28	4.2	5050

Finally, the perfusion pressure in the baby's brain will not be in any way affected. There is thus no evidence and little rational argument on the selection of the baby's position. It is much more important that the baby should be nursed in a way which aids the process of intubation, so that there is as little delay as possible in relieving the asphyxia.

Despite improvements in obstetric care, babies continue to be born who are brain damaged as a result of perinatal asphyxia. On some occasions this may be inevitable. It is, however, totally unacceptable that any brain damage should arise from a lack of facilities or appropriate action once the baby has been born.

References

ADAMSON, K. JR, BEHRMAN, R., DAWES, G. S. and JAMES, L. S. (1964) Resuscitation of rhesus monkeys ι sphyxiated at birth by positive pressure ventilation and tri-hydroxymethyl aminomethane. *Journal of Pediatrics*, **65**, 807–818

AHFIELD, F. (1888) Uber bisher noch nicht beschriebene intrauterine Bewegunger des Kindes Verh. *Deutsch Gesellschaft fuer Gynaekology*, **2**, 203

AKERREN, Y. and FURSTENBERG, N. (1950) Gastrointestinal administration of oxygen in treatment of asphyxia in the newborn. *Journal of Obstetrics and Gynaecology of the British Empire*, **57**, 705–713

BILLARD, C. M. (1828) *A Treatise on the Diseases of Infants*, pp. 399–402. Churchill: London

BISCOE, T. J., PURVES, M. J. and SAMPSON, S. R. (1969) Types of nervous activity which may be recorded from the carotid sinus nerve in the sheep fetus. *Journal of Physiology*, **202**, 1–23

BLAIKLEY, J. B. and GIBBERD, G. F. (1935) Asphyxia neonatorum. *Lancet*, **i**, 736–739

BODDY, K. and ROBINSON, J. S. (1971) External method for detection of fetal breathing *in utero*. *Lancet*, **ii**, 1231–1233

BOON, A. W., MILNER, A. D. and HOPKIN, I. E. (1979) Physiological responses of the newborn infant to resuscitation. *Archives of Disease in Childhood*, **54**, 492

BOYLE, R. (1670) Pneumatical experiments about respiration. *Philosophical Times*, **5**, 360–361

CASSIN, S., SWANN, H. G. and CASSIN, B. (1960) Respiratory and cardiovascular alterations during the process of anoxic death in the newborn. *Journal of Applied Physiology*, **15**, 249–252

CHERNICK, V., MADANSKY, D. L. and LAWSON, E. E. (1980) Naloxone decreases the duration of primary apnoea with neonatal asphyxia. *Pediatric Research*, **14**, 357–359

CLEMENT SMITH (1967) The Valley of the Shadow of Birth. *American Journal of Diseases in Children*, 171–201

COCKBURN, F., DANIEL, S. S., DAWES, G. S., JAMES, L. S., MYERS, R. E., NIEMANN, W. *et al.* (1969) The effect of pentobarbital anaesthesia on resuscitation and brain damage in fetal rhesus monkeys asphyxiated on delivery. *Journal of Pediatrics*, **75**, 281–291

CORDORELLI, S. and CARPELLI, E. M. (1975) Somatic-respiratory reflex and onset of regular breathing movements in the lamb fetus *in utero*. *Pediatric Research*, **9**, 879–884

COXON, R. V. (1960) The effect of intragastric oxygen on the oxygenation of arterial and portal blood in hypoxic animals. *Lancet*, **i**, 1315–1317

DAWES, G. S. (1968) *Fetal and Neonatal Physiology*. Chicago: Year Book Medical Publishers, Inc.

DAWES, G. S., FOX, H. E., LEDUC, M. B., LIGGINS, G. C. and RICHARDS, R. T. (1972) Respiratory movements and rapid eye movement sleep in the fetal lamb. *Journal of Physiology (London)*, **220**, 119–143

DAWES, G. S., JACOBSON, H. N., MOTT, J. C., SHELLEY, H. J. and STAFFORD, A. (1963) The treatment of asphyxiated mature fetal lambs and rhesus monkeys with intravenous glucose and sodium bicarbonate. *Journal of Physiology (London)*, **169**, 167–184

DOE, E. (1889) Apparatus for resuscitating asphyxiated children. *Boston Medical and Surgical Journal*, **120**, 9

ELIOT, R. J., LAM, R., LEAKE, R., HOBEL, C. J. and FISHER, D. A. (1980) Plasma catecholamine concentrations in infants at birth and during first 48 hours of life. *Journal of Pediatrics*, **96**, 311

EVANSON, R. T. and MAUNSELL, H. (1842) *Practical Treatise on the Management of Children*, pp. 194–200. Dublin: Fanin and Co.

FAULCONER, A. and KEYS, T. E. (1965) *Foundation of Anesthesiology*, Vol. 1. Springfield, Illinois: Charles C. Thomas

FLAGG, P. J. (1928) *Journal of American Medical Association*, **91**, 788–791

HARNED, H. S. JR, MCKINNEY, L. G., BERRYHILL, W. S. JR and HOMES, C. K. (1966) Effects of hypoxia and acidity on the initiation of breathing in the fetal lamb at birth. *American Journal of Diseases of Children*, **112**, 334–342

HEY, E. and LENNEY, W. (1973) Letter to the Editor. *Lancet*, **ii**, 103–104

HULL, D. (1969) Lung expansion and ventilation during resuscitation of asphyxiated newborn infants. *Journal of Pediatrics*, **75**, 47–58

HULL, D. (1971) Asphyxia neonatorum. In *Recent Advances in Pediatrics*, 4th edn. Eds D. Gairdner and D. Hull, pp. 63–87. London: J. A. Churchill

IOFFE, S., JANSEN, A. H., RUSSELL, B. J. and CHERNICK, V. (1980) Sleep, wakefulness and monosynaptic reflex in fetal and newborn lambs. *Pfluegers Archives*, **388**, 149–157

JANSEN, A. H., IOFFE, S., RUSSELL, B. J. and CHERNICK, V. (1981) Effect of carotid chemoreceptor denervation on breathing *in utero* and after birth. *Journal of Applied Physiology*, **51**, 630–633

KARLBERG, P., CHERRY, R. B., ESCARDO, F. E. and KOCH, G. (1962) Pulmonary ventilation and mechanics of breathing in the first minutes of life, including the onset of respirations. *Acta Pediatrica*, **51**, 121–136

LAGERCRANTZ, H. and BISTOLETTI, P. (1977) Catecholamine release in the newborn infant at birth. *Pediatric Research,* **11,** 889

LAGERCRANTZ, H., BISTOLETTI, P. and NYLUND, L. (1981) Sympathoadrenal activity in the fetus during delivery and at birth in intensive care in the newborn. In *Intensive Care of the Newborn,* Eds L. Stern, B. Salle and B. Friis-Hansen, pp. 1–11. New York: Masson Inc.

LUCEY, J. F. and DANGMAN, B. (1984) Re-examination of the role of oxygen in retrolental fibroplasia. *Pediatrics,* **73,** 82–96

MILNER, A. D. and VYAS, H. (1982) Lung expansion at birth. *Journal of Pediatrics,* **101,** 879–886

MILNER, A. D., VYAS, H. and HOPKIN, I. E. (1983) Face mask resuscitation: does it lead to gastric distension? *Archives of Disease in Childhood,* **58,** 373–375

O'DWYER, J. (1887) Fifty cases of croup in private practice treated by intubation of the larynx, with a description of the method and of the danger incident thereto. *Medical Records,* **32,** 557

PATRICK, J., CAMPBELL, K., CARMICHAEL, L., NATALE, R. and RICHARDSON, B. (1980) Patterns of human fetal breathing during the last 10 weeks of pregnancy. *Journal of Obstetrics and Gynaecology of the British Commonwealth,* **56,** 24–30

PATRICK, J., FETHERSTON, W., VICK, H. and VOEGELIN, R. (1978) Human fetal breathing movements and gross fetal body movements at weeks 34–35 of gestation. *American Journal of Obstetrics and Gynecology,* **130,** 693–699

PATRICK, J., NATALE, R. and RICHARDSON, B. (1978) Patterns of human fetal activity at 34 to 35 weeks gestational age. *American Journal of Obstetrics and Gynecology,* **132,** 507–513

ROBSON, F. and HEY, E. N. (1982) Resuscitation of preterm babies at birth reduces the rate of death from hyaline membrane disease. *Archives of Disease in Childhood,* **57,** 184–186

ROSEN, M. and LAURENCE, K. M. (1965) Expansion pressures and rupture pressures in the newborn lung. *Lancet,* **ii,** 721–722

ROYAL HUMANE SOCIETY (1812) Breathing into the mouth. *Annual Report,* **27**

SALING, E. (1964) Die Blutgasverhaltnisse und der Saure-Basen-hausalt des feteb bei ungestortem Geburtsablauf. *Zeitschrift fuer Geburtsch und Gynakologie,* **161,** 261–292

SCOTT, H. (1976) Outcome of very severe birth asphyxia. *Archives of Disease in Childhood,* **51,** 712–716

TRUEHEAD (1869–1872) Ein Apparat zur Kunstlichen Respiration bei Asphyxia, mitth. a.d sitzprotok, *Gesselschaft für Gebertsch,* **2,** 154–156. Berlin: T2 Berlin Obstetric Society

VYAS, H., MILNER, A. D. and HOPKIN, I. E. (1981) Physiological responses to prolonged and slow rise inflation. *Journal of Pediatrics,* **99,** 635

2
Regulation of respiratory muscles in infants and children

Waldemar A. Carlo and Richard J. Martin

In recent years there has been increased interest in the role played by respiratory muscles in the maintenance of ventilatory homeostasis. This has greatly enhanced our understanding of the inter-relationship of upper airway and chest wall muscles under various conditions of altered respiratory drive. The role of upper airway muscles in modifying airflow patterns and maintaining airway patency, the effect of sleep state on the control of respiratory muscles and the role of muscle fatigue in respiratory failure are all being clarified.

It is now widely accepted that various accessory muscles of the chest wall and muscles of the upper airway are activated in synchrony with either the inspiratory or expiratory phase of the respiratory cycle. Furthermore, the physiological roles ascribed to activation of these muscles are being characterized. The purpose of this chapter is to review the role of various respiratory muscles, with particular emphasis on those of the upper airway, in both health and disease states pertaining to the human infant. In areas where limited neonatal data exist, the relevant animal and adult human studies will be addressed.

THE RESPIRATORY MUSCLES

Chest wall muscles

In terms of respiratory physiology, the chest wall comprises the rib cage, abdomen and intervening diaphragm (DIA). The DIA is the major respiratory muscle, and serves as an interface between these other two components of the chest wall. Intercostals (IC), accessory and abdominal (ABD) muscles variably supplement diaphragmatic activity in order to accomplish the necessary chest wall excursions.

The diaphragm

The diaphragm, a dome-shaped muscle, consists of distinct costal and crural components (De Troyer *et al.*, 1981). Contraction of either part of the DIA results in caudal and anterior displacement of the abdominal contents. By way of its attachment to the rib cage, the costal DIA can also elevate the ribs, especially when there is accompanying ABD muscle contraction (Goldman and Mead, 1973). Both of these actions contribute to the development of negative pleural pressures that result in lung inflation. The total pressure generated by diaphragmatic contraction, or transdiaphragmatic pressure, may be expressed as the difference between abdominal and pleural pressure. As for any muscle, the ability of the DIA to generate this pressure is partly dependent on the resting length of its fibers (Pengelly, Alderson and Milic-Emili, 1971). When this length is shortened (as during conditions of increased lung volume), the force generated by the muscle decreases according to Starling's law (Grassino *et al.*, 1978).

The intercostal muscles

As in the case of other accessory muscles, the intercostal muscles are frequently quiet during resting breathing, but recruited under circumstances of increased respiratory drive. The external IC muscles elevate the ribs and move them forward. This enlarges the chest cavity, thus creating negative pleural pressures and promoting lung inflation. The effectiveness of external IC muscle contraction is dependent on DIA activation since, without the latter, there would be upward displacement of abdominal contents, reducing the pressure-generating ability of the IC muscles. The external IC muscles also prevent bulging of the intercostal spaces during expiration. The internal IC may be activated during forced expirations. Their action, although still a matter of controversy, may be inspiratory or expiratory, and contributes to stability of the intercostal spaces.

Harding, Johnson and McClelland (1980) showed that, despite the absence of IC muscle activity in fetal lambs, inspiratory IC activation was observed immediately after birth. Sleep state also modulates IC muscle activity in the neonatal period, as will be discussed later. Inspiratory IC muscle activity is of particular importance in newborn infants, who typically have a highly compliant rib cage. Prevention of paradoxical or asynchronous inward motion of the rib cage during inspiration will enhance the pressure-generating capability of the DIA.

The abdominal muscles

Although the primary role of the abdominal muscles is to compress the visceral contents, Campbell (1952) has shown that during spontaneous breathing healthy adults may exhibit inspiratory and expiratory ABD muscle activity which is increased during forced breathing. Inspiratory activity of the ABD muscles may facilitate lung expansion by displacing the DIA upwards and consequently lengthening the muscle as well as diminishing its radius of curvature, both of which increase its pressure-generating capability.

Respiratory activity of ABD muscles is seen more commonly in patients with obstructive sleep apnea than in normal children (Jeffries, Brouillette and Hunt, 1983). In newborn infants ABD muscle activity that is in synchrony with inspiration decreases when the infant is moved from the upright to the supine position (Prechtl, Van Eykern and O'Brien, 1977). Since infants are usually nursed in the supine position this lack of abdominal support may impair their ability to generate inspiratory pressures. Fleming *et al.* (1979) applied abdominal loading to a group of preterm and term infants and immediately reduced or eliminated rib cage distortion. The magnitude of the load was small, resulting in an increase in gastric pressure of only 1–2 cm H_2O and did not interfere with the inspired tidal volumes or DIA electromyogram, suggesting that increase in respiratory drive and consequent recruitment of other respiratory muscles did not occur. It is possible that the ABD muscles contribute to chest wall stability and ventilation in the neonate by altering the configuration of the chest wall or DIA and enhancing the efficiency of respiratory muscles.

Upper airway muscles

Although multiple muscles of the upper airway are known to be activated in synchrony with either phase of the respiratory cycle (Ogawa *et al.*, 1960; Rothstein *et al.*, 1983), it is only in recent years that the significance of their action in relation to the respiratory system has been demonstrated.

Genioglossus

The genioglossus (GG) is primarily involved in movements of the tongue. Since it is attached anteriorly to the mandible, its contraction moves the tongue forward, preventing it from obstructing the pharyngeal space.

The laryngeal muscles

The main function of the laryngeal muscles is to ensure motion of the vocal cords. The posterior cricoarytenoid, innervated by the vagus, is the abductor of the vocal cords. The cricothyroid and the thyroarytenoid are the main cord adductors. The laryngeal muscles play an important role in controlling upper airway resistance and, in particular, in modifying expiratory airflow.

Alae nasi

The alae nasi (AN) cause enlargement of the nostrils. In both humans and animals of many species dilation of the nares is observed during deep inspiration. Dilation of the nares causes marked reduction in nasal resistance.

Other accessory muscles

The sternocleidomastoid muscles, apart from their ability to rotate the head, have an inspiratory function by elevating the sternum and the ribs when the head is fixed on the neck by other muscles (De Troyer and Kelly, 1984). These muscles are more frequently active in children with obstructive sleep apnea than in normal controls (Jeffries, Brouillette and Hunt, 1983), although their specific role in patients with airway obstruction is unclear. The scalene muscles consist of a group of three muscles (anterior, medial and posterior) that insert on the first two ribs and also elevate the rib cage during inspiration (De Troyer and Kelly, 1984).

CONTROL OF THE RESPIRATORY MUSCLES

Sequence of activation

A specific sequential pattern of activation of the respiratory muscles (and their innervation) has emerged. This is characterized by activation of upper airway muscles (or nerves) before that of the DIA (or phrenic) and onset of inspiratory airflow.

Önal, Lopata and O'Connor (1981a) observed that, in awake adults, the onset of the genioglossus electromyogram (EMG) preceded that of the diaphragm (DIA) by an average of 70 ms and the genioglossus EMG had a characteristic rapid rate of rise with an early peak. Although in cats the relationship between onsets of hypoglossal and phrenic discharges was variable during resting breathing, with increased drive caused by chemoreceptor stimulation, hypoglossal activity commenced earlier (Hwang, St John and Bartlett, 1983). Cohen (1975) has shown that in cats the onset of activity of the recurrent laryngeal nerve, another upper airway nerve, preceded that of the phrenic nerve and that peak activity occurred early in the inspiratory phase. He also observed that laryngeal nerve activity persisted throughout or beyond the total inspiratory cycle, which may reflect possible expiratory roles of laryngeal muscles. In contrast, Harding, Johnson and McClelland (1980) and Sherrey and Megirian (1977, 1980) have observed that posterior cricoarytenoid and cricothyroid EMGs have their onset coincident with that of the DIA. Nonetheless, Sherrey and Megirian (1980) also observed that, when the expiratory activity of these laryngeal muscles was decreased with pentobarbital anaesthesia, the onset of both EMGs preceded that of the DIA, suggesting that underlying expiratory activity may have masked the early activation of the laryngeal muscles.

In awake adults Strohl et al. (1980) found an average of 90 ms between the onset of alae nasi EMG and inspiratory airflow and this delay increased several-fold during sleep and hypercapnia. In preterm infants we have observed (Carlo et al., 1983a) that AN activity precedes that of the DIA by 40–50 ms and precedes airflow by approximately 100 ms (*Figure 2.1*). In addition, alae nasi EMG peaked and ended before both diaphragm EMG and airflow. During hypercapnia diaphragm EMG was observed to extend into the expiratory phase. Although these timing relationships were generally present, at times there was marked variability even on consecutive breaths (*Figure 2.2*). The onset of the diaphragm EMG, prior to airflow, and its persistence during the initial phase of expiration, are consistent with similar findings in human adults (Agostoni, Sant'Ambrogio and del Portillo Carrasco, 1960; Petit, Milic-Emili and Delhez, 1960). The expiratory diaphragm EMG, which we observed most consistently during CO_2 breathing, may constitute an active expiratory breaking mechanism in these infants. Possible mechanisms for the time delays between upper airway muscles and DIA include differences in central control of the various respiratory muscles or in motor neurone thresholds. In anesthetized cats, using stimulation of the central tegmental field, Orem, Lydic and Norris (1977) observed that the latency in activation of the posterior cricoarytenoid was approximately 100 ms less than that of the DIA. The early activation of the upper airway muscles may be important in facilitating ventilation by reducing upper airway resistance early during inspiration and at the time of peak airflow.

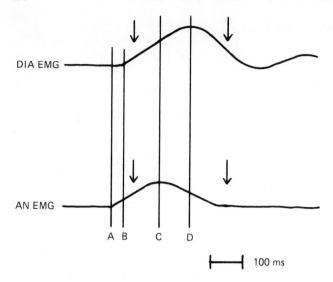

Figure 2.1 Output of electronic ensemble averager of the alae nasi (AN) and diaphragm (DIA) EMG moving averaged signals for 10 consecutive breaths is shown for one infant during quiet sleep while breathing 4% CO_2. Lines A and B indicate onset of alae nasi and diaphragm (DIA) EMGs, respectively. Lines C and D indicate peak alae nasi and diaphragm EMGs, respectively. Arrows mark onset and end of inspiratory airflow. (Reproduced from Carlo *et al.*, 1983a, by courtesy of the Editor and Publisher, *Journal of Applied Physiology: Respiratory, Environmental and Exercise Physiology*)

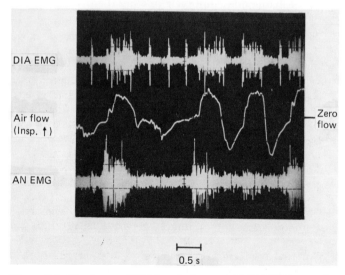

Figure 2.2 Diaphragm (DIA) and alae nasi (AN) EMGs are shown in relation to airflow in one infant during active sleep while breathing 4% CO_2. Onset of alae nasi EMG precedes that of diaphragm EMG and onset of inspiratory airflow. Note variability in temporal relationships of these signals and in magnitude of alae nasi EMG. Electrocardiographic artifact occurs in diaphragm. (Reproduced from Carlo *et al.*, 1983a, by courtesy of the Editor and Publisher, *Journal of Applied Physiology: Respiratory, Environmental and Exercise Physiology*)

Sleep state

Following the observations that behavioral states may markedly modify the regulation of breathing, many studies have focused on the effect of sleep state on the control of the respiratory muscles. Review of previous work is complicated by the different criteria frequently used to categorize sleep state. In addition, maturational and interspecies differences may modify these criteria as well as the behavior of the respiratory muscle groups themselves.

Sleep in infants may be classified using behavioral and/or electroencephalographic criteria. Parmelee and Stern (1972) have classified sleep states into active or rapid eye movement sleep (AS) and quiet sleep (QS) using simple behavioral criteria. AS is characterized by the presence of eye and body movements with irregular respiration. In contrast, during QS there is absence of eye or body movements (apart from occasional startles) and respiration is regular. The electroencephalogram shows continuous irregular low voltages in preterm and term infants during AS and a pattern of discontinuity in preterm infants during QS that evolves into typical trace alternans in the term neonate (Dreyfus-Brisac, 1970; Werner, Stockard and Bickford, 1977). Nonetheless, in the preterm infant classification of sleep states may be difficult, particularly prior to 32 weeks' postconceptual age and extensive periods frequently have to be classified as indeterminate or transitional.

Respiration during AS in neonates is characterized by a decreased functional residual capacity (Henderson-Smart and Read, 1979), asynchronous chest wall movements (Prechtl, Van Eykern and O'Brien, 1977; Curzi-Dascalova, 1978; Martin, Okken and Rubin, 1979) and increased frequency of apneic episodes (Drefus-Brisac, 1970; Gabriel, Albani and Schulte, 1976; Curzi-Dascalova, 1978).

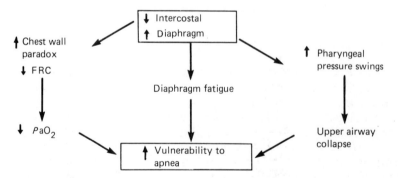

Figure 2.3 Mechanisms that may mediate the increased vulnerability to apnea in active sleep. (Reproduced from Miller, Martin and Carlo, 1984, by courtesy of the Editor and Publisher, Churchill Livingstone Inc.)

Figure 2.3 demonstrates some of the mechanisms that have been proposed to increase the vulnerability to apnea in AS. There is also greater variability in respiratory rate and tidal volume and usually an increased minute ventilation that manifests with lower levels of transcutaneous and alveolar P_{CO_2} (Davi *et al.*, 1979; Martin, Herrell and Pultusker, 1981). Oxygen consumption is slightly increased in AS (Stothers and Warner, 1978) and transcutaneous P_{O_2} is decreased by approximately 5–10 mmHg. The mechanisms underlying these effects are largely mediated by alterations in the control of the respiratory muscles. It has been postulated that during AS there are motor neurone inhibitory influences that interfere with breathing regularity, thus producing central apneas (Pompeiano, 1966). The increased DIA activity during AS (Bryan, 1979; Muller *et al.*, 1979b; Carlo *et al.*, 1983a) may serve as a compensatory mechanism for the decreased IC muscle activity observed in this sleep state, in both preterm and term infants (Hagan *et al.*, 1977; Prechtl, Van Eykern and O'Brien, 1977; Curzi-Dascalova, 1982).

It is now clear from observations in various human and animal studies that the upper airway muscles are also modulated by sleep state. Healthy adults have comparable genioglossus (GG) activity during wakefulness and QS but a marked reduction and even cessation of both phasic and tonic activity during AS (Sauerland and Harper, 1976). Decreased activity of two laryngeal muscles, the posterior cricoarytenoid and cricothyroid, has also been observed in adult rats (Sherrey and Megirian, 1980) and cats (Orem and Lydic, 1978) during AS. Harding, Johnson and McClelland (1980) have evaluated the effect of maturation on the control of laryngeal muscles during sleep and wakefulness. In anesthetized fetal sheep they observed that, while activity of the posterior cricoarythenoid and cricothyroid was decreased during a fetal sleep state similar to AS, thyroarytenoid activity was higher in the same sleep state. Increased activity of another group of upper airway muscles, the nasolabialis, has been observed in rats during AS (Sherrey and Megirian, 1977). Interestingly, we have shown that the AN also has increased activity during AS in human infants (Carlo *et al.*, 1983a). These observations indicate that the effect of sleep state or neural control of the respiratory muscles may depend on the specific muscle group under consideration.

Role of chemoreceptors

Whereas adult animals and humans respond with sustained hyperventilation to chemical stimuli such as hypoxia or hypercapnia, the response of the newborn of most species is affected by the maturational process. The preterm and term infant respond to hypoxia in the first days of life with a biphasic ventilatory behavior. This is characterized by an early increase in ventilation during the first 1 or 2 min of the stimulus with a late (4–5 min) return of ventilation to baseline or even below. In contrast, the ventilatory response during hypercapnia is sustained hyperventilation, although the slope of the response increases with postnatal age (Rigatto, Brady and de la Torre Verduzco, 1975). Krauss *et al.* (1975) observed that, with advancing gestational age, the improved CO_2 sensitivity was accompanied by increased lung compliance. They postulated that mechanical factors could in part explain the maturational change in the ventilatory response to hypercapnia. Furthermore, the response to hypercapnia is affected by the level of oxygenation (Rigatto, de la Torre Verduzco and Cates, 1975) such that improved oxygenation enhances CO_2 sensitivity in neonates. These changing ventilatory responses to chemical stimuli clearly reflect to some degree alterations in respiratory muscle behavior.

We have shown in preterm infants that peak DIA activity increased proportionately to changes in end-tidal P_{CO_2} induced by hypercapnic stimulation (Carlo *et al.*, 1983a). These increases in DIA activity paralleled the corresponding changes in tidal volume. Peak DIA activity prior to CO_2 exposure was higher in AS than QS, but in response to hypercapnia EMG increased during both sleep states. Moriette *et al.* (1984) have also shown that in response to hypercapnia there was an increase in diaphragm EMG that correlated with the corresponding ventilatory response. In response to hypercapnia, human adults increase IC muscle activity more than that of the DIA (D'Angelo, 1982). The IC muscle response to hypercapnia has not been appropriately measured in newborn infants. As the asynchronous or paradoxical breathing pattern is frequently converted to synchronous rib cage and abdominal movements, it can be inferred that hypercapnia enhances IC muscle activity in infants.

Several studies have described the response of upper airway muscles (or their innervation) to hypercapnic stimulation, usually in comparison to the changes in DIA or phrenic nerve activity. A curvilinear response (small increases initially followed by marked augmentation at higher CO_2 levels) of the GG muscle or hypoglossal nerve during hypercapnia has been observed in anesthetized adult rabbits (Brouillette and Thach, 1980), cats (Bruce, Mitra and Cherniack, 1982), and dogs (Weiner *et al.*, 1982). These observations contrast markedly with the proportionate or linear change in DIA or phrenic activity found by the same investigators. Hwang, St John and Bartlett (1983) observed that anesthesia in cats depressed hypoglossal activity more than that of the phrenic nerve. These findings led them to conclude that the reported curvilinear activation of upper airway muscles during both hypercapnia and hypoxia could be secondary to the level of anesthesia. This could also explain the predisposition of some patients to develop obstructive apnea following sedation and/or anesthesia. Most recently, Haxhiu *et al.* (1984) have measured respiratory muscle activity in awake cats with chronically implanted electrodes. They observed that with increasing hypercapnia the relationship between genioglossus and diaphragm EMG changes was indeed curvilinear, with preferential increases in GG activity occurring at high levels of $P\text{CO}_2$. Furthermore, the transient responses of these EMGs to CO_2 inhalation differed substantially, with the DIA reaching a new steady state earlier than the GG.

Consistent with these findings, hyperventilation and hypocapnia caused the genioglossus EMG to be abolished before the development of diaphragmatic apnea (Brouillette and Thach, 1980). Bruce, Mitra and Cherniack (1982) have demonstrated that the respiratory muscle response to hypercapnia is differentially affected by sectioning the carotid sinus nerve or inhibition of the intermediate area of the ventral medullary surface in anesthetized cats. They observed that hypoglossal nerve activity was more dependent on peripheral chemoreceptor activity (carotid sinus nerve), while phrenic activity depended more on central chemoreceptors at the medulla. These findings are supported by the tendency for carotid body chemoreceptor activity to increase curvilinearly in relation to $P\text{CO}_2$ (Fitzgerald and Parks, 1971). Another upper airway muscle, the posterior cricoarytenoid, and its nerve supply, the recurrent laryngeal nerve, have linear responses that parallel those of the DIA in both anesthetized (Weiner *et al.*, 1982) and unanesthetized (Haxhiu *et al.*, 1984) animals.

Consistent with the curvilinear activation of upper airway muscles in response to hypercapnia in these animal studies, we have observed in preterm infants that while 2% CO_2 inhalation variably altered AN activity, 4% CO_2 enhanced alae nasi EMG in all infants during both AS and QS (Carlo *et al.*, 1983a). It is possible that an absent or small response of upper airway muscles when accompanied by a linear increase in chest wall muscle activity during increasing hypercapnia may result in ventilatory instability (*Figure 2.4*).

In contrast to the observation in animals and human infants, in the sleeping or awake human adult AN and GG responses to hypercapnia are linear, paralleling those of the DIA (Strohl *et al.*, 1980; Önal, Lopata and O'Connor, 1981a; Parker *et al.*, 1981). In a recent preliminary report, Jeffries, Brouillette and Hunt (1983) presented preliminary data on measurements of GG activity in children. They observed increased EMG during hypercapnia and hypoxia, but did not compare these respones to those of the DIA.

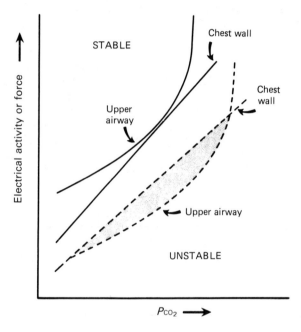

Figure 2.4 Schematic representation used in the model of the electrical activity or effective force of upper airway and chest wall muscles and P_{CO_2}. Solid lines show relationships during upper airway stability, broken lines during instability. Shaded area indicates that there is a range of P_{CO_2} in which upper airway obstruction can occur. (Modified from Longobardo *et al.*, 1982)

Lawson and Long (1983) have shown that the characteristic biphasic ventilatory response to hypoxia in newborn piglets is accompanied by biphasic changes in minute phrenic nerve activity. These data suggest that central mechanisms at least partially mediate the ventilatory changes that accompany hypoxia in the newborn piglet. In contrast, the adult human responds to isocapnic hypoxia with persistent elevation of upper airway muscle activity (Önal, Lopata and O'Connor, 1981b). Furthermore, these investigators reported a linear relationship between changes in oxygen saturation and both DIA and GG electromyograms. Respiratory muscle responses have not yet been correlated with the ventilatory changes induced by hypoxia in human infants.

Role of mechanoreceptors

In their classical studies, Hering and Breuer demonstrated in 1868 that lung inflation was followed by decreased respiratory frequency primarily due to a prolongation of expiratory time. This reflex, first described in animals, is weak or absent in human adults but appears quite active in the newborn infant (Bodegard *et al.*, 1969; Cross *et al.*, 1980). It originates within the pulmonary stretch receptors in the smooth muscles of the airway, and large myelinated fibers in the vagus nerve carry the afferent input to the medulla. It is considered to be a slowly adapting reflex since it shows sustaining discharges during prolonged inflation.

Mechanoreceptors play a key role in modulating the control of respiratory muscles. During early inspiration there is a positive volume-related vagally mediated feedback mechanism that increases phrenic activity in anesthetized animals (Bartoli *et al.*, 1975; Cross, Jones and Guz, 1980; DiMarco *et al.*, 1981). In addition, during late inspiration lung inflation is accompanied by a graded inhibition of inspiratory muscle activity (Younes, Remmers and Baker, 1978). All these responses have been completely eliminated by vagotomy and are thus vagally mediated.

The effect of volume-related feedback on the relative activities of upper airway and chest wall muscles (or their nerve supply) has been evaluated. Bradley (1972) performed end-expiratory occlusion on anesthetized adult cats and compared diaphragm and intercostal EMGs of control and occluded breaths. Both diaphragm and intercostal EMGs had a higher peak during occlusion without change in the rate of rise and the response was eliminated by vagotomy. This suggested that the effect was due to a timing mechanism associated with a release of inhibition present during spontaneous breathing rather than enhanced activation. Cohen (1975) showed that in adult anesthetized cats inhibition of both phrenic and recurrent laryngeal nerve activity occurred during spontaneous breathing. Inhibition of the recurrent laryngeal nerve was, however, greater and started earlier during inspiration. Similarly, greater inhibition of upper airway nerves and muscles has been observed by both Weiner *et al.* (1982) and van Lunteren *et al.* (1984a) in anesthetized adult dogs. In contrast, Brouillette and Thach (1980) observed in anesthetized adult rabbits similar increases in peak diaphragm and genioglossus EMGs in response to end-expiratory airway occlusion. The responses of both upper airway and chest wall muscles and nerves to occlusion were eliminated by vagotomy (Cohen, 1975; Brouillette and Thach, 1980; Weiner *et al.*, 1982; van Lunteren *et al.*, 1984).

Using the technique of end-expiratory airway occlusion, we have evaluated the strength of this volume-related inspiratory inhibition in healthy preterm infants during sleep (Carlo, Miller and Martin, 1984). We have observed a greater than 100% increase in peak submental EMG during occlusion, while peak diaphragm EMG was not significantly altered. Rate of rise of both EMGs was unaffected. Our data thus indicate that the EMG of the submental area (probably reflecting the GG muscle) is subjected to greater inhibition than the DIA during spontaneous breathing. It is clear from these studies that mechanoreceptors alter respiratory muscle behavior, with a likely preferential effect on upper airway muscles. The animal data indicate that this volume-related feedback is vagally mediated. In contrast, in kittens during the first week of life, two chest wall muscles, the DIA and IC, exhibit parallel EMG responses during occlusion (Trippenbach and Kelly,

1983). It is still unclear whether the volume-related preferential inhibition of accessory respiratory muscles is limited to these upper airway muscles.

Several investigators have altered stimulation of mechanoreceptors in the isolated airway and observed the effect on respiratory muscles. Abu-Osba, Mathew and Thach (1981) have shown that deviation of airflow from the upper airway through a tracheostomy decreased genioglossus EMG. Furthermore, GG activity in rabbits and dogs is increased by a constant negative pressure or pressure fluctuation applied to the isolated upper airway (Mathew, Abu-Osba and Thach, 1982; van Lunteren *et al.*, 1984) and decreased by positive pressure on the isolated airway (Mathew, Abu-Osba and Thach, 1982). Negative pressure applied to the isolated upper airway also increases the EMG of the airway muscles including the cricothyroid, posterior cricoarytenoid, nasolabial, sternohyoid, alae nasi (Abu-Osba, Mathew and Thach, 1981; Mathew, Abu-Osba and Thach, 1982; Mathew, 1984; van Lunteren *et al.*, 1984b). In contrast, Al-Shway and Mortola (1982) have proposed that flow rather than pressure changes in the upper airway influence ventilation in newborn animals. Alterations in respiratory control in the three previous studies were eliminated by the application of local anesthesia, suggesting that local mechanoreceptors in the upper airway mediate these responses.

Other mechanoreceptor reflexes may regulate respiratory activity in infants. Although newborn infants usually respond to end-expiratory occlusion with a prolonged inspiratory effort, at times this effort is shorter than the preceding inspiration (Knill and Bryan, 1976; Martin *et al.*, 1977; Thach *et al.*, 1978; Gerhardt and Bancalari, 1981). This reflex response occurs more frequently in preterm infants and, with advancing intrauterine or extrauterine maturation, prolongation of inspiratory efforts usually occurs (Kirkpatrick *et al.*, 1976; Gerhardt and Bancalari, 1981). Rapid compression of the chest at end expiration or chest wall vibration also produced shortening of inspiratory time while continuous positive airway pressure (CPAP) reduced chest wall asynchrony and prolonged inspiratory time (Knill and Bryan, 1976; Hagan *et al.*, 1977). These investigators proposed that chest wall distortion might stimulate stretch receptors in the vicinity of the IC muscles, resulting in an intercostal–phrenic inhibitory reflex. As chest wall distortion might be accompanied by compression of underlying lung, vagal afferents originating in pulmonary tissues cannot be excluded in this response. In fact, Trippenbach, Zinman and Mozes (1981) have shown that in kittens this response disappeared after vagotomy. Studies on the direct effect of this and other mechanoreflexes on control of respiratory muscles have not been performed.

CLINICAL IMPLICATIONS

Obstructive apnea

Following initial reports of the occurrence of obstructive sleep apnea in adults, obstructive apnea was also described in some patients with near-miss sudden infant death syndrome (Guilleminault *et al.*, 1976a; Guilleminault *et al.*, 1979), in children (Guilleminault *et al.*, 1976b; Brouillette, Fernbach and Hunt, 1982) and in preterm infants (Stark and Thach, 1976; Milner *et al.*, 1980). In fact, recent studies suggest that most apneic episodes in neonates have obstructive components (Mathew, Roberts and Thach, 1982; Dransfield, Spitzer and Fox, 1983; Miller, Carlo and Martin, 1984). Negative pharyngeal pressures, decreased upper airway muscle tone and neck flexion variably contribute to the development of airway obstruction (*Figure 2.5*). In rabbits, Brouillette and Thach (1980) have shown that airway patency is at least partially dependent on the ability of the GG muscle to maintain pharyngeal patency. A decrease in genioglossus EMG has been observed at the time of upper airway obstruction in adults, while re-establishment of patency coincided with a burst of GG activity (Remmers *et al.*, 1978; Önal, Lopaka and O'Connor, 1982). Similar observations have not yet been reported in infants or

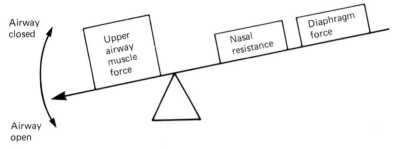

Figure 2.5 A model of pharyngeal airway maintenance. Nasal resistance and diaphragm contractile force, which together determine the inspiratory drop in transpharyngeal pressure, are pictured on one side of a fulcrum. On the other side is the contractile force of airway dilating muscles which opposes the airway constricting effect of reduced airway pressure. The balance of these various forces determines airway caliber. This model is supported by a number of clinical and laboratory observations. (Reproduced from Thach, 1983, by courtesy of the Editor and Publisher, Academic Press)

children, although Jeffries, Brouillette and Hunt (1983) have presented preliminary data suggesting that infants and children with obstructive apnea have increased activation of their GG muscles as well as other accessory muscles of respiration. It is possible that such infants need high levels of upper airway muscle activity in order to maintain pharyngeal patency. Control of the GG thus seems to be of considerable importance in the development of obstructive apnea. As already noted, studies have now documented that in response to hypercapnia the activity of many upper airway muscles increases in a curvilinear manner in comparison to the linear increase in diaphragmatic activity. It has thus been hypothesized that an absent response of the upper airway muscles during initial hypercapnia, if accompanied by a high level of DIA activity, may result in partial or complete airway obstruction (Cherniack, 1981; Longobardo *et al.*, 1982).

Inspiratory muscle fatigue

Fatigue of a muscle implies its inability to generate the necessary contractile force and pressure. In the case of the DIA this pressure is the transdiaphragmatic pressure, and fatigue translates into impairment of ventilation. The problem of muscle fatigue may originate in the muscle itself or be mediated through its neural control. It has been proposed that respiratory muscle fatigue occurs when there is excessive work of breathing and a shortage of substrate (Roussos and Macklem, 1982). In newborns and children, increased work of breathing may be due to lung disease such as respiratory distress syndrome and bronchial asthma. Hypoxemia, low cardiac output and a catabolic state are some of the commonly occurring factors that may limit the supply of oxygen or energy to the muscles. Furthermore, the diaphragm and intercostal muscles of preterm infants have decreased low-oxidative fatigue resistant muscle fibers (Keens *et al.*, 1978). The percentage of low-oxidative fibers increases to adult levels during the first year of life. These investigators thus proposed that newborns may be particularly susceptible to respiratory muscle fatigue.

Although the diagnosis of DIA fatigue ultimately depends on the demonstrated inability to generate an adequate transdiaphragmatic pressure, it has been known since early in this century that EMG changes accompany muscle fatigue. These changes include an increase in the power or amount of low-frequency components with a decrease in the high-frequency components. Muller *et al.* (1979a) have shown that similar changes in the power spectrum of the diaphragm EMG occur in preterm infants during asynchronous chest wall movements. Furthermore, these investigators observed that after some infants were weaned from ventilators, a decrease in the high-to-low frequency components of more than 20% frequently preceded CO_2 retention and apneic episodes that required assisted ventilation to be reinstituted (*Figure 2.6*) (Muller *et al.*, 1979a,b).

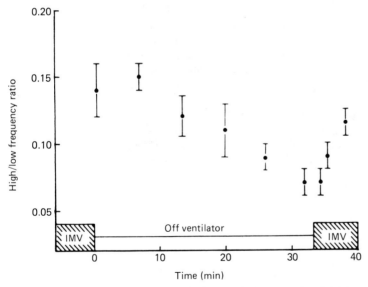

Figure 2.6 High/low frequency ratio in one infant. During initial IMV period frequency spectrum was normal. During the period off the ventilator, the changes in the high/low frequency ratio that developed are characteristic of muscle fatigue. (Reproduced from Muller *et al.*, 1979a, by courtesy of the Editor and Publisher of *Journal of Applied Physiology: Respiratory, Environmental and Exercise Physiology*)

It is interesting that aminophylline has been found to improve diaphragm contractility in man (Aubier *et al.*, 1981), since in newborns it increases CO_2 sensitivity and is highly effective in the treatment of apnea. Further studies need to be performed in order to confirm the significance of respiratory muscle fatigue in the newborn period.

Airway resistance in the newborn period

Nasal resistance contributes from approximately 30 to 50% of the total lung resistance. Since newborns are considered to be obligate nose breathers, nasal resistance is a major determinant of airflow to the lungs. Nasal resistance is known to undergo marked spontaneous variability in neonates. We attempted to determine if changes in the activation of the AN, the dilator of the nostrils, altered nasal resistance in preterm infants. The presence of a tonic or phasic alae nasi EMG was accompanied by a significant decrease in nasal resistance (*Figure 2.7*) (Carlo *et al.*, 1983b). A reduction in nasal resistance is important because the work of breathing is decreased. Furthermore, a decrease in nasal resistance may reduce negative inspiratory pharyngeal pressure and thus protect against airway obstruction. Infant studies have shown that impairment of nasal patency results in augmented negative pharyngeal pressures during inspiration (Tonkin *et al.*, 1979).

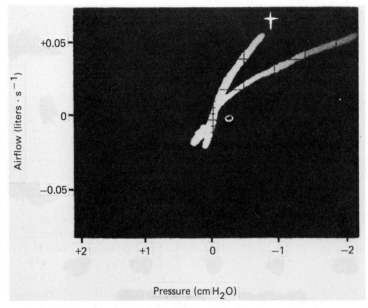

Figure 2.7 Effect of alae nasi (AN) activation on nasal resistance in one infant during quiet sleep shown by relationship between airflow and transnasal pressure of two consecutive breaths, only one (indicated by dagger) of which was accompanied by AN activity. At peak inspiration nasal resistance decreased from approximately 40 to $15\,cm\,H_2O\cdot l^{-1}\cdot s^{-1}$. (Reproduced from Carlo *et al.*, 1983b, by courtesy of the Editor and Publisher of *Paediatrics*; copyright of the American Academy of Pediatrics, 1983)

Upper airway flows may also be modified by the laryngeal muscles. It has been shown in anesthetized cats that laryngeal resistance may be actively controlled by adduction of the vocal cords (Bartlett, Remmers and Gautier, 1973; Gautier, 1973; Bartlett, 1979). Similar observations have been made in adults, and in addition it has been found that hypercapnia or exercise enlarge the glottis during expiration while hypoxia narrows it (England and Bartlett, 1982; England, Bartlett and Daubenspeck, 1982).

The common grunting of the neonate serves to delay expiratory flows, prolong expiration, and maintain functional residual capacity. It is mediated via laryngeal muscles and eliminated with endotracheal intubation. The precise role played by the laryngeal muscles in controlling expiration during spontaneous breathing in healthy neonates is unclear.

Asynchrony of chest wall movements

Asynchronous (out of phase, paradoxical) chest wall movements are observed most commonly during active sleep and thought to be secondary to decreased intercostal muscle activity. As discussed before, it is possible that lack of abdominal muscle tone also contributes to the asynchrony of chest wall muscles. Asynchrony occurs more frequently in the young preterm infant without respiratory distress syndrome (Carlo *et al.*, 1982). It has also been reported that asynchronous chest wall movements occur simultaneously with DIA fatigue (Muller *et al.*, 1979c). While asynchronous chest wall movements would clearly appear to be a handicap in sustaining adequate ventilation, their precise implications have not yet been determined.

Relationship to sucking, swallowing and feeding

Sucking and swallowing are both vital neonatal functions that are developing prenatally but must be carefully coordinated with respiration following birth. With advancing post-conceptional age, non-nutritive sucking bursts become increasingly prolonged and are accompanied by intermittent swallows. Wilson *et al.* (1981) have documented that spontaneous non-feeding swallows in preterm infants interrupt either inspiratory or expiratory airflow by closing off the airway for approximately 1 second. These periods of absent airflow were frequently accompanied by obstructed inspiratory efforts. Nonetheless, Paludetto *et al.* (1984) have recently observed that oxygenation of preterm infants (as measured via transcutaneous Po_2) is actually improved by approximately 2–4 mmHg during non-nutritive sucking. This effect was apparent between 32 to 35 weeks' postconceptional age and was not due to a change in sleep state or respiratory frequency. It is possible that ventilation is facilitated secondary to a reflex activation of upper airway muscles that might lower upper airway resistance during non-nutritive sucking. The common clinical observation that nasal flaring frequently accompanied sucking would support this concept.

During oral feeding, on the other hand, sucking and swallowing must be precisely coordinated with breathing in order to prevent milk from being aspirated into the airway. Harding *et al.* (1978) observed that during feeding, newborn lambs exhibited an initial period of continuous sucking followed by a period of intermittent sucking bursts of variable duration. They noted that effective breathing movements tended to be absent in the lambs for the first 10–20 s of sucking, and after 30 s Pao_2 had fallen an average of 23 mmHg. There was subsequently a gradual recovery of breathing as feeding continued. We have recently observed a 40–50% fall in minute ventilation during the initial period of continuous sucking that occurs when preterm infants are nipple fed (Shivpuri *et al.*, 1983). During the subsequent period of intermittent sucking, ventilation only recovered in those infants 36 weeks' postconceptional age. Continuous sucking was associated with a fall in both tidal volume and inspiratory time, while mean inspiratory flow did not change significantly. These data suggest that, unlike term infants (Durand *et al.*, 1981), preterm neonates are unable to increase inspiratory drive and maintain ventilation during feeding, when inspiratory time is frequently shortened.

These data indicate that respiratory muscle behavior is influenced by a wide diversity of factors that extend beyond traditional chemical and mechanoreceptor control mechanisms. An understanding of the interaction between muscles of the upper airway and chest wall is important if we are to appreciate the role of respiration during normal homeostatic mechanisms for ventilatory control. Evaluation of these interactions during normal postnatal maturation should result in greater understanding of respiratory muscle control in both healthy and apneic human infants.

Acknowledgements

This work was supported in part by the National Institutes of Health Grants HL-31173 and HL-25830.

References

ABU-OSBA, Y.K., MATHEW, O.P. and THACH, B.T. (1981) An animal model for airway sensory deprivation producing obstructive apnea with postmortem findings of sudden infant death syndrome. *Pediatrics*, **68**, 796–801

AGOSTONI, E., SANT'AMBROGIO, G. and DEL PORTILLO CARRASCO, H. (1960) Electromyography of the diaphragm in man and transdiaphragmatic pressure. *Journal of Applied Physiology*, **15**, 1093–1097

AL-SHWAY, S. F. and MORTOLA, J. P. (1982) Respiratory effects of airflow through the upper airways in newborn kittens and puppies. *Journal of Applied Physiology: Respiratory, Environmental and Exercise Physiology*, **53**, 805–814

AUBIER, M., DE TROYER, A., SAMPSON, M., MACKLEM, P. T. and ROUSSOS, C. (1981) Aminophylline improves diaphragmatic contractility. *New England Journal of Medicine*, **305**, 249–252

BARTLETT, D. JR (1979) Effects of hypercapnia and hypoxia on laryngeal resistance to airflow. *Respiration Physiology*, **37**, 293–302

BARTLETT, D. JR, REMMERS, J. E. and GAUTIER, H. (1973) Laryngeal regulation of respiratory airflow. *Respiration Physiology*, **18**, 194–204

BARTOLI, A., CROSS, B. A., GUZ, A., HUSZCZUK, A. and JEFFERIES, R. (1975) The effect of varying tidal volume on the associated phrenic motoneuron output: studies of vagal and chemical feedback. *Respiration Physiology*, **25**, 135–155

BODEGARD, G., SCHWIELER, G. H., SKOGLUND, S. and ZETTERSTROM, R. (1969) Control of respiration in newborn babies. I. The development of the Hering–Breuer inflation reflex. *Acta Paediatrica Scandinavica*, **58**, 567–571

BRADLEY, G. W. (1972) The response of the respiratory system to elastic loading in cats. *Respiration Physiology*, **16**, 142–160

BROUILLETTE, R. T., FERNBACH, S. K. and HUNT, C. E. (1982) Obstructive sleep apnea in infants and children. *Pediatrics*, **100**, 31–40

BROUILLETTE, R. T. and THACH, B. T. (1980) Control of genioglossus muscle inspiratory activity. *Journal of Applied Physiology: Respiratory, Environmental and Exercise Physiology*, **49**, 801–808

BRUCE, E. N., MITRA, J. and CHERNIACK, N. S. (1982) Central and peripheral chemoreceptor inputs to phrenic and hypoglossal motoneurons. *Journal of Applied Physiology: Respiratory, Environmental and Exercise Physiology*, **53**, 1504–1511

BRYAN, M. H. (1979) The work of breathing during sleep in newborns. *American Review of Respiratory Diseases*, **119**, 137–138

CAMPBELL, E. J. M. (1952) An electromyographic study of the role of the abdominal muscles in breathing. *Journal of Physiology*, **117**, 222–233

CARLO, W. A., MARTIN, R. J., ABBOUD, E. F., BRUCE, E. N. and STROHL, K. P. (1983a) Effect of sleep state and hypercapnia on alae nasi and diaphragm EMGs in preterm infants. *Journal of Applied Physiology: Respiratory, Environmental and Exercise Physiology*, **54**, 1590–1596

CARLO, W. A., MARTIN, R. J., BRUCE, E. N., STROHL, K. P. and FANAROFF, A. A. (1983b) Alae nasi activation (nasal flaring) decreases nasal resistance in preterm infants. *Pediatrics*, **72**, 338–343

CARLO, W. A., MARTIN, R. J., VERSTEEGH, F. G. A., GOLDMAN, M. D., ROBERTSON, S. S. and FANAROFF, A. A. (1982) The effect of respiratory distress syndrome on chest wall movements and respiratory pauses in preterm infants. *American Review of Respiratory Diseases*, **126**, 103–107

CARLO, W. A., MILLER, M. J. and MARTIN, R. J. (1984) Release of upper airway muscle inhibition during airway occlusion. *Pediatric Research* (Abstract), **18**, 388A

CHERNIACK, N. S. (1981) Respiratory dysrrhythmias during sleep. *New England Journal of Medicine*, **305**, 325–330

CLARK, F. J. and VON EULER, C. (1972) On the regulation of depth and rate of breathing. *Journal of Physiology*, **222**, 267–295

COHEN, M. I. (1975) Phrenic and recurrent laryngeal discharge patterns and the Hering–Breuer reflex. *American Journal of Physiology*, **228**, 1489–1496

CROSS, B. A., JONES, P. W. and GUZ, A. (1980) The role of vagal afferent information during inspiration in determining phrenic motoneurone output. *Respiration Physiology*, **39**, 149–167

CROSS, K. W., KLAUS, M., TOOLEY, W. H. and WEISSER, K. (1980) The response of the new-born baby to inflation of the lungs. *Journal of Physiology*, **151**, 551–565

CURZI-DASCALOVA, L. (1978) Thoracico-abdominal respiratory correlations in infants: constancy and variability in different sleep states. *Early Human Development*, **2**, 25–38

CURZI-DASCALOVA, L. (1982) Phase relationships between thoracic and abdominal respiratory movement during sleep in 31–38 weeks CA normal infants. Comparison with full-term (39–41 weeks) newborns. *Neuropediatrics*, **13** (Suppl.), 15–20

D'ANGELO, E. (1982) Inspiratory muscle activity during rebreathing in intact and vagotomized rabbits. *Respiration Physiology*, **47**, 193–218

DAVI, M., SANKARAN, K., MACCALLUM, M., CATES, D. and RIGATTO, H. (1979) Effect of sleep state on chest distortion and on the ventilatory response to CO_2 in neonates. *Pediatric Research*, **13**, 982–986

DE TROYER, A. and KELLY, Z. (1984) Action of neck accessory muscles on rib cage in dogs. *Journal of Applied Physiology: Respiratory, Environmental and Exercise Physiology*, **56**, 326–332

DE TROYER, A., SAMPSON, M., SIGRIST, S. and MACKLEM, P. T. (1981) The diaphragm: two muscles. *Science*, **213**, 237–238

DIMARCO, A. F., VON EULER, C., ROMANIUK, J. R. and YAMAMOTO, Y. (1981) Positive feedback facilitation of external intercostal and phrenic inspiratory activity by pulmonary stretch receptors. *Acta Physiologica Scandinavica*, **113**, 375–386

DRANSFIELD, D. A., SPITZER, A. R. and FOX, W. W. (1983) Episodic airway obstruction in premature infants. *American Journal of Diseases of Children*, **137**, 441–443

DREYFUS-BRISAC, C. (1970) Ontogenesis of sleep in human premature after 32 weeks of conceptional age. *Developmental Psychobiology*, **3**, 91–121

DURAND, M., LEAHY, F. N., MacCALLUM, M., CATES, D. B., RIGATTO, H. and CHERNICK, V. (1981) Effect of feeding on the chemical control of breathing in the newborn infant. *Pediatric Research*, **15**, 1509–1512

ENGLAND, S. J. and BARTLETT, D. JR (1982) Changes in respiratory movements of the human vocal cords during hypercapnea. *Journal of Applied Physiology: Respiratory, Environmental and Exercise Physiology*, **52**, 780–785

ENGLAND, S. J., BARTLETT, D. JR and DAUBENSPECK, J. A. (1982) Influence of human vocal cord movements on airflow and resistance during eupnea. *Journal of Applied Physiology: Respiratory, Environmental and Exercise Physiology*, **53**, 81–86

FITZGERALD, R. S. and PARKS, D. C. (1971) Effect of hypoxia on carotid chemoreceptor response to carbon dioxide in cats. *Respiration Physiology*, **12**, 218–229

FLEMING, P. J., MULLER, N. L., BRYAN, M. H. and BRYAN, A. C. (1979) The effects of abdominal loading on rib cage distortion in premature infants. *Pediatrics*, **64**, 425–428

GABRIEL, M., ALBANI, M. and SCHULTE, F. J. (1976) Apneic spells and sleep states in preterm infants. *Pediatrics*, **57**, 142–147

GAUTIER, H., REMMERS, J. E. and BARTLETT, D. JR (1973) Control of the duration of expiration. *Respiration Physiology*, **18**, 205–221

GERHARDT, T. and BANCALARI, E. (1981) Maturational changes of reflexes influencing inspiratory timing in newborns. *Journal of Applied Physiology: Respiratory, Environmental and Exercise Physiology*, **50**, 1282–1285

GIMBY, G., GOLDMAN, M. and MEAD, J. (1976) Respiratory muscle action inferred from rib cage and abdominal V–P partitioning. *Journal of Applied Physiology,* **41,** 739–751

GOLDMAN, M. D. and MEAD, J. (1973) Mechanical interaction between the diaphragm and rib cage. *Journal of Applied Physiology,* **35,** 197–204

GRASSINO, A., GOLDMAN, M. D., MEAD, J. and SEARS, T. A. (1978) Mechanics of the human diaphragm during voluntary contraction. *Journal of Applied Physiology: Respiratory, Environmental and Exercise Physiology,* **42,** 829–839

GUILLEMINAULT, C., ARIAGNO, R., KOROHKIN, R. *et al.* (1979) Mixed and obstructive sleep apnea and near-miss for Sudden Infant Death. 2. Comparison of near-miss and normal control infants by age. *Pediatrics,* **64,** 882–891

GUILLEMINAULT, C., ARIAGNO, R., SOUQUET, M. and DEMENT, W. C. (1976a) Abnormal polygraphic findings in near-miss Sudden Infant Death. *Lancet,* **i,** 1326–1327

GUILLEMINAULT, C., ELDRIDGE, F. L., SIMMONS, F. B. and DEMENT, W. C. (1976b) Sleep apnea in eight children. *Pediatrics,* **58,** 23–31

HAGAN, R., BRYAN, A. C., BRYAN, M. H. and GULSTON, G. (1977) Neonatal chest wall afferents and regulation of respiration. *Journal of Applied Physiology: Respiratory, Environmental and Exercise Physiology,* **42,** 362–367

HARDING, R., JOHNSON, P. and MCCLELLAND, M. E. (1980) Respiratory function of the larynx in developing sheep and the influence of sleep state. *Respiration Physiology,* **40,** 165–179

HARDING, R., JOHNSON, P., MCCLELLAND, M. E., MCLEOD, C. N., WHYTE, P. L. and WILKINSON, A. R. (1978) Respiratory and cardiovascular responses to feeding in lambs. *Journal of Physiology,* **275,** 40P–41P

HAXHIU, M. A., CHERNIACK, N. S., ALTOSE, M. D. and KELSEN, S. G. (1983) Effect of respiratory loading on the relationship between occlusion pressure and diaphragm EMG during hypoxia and hypercapnia. *American Review of Respiratory Diseases,* **127,** 185–188

HAXHIU, M. A., VAN LUNTEREN, E., MITRA, J. and CHERNIACK, N. S. (1984) Responses to chemical stimulation of upper airway muscles and diaphragm in awake cats. *Journal of Applied Physiology: Respiratory, Environmental and Exercise Physiology,* **56,** 397–403

HENDERSON-SMART, D. J. and READ, D. J. C. (1979) Reduced lung volume during behavioral active sleep in the newborn. *Journal of Applied Physiology: Respiratory, Environmental and Exercise Physiology,* **46,** 1081–1085

HWANG, J. C., ST JOHN, W. M. and BARTLETT, D. JR (1983) Respiratory-related hypoglossal nerve activity: influence of anesthetics. *Journal of Applied Physiology: Respiratory, Environmental and Exercise Physiology,* **55,** 785–792

JEFFRIES, B., BROUILLETTE, R. T. and HUNT, C. F. (1983) Electromyography of accessory muscles of respiration in children referred for obstructive sleep apnea. *Pediatric Research* (Abstract), **17,** 379A

KEENS, T. G., BRYAN, A. C., LEVISON, H. and IANUZZO, C. D. (1978) Developmental pattern of muscle fiber types in human ventilatory muscles. *Journal of Applied Physiology: Respiratory, Environmental and Exercise Physiology,* **44,** 909–913

KIRKPATRICK, S. M. L., OLINSKY, A., BRYAN, M. H. and BRYAN, A. C. (1976) Effect of premature delivery on the maturation of the Hering–Breuer inspiratory inhibitory reflex in human infants. *Journal of Pediatrics,* **88,** 1010–1014

KNILL, R. and BRYAN, A. C. (1976) An intercostal–phrenic inhibitory reflex in human newborn infants. *Journal of Applied Physiology,* **40,** 352–356

KRAUSS, A. N., KLAIN, D. B., WALDMAN, S. and AULD, P. A. M. (1975) Ventilatory response to carbon dioxide in newborn infants. *Pediatric Research,* **9,** 46–50

LAWSON, E. E. and LONG, W. A. (1983) Central origin of biphasic breathing pattern during hypoxia in newborns. *Journal of Applied Physiology: Respiratory, Environmental and Exercise Physiology,* **55,** 483–488

LONGOBARDO, G. S., GOTHE, B., GOLDMAN, M. D. and CHERNIACK, N. S. (1982) Sleep apnea considered as a control system instability. *Respiration Physiology,* **50,** 311–333

MARTIN, R. J., HERRELL, N. and PULTUSKER, M. (1981) Transcutaneous measurement of carbon dioxide tension: effect of sleep state in term infants. *Pediatrics,* **67,** 622–625

MARTIN, R. J., NEARMAN, H. S., KATONA, P. G. and KLAUS, M. H. (1977) The effect of a low continuous positive airway pressure on the reflex control of respiration in the preterm infant. *Journal of Pediatrics,* **90,** 976–981

MARTIN, R. J., OKKEN, A. and RUBIN, D. (1979) Arterial oxygen tension during active and quiet sleep in the normal neonate. *Journal of Pediatrics,* **94,** 271–274

MATHEW, O. P. (1984) Upper airway negative-pressure effects on respiratory activity of upper airway muscles. *Journal of Applied Physiology: Respiratory, Environmental and Exercise Physiology,* **56,** 500–505

MATHEW, O. P., ABU-OSBA, Y. K. and THACH, B. T. (1982) Genioglossus muscle responses to upper airway pressure changes: afferent pathways. *Journal of Applied Physiology: Respiratory, Environmental and Exercise Physiology*, **52**, 445–450

MATHEW, O. P., ROBERTS, J. L. and THACH, B. T. (1982) Pharyngeal airway obstruction in preterm infants during mixed and obstructive apnea. *Journal of Pediatrics*, **100**, 964–970

MILLER, M. J., CARLO, W. A. and MARTIN, R. J. (1985) Continuous positive airway pressure selectively reduces obstructive apnea in preterm infants. *Journal of Pediatrics*, **106**, 91–94

MILLER, M. J., MARTIN, R. J. and CARLO, W. A. (1984) Apnea: a disorder of respiratory control in newborn infants. In *Contemporary Issues in Pulmonary Disease-Sleep and Breathing*, Eds N. S. Cherniack and N. H. Edelman. New York: Churchill Livingstone Inc. (in press)

MILNER, A. D., BOON, A. W., SAUNDERS, R. A. and HOPKIN, I. E. (1980) Upper airways obstruction and apnea in preterm babies. *Archives of Disease in Childhood*, **55**, 22–25

MORIETTE, G., VAN REEMPTS, P., MOORE, M., CATES, D. and RIGATTO, H. (1984) The effect of rebreathing CO_2 on ventilation and diaphragmatic electromyography in newborn infants. *Federation Proceedings* (Abstract), **43**, 1008

MULLER, N., GULSTON, G., CADE, D. *et al.* (1979a) Diaphragmatic muscle fatigue in the newborn. *Journal of Applied Physiology: Respiratory, Environmental and Exercise Physiology*, **46**, 688–695

MULLER, N., VOLGYESI, G., BECKER, L., BRYAN, M. H. and BRYAN, A. C. (1979b) Diaphragmatic muscle tone. *Journal of Applied Physiology: Respiratory, Environmental and Exercise Physiology*, **47**, 279–284

MULLER, N., VOLGYESI, G., BRYAN, M. H. and BRYAN, A. C. (1979c) The consequences of diaphragmatic muscle fatigue in the newborn infant. *Pediatrics*, **95**, 793–797

OGAWA, T., JEFFERSON, N. C., TOMAN, J. E., CHILES, T., ZAMBETOGLOU, A. and NECHELES, H. (1960) Action potentials of accessory respiratory muscles in dogs. *American Journal of Physiology*, **199**, 569–572

ÖNAL, E., LOPATA, M. and O'CONNOR, T. D. (1981a) Diaphragmatic and genioglossal electromyogram responses to CO_2 rebreathing in humans. *Journal of Applied Physiology: Respiratory, Environmental and Exercise Physiology*, **50**, 1052–1055

ÖNAL, E., LOPATA, M. and O'CONNOR, T. D. (1981b) Diaphragmatic and genioglossal electromyogram responses to isocapnic hypoxia in humans. *American Review of Respiratory Diseases*, **124**, 215–217

ÖNAL, E., LOPATA, M. and O'CONNOR, T. (1982) Pathogenesis of apneas in hypersomnia – sleep apnea syndrome. *American Review of Respiratory Diseases*, **125**, 167–174

OREM, J. and LYDIC, R. (1978) Upper airway function during sleep and wakefulness: experimental studies on normal and anesthetized cats. *Sleep*, **1**, 49–68

OREM, J., LYDIC, R. and NORRIS, P. (1977) Experimental control of the diaphragm and laryngeal abductor muscles by brain stem arousal systems. *Respiration Physiology*, **38**, 203–221

PALUDETTO, R., ROBERTSON, S. S., HACK, M., SHIVPURI, C. and MARTIN, R. J. (1984) Transcutaneous oxygen tension during non-nutritive sucking in preterm infants. *Pediatrics*, **74**, 539–542

PARKER, D., STROHL, K., MITRA, J., SALAMONE, J. and CHERNIAK, N. S. (1981) Effect of CO_2 and tidal volumes on upper airway muscles. *Federation Proceedings* (Abstract), **40**, 481

PARMELEE, A. N. and STERN, E. (1972) Development of states in infants. In *Sleep and the Maturing Nervous System*, Ed. E. D. Clemente, pp. 199–228. New York: Academic Press

PENGELLY, L. D., ALDERSON, A. M. and MILIC-EMILI, J. (1971) Mechanics of the diaphragm. *Journal of Applied Physiology*, **30**, 797–805

PETIT, J. M., MILIC-EMILI, G. and DELHEZ, L. (1960) Role of the diaphragm in breathing in conscious normal man: an electromyographic study. *Journal of Applied Physiology*, **15**, 1101–1106

POMPEIANO, O. (1966) Muscular afferents and motor control during sleep. In *Muscular Afferents and Motor Control*, Ed. R. Grani, p. 415. Stockholm: Almquist and Wiskell

PRECTL, H. F. R., VAN EYKERN, L. A. and O'BRIEN, M. J. (1977) Respiratory muscle EMG in newborn: A non-intrusive method. *Early Human Development*, **1**, 265–283

REMMERS, J. E., DEGROOT, W. J., SAUERLAND, E. K. and ANCH, A. M. (1978) *Journal of Applied Physiology: Respiratory, Environmental and Exercise Physiology*, **44**, 931–938

RIGATTO, H., BRADY, J. P. and DE LA TORRE VERDUZCO, R. (1975) Chemoreceptor reflexes in preterm infants. II. The effect of gestational and postnatal age on the ventilatory response to inhaled carbon dioxide. *Pediatrics*, **55**, 614–620

RIGATTO, H., DE LA TORRE VERDUZCO and CATES, D. B. (1975) Effects of O_2 on the ventilatory response to CO_2 in preterm infants. *Journal of Applied Physiology*, **39**, 896–899

ROTHSTEIN, R. J., NARCE, S. L., DEBERRY-BOROWIECKI, B. and BLANKS, R. H. I. (1983) Respiratory-related activity of upper airway muscles in anesthetized rabbit. *Journal of Applied Physiology: Respiratory, Environmental and Exercise Physiology*, **55**, 1830–1836

ROUSSOS, C. and MACKLEM, P. T. (1982) The respiratory muscles. *New England Journal of Medicine*, **307**, 786–797

SAUERLAND, E. K. and HARPER, R. M. (1976) The human tongue during sleep: electromyographic activity of the genioglossus muscle. *Experimental Neurology,* **51,** 160–170

SHERREY, J. H. and MEGIRIAN, D. (1977) State dependence of upper airway respiratory motoneurons: functions of the cricothyroid and nasolabial muscles of the unanesthetized rat. *Electroencephalography and Clinical Neurophysiology,* **43,** 218–228

SHERREY, J. H. and MEGIRIAN, D. (1980) Respiratory EMG activity of the posterior cricoarytenoid, cricothyroid and diaphragm muscles during sleep. *Respiration Physiology,* **39,** 355–365

SHIVPURI, C. R., MARTIN, R. J., CARLO, W. A. and FANAROFF, A. A. (1983) Decreased ventilation in preterm infants during oral feeding. *Journal of Pediatrics,* **103,** 285–289

STARK, A. R. and THACH, B. T. (1976)Mechanistics of airway obstruction leading to apnea in newborn infants. *Journal of Pediatrics,* **89,** 982–985

STOTHERS, J. K. and WARNER, R. M. (1978) Oxygen consumption and neonatal sleep state. *Journal of Physiology,* **278,** 435–440

STROHL, K. P., HENSLEY, M. J., HALLETT, M., SAUNDERS, N. A. and INGRAM, R. H. JR (1980) Activation of upper airway muscles before onset of inspiration in normal humans. *Journal of Applied Physiology: Respiratory, Environmental and Exercise Physiology,* **49,** 638–642

STROHL, K. P., O'CAIN, C. F. and SLUTSKY, A. S. (1982) Alae nasi activation and nasal resistance in healthy subjects. *Journal of Applied Physiology: Respiratory, Environmental and Exercise Physiology,* **52,** 1432–1437

THACH, B. T. (1983) The role of pharyngeal airway obstruction in prolonging infantile apneic spells. In *Sudden Infant Death Syndrome,* Eds J. T. Tildon, L. M. Roeder and A. Steinschneider, pp. 279–292. New York: Academic Press

THACH, B. T., FRANTZ, I. D. III, ADLER, S. M. and TAEUSCH, H. W. (1978) Maturation of reflexes influencing inspiratory duration in human infants. *Journal of Applied Physiology: Respiratory, Environmental and Exercise Physiology,* **45,** 203–211

THACH, B. T. and STARK, A. R. (1979) Spontaneous neck flexion and airway obstruction during apneic spells in preterm infants. *Journal of Pediatrics,* **94,** 275–281

TONKIN, S. L., PARTRIDGE, J., BEACH, D. and WHITENEY, S. (1979) The pharyngeal effect of partial nasal obstruction. *Pediatrics,* **63,** 261–271

TRIPPENBACH, T. and KELLY, G. (1983) Phrenic activity and intercostal muscle EMG during inspiratory loading in newborn kittens. *Journal of Applied Physiology: Respiratory, Environmental and Exercise Physiology,* **54,** 496–501

TRIPPENBACH, T., ZINMAN, R. and MOZES, R. (1981) Effects of airway occlusion at functional residual capacity in pentobarbital-anesthetized kittens. *Journal of Applied Physiology: Respiratory, Environmental and Exercise Physiology,* **51,** 143–147

VAN LUNTEREN, E., STROHL, K. P., PARKER, D. M., BRUCE, E. N., VAN DE GRAAFF, W. B. and CHERNIACK, N. S. (1984a) Phasic volume-related feedback on upper airway muscle activity. *Journal of Applied Physiology: Respiratory, and Environmental Exercise Physiology,* **56,** 730–736

VAN LUNTEREN, E., VAN DE GRAAFF, W. B., PARKER, D. M. *et al.* (1984b) Nasal and laryngeal reflex responses to negative upper airway pressure. *Journal of Applied Physiology: Respiratory, Environmental and Exercise Physiology,* **56,** 746–752

WEINER, D., MITRA, J., SALAMONE, J. and CHERNIAK, N. S. (1982) Effect of chemical stimuli on nerves supplying upper airway muscles. *Journal of Applied Physiology: Respiratory, Environmental and Exercise Physiology,* **52,** 530–536

WERNER, S. S., STOCKARD, J. E. and BICKFORD, R. G. (1977) *Atlas of Neonatal Electroencephalography,* pp. 47–91. New York: Raven Press

WILSON, S. L., THACH, B. T., BOUILLETTE, R. T. and ABU-OSBA, Y. K. (1981) Coordination of breathing and swallowing in human infants. *Journal of Applied Physiology: Respiratory, Environmental and Exercise Physiology,* **50,** 851–858

YOUNES, M. K., REMMERS, J. E. and BAKER, J. (1978) Characteristics of inspiratory inhibition by phasic volume feedback in cats. *Journal of Applied Physiology: Respiratory, Environmental and Exercise Physiology,* **45,** 80–86

3
High frequency ventilation

Ivan D. Frantz III

Newer forms of assisted ventilation have centered around the use of faster than usual respiratory rates and have generated considerable recent interest. In some cases these rates are within or close to the range that a patient with respiratory distress may spontaneously achieve, but they may be as high as several thousand cycles per minute. More important than the rate used, however, is the size of the tidal volume in relation to dead space volume, for this dictates whether gas exchange is primarily through conventional mechanisms or whether additional mechanisms must be invoked.

Because all the various new techniques have been called 'high frequency ventilation' (HFV), confusion exists in differentiating one from another. I will discuss them in three categories: high frequency positive pressure ventilation (HFPPV), high frequency jet ventilation (HFJV) and high frequency oscillation (HFO). The first two categories resemble one another and conventional techniques in that tidal volume is greater than dead space volume, while the third makes a substantial departure from conventional techniques in that tidal volume is close to or less than dead space volume.

HIGH FREQUENCY POSITIVE PRESSURE VENTILATION

High frequency positive pressure ventilation was first described in Sweden by workers in the laboratory of Sjostrand (Jonzon et al., 1970, 1971; Heijman et al., 1972; Sjostrand et al., 1973; Borg et al., 1977; Eriksson and Sjostrand, 1977; Sjostrand, 1980). Their original rationale was to develop a technique for ventilation that would eliminate changes in blood pressure synchronous with respiration (Sjostrand et al., 1973; Sjostrand, 1977). They later postulated that the technique might have other advantages over conventional ventilatory techniques, particularly the need for lower respiratory pressures. The frequencies used by Sjostrand and coworkers were 60–120 min^{-1}.

In Sjostrand's original animal work tidal volume was provided through an insufflation catheter placed in the endotracheal tube. For clinical application, they developed a pneumatic valve system (Sjostrand, 1977) that delivered a pulse of compressed gas through a side-arm of the endotracheal tube adapter. Meanwhile,

37

Bland *et al.* (1980) have advocated rates similar to those used by Sjostrand for ventilation of infants with respiratory distress syndrome (RDS). They demonstrated good survival in a group of infants with RDS but did not include a control group, so it is impossible to determine if the technique is superior to ventilation at more conventional frequencies. Use of such rates, whether with a ventilator or by manual ventilation with an anesthesia bag, has nonetheless become common for a variety of lung diseases in infancy.

The tidal volumes delivered with HFPPV have not been carefully quantified, but are probably smaller than with conventional techniques, although larger than the subject's dead space volume. For this reason one need not invoke new mechanisms for gas exchange.

The principal indication for HFPPV has been during bronchoscopy, when both surgeon and anesthesiologist require simultaneous access to the airway (Borg *et al.*, 1977; Eriksson and Sjostrand, 1977). Otherwise, it has had little adult clinical application. In infants, on the other hand, it represents only a small modification of conventional ventilatory techniques and has been widely practised, although seldom referred to as HFPPV.

HIGH FREQUENCY JET VENTILATION

Of the techniques included in the general category of HFV, jet ventilation has had the widest use (Carlon *et al.*, 1982; Smith, 1982; Gallagher, 1983). The frequencies used clinically have been up to $250\,min^{-1}$; however, faster rates have been used in animal studies. Tidal volumes are larger than dead space volume and accordingly conventional mechanisms can account for gas exchange (Carlon *et al.*, 1983a; Frantz and Close, 1985a).

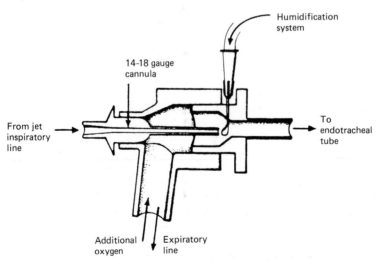

Figure 3.1 Diagram of jet injector system as used by Carlon *et al.* (1981a). Jet pulses are injected through the cannula which, in this case, is placed just outside the endotracheal tube. Fresh gas is entrained and expired gas eliminated through a second line. (Reproduced from Carlon *et al.*, 1981a, by courtesy of the Editors and Publisher, *Critical Care Medicine*)

The technique relies on the release of a pulse of gas under high pressure through a small-bore cannula in a venturi (*Figure 3.1*). The delivered tidal volume is the sum of the pulse of gas plus an additional amount entrained in the venturi. Although the technique has had a good deal of animal and human application, many of its parameters have not been characterized. For instance, the tidal volume depends on the relative sizes of the jet cannula and venturi, the driving pressure, and the duration of the pulse (Carlon *et al.*, 1983a). In addition, whether the cannula tip is distal to the endotracheal tube, within the tube or outside the tube will influence the amount of gas entrainment and the composition of the entrained gas (Davey, Lay and Leigh, 1982; Woo and Eurenius, 1982). All of these factors will also affect to what degree, if any, lung volume may be increased during jet ventilation (Frantz and Close, 1985a).

The most clinical experience has been acquired with jet ventilation in the operating room where, like HFPPV, it has been especially useful during bronchoscopy (Sanders, 1967; Gillespie, 1983). Some have also found it to be of advantage during thoracic surgery, where respiratory motion may be a problem (El-Baz *et al.*, 1982). Success has also been reported when the technique was used in patients with bronchopleural fistula, but conclusive data of superiority over conventional techniques are not available (Carlon *et al.*, 1980; Turnbull *et al.*, 1980). Jet ventilation has been used in adults with respiratory failure from a variety of causes. Schuster *et al.* (1981) presented a single case of a man with pulmonary edema who appeared to have had improved oxygenation during jet ventilation. It is not clear whether other factors, particularly mean airway pressure, were maintained constant during both jet and conventional ventilation. The same investigators treated a group of adults with respiratory failure due to pneumonia, adult respiratory distress syndrome and bronchospasm (Schuster, Klain and Snyder, 1982). In these patients, oxygenation comparable with conventional ventilation could be maintained. Mean pressures measured in the ventilator circuit were comparable, and peak pressures on jet ventilation were lower. The ventilator circuit may not, however, be the appropriate place for pressure measurement during jet ventilation (Close and Manchester, 1983; Frantz and Close, 1985a).

Rouby *et al.* (1983) used jet ventilation in 24 patients with respiratory failure due to such causes as pneumonia, acute respiratory distress syndrome, pulmonary contusion and fat embolism. They demonstrated adequate oxygenation at rates of from 100 to 600 min^{-1}. Their most significant observation was a marked increase in end-expiratory volume (EEV) during jet ventilation. Oxygenation appeared to be related to this increase in EEV. The EEV increase was greater both when inspiration made up a larger portion of the respiratory cycle and at higher rates, and was secondary to an increase in mean alveolar pressure. The authors correctly point out that the nature of the patient's lung disease will influence the degree of EEV change, the increase being greater in those patients with long respiratory time constants. Carbon dioxide elimination appeared to be related to both frequency and tidal volume, although tidal volume was not determined in this study.

Carlon *et al.* (1983) randomly assigned 309 patients with respiratory failure to treatment with either conventional or jet ventilation. There was no difference in survival or duration of stay within the intensive care unit between the two groups. There were also no substantial differences in gas exchange. More jet ventilator treated patients reached predetermined end points for ventilation; however, different end points were chosen for the two therapeutic groups. Lower peak inspiratory pressures were required for jet ventilation, although it appears that the pressures were measured in the ventilator circuit, not in the airway, and thus may not be meaningful. The investigators concluded that while jet ventilation was safe and reliable it did not have obvious benefits over conventional ventilation.

Pokora and coworkers have employed jet ventilation to treat ten neonates with complications of respiratory distress syndrome including pulmonary interstitial emphysema and bronchopleural fistula (Pokora *et al.*, 1983). Although radiological appearance of pulmonary air leak decreased in seven of the infants, only five survived. Three of the six patients treated for 20 or more hours developed tracheal obstruction. This obstruction was attributed to inadequate humidification, but may also have been the result of direct tracheal trauma due to the jet stream of gas or water particles.

Chatburn and co-workers appear to have solved the humidification problem during jet ventilation, and have applied the technique on a short-term basis to 12 infants with respiratory distress syndrome (Chatburn and McClellan, 1982; Carlo *et al.*, 1984). They achieved gas exchange at a rate of $250\,min^{-1}$ as good as or better than that with conventional ventilation with lower peak and mean tracheal pressures. The results of this study are encouraging, and may indicate that larger scale, longer term clinical trials are indicated.

Another potential advantage of jet ventilation is the possibility for its use via transtracheal puncture (Klain and Smith, 1977). This application may be of value in emergency situations where tracheal intubation is not possible or when skilled personnel are not available. Its practitioners must be aware, however, of the potential for tracheal damage due to impact of the jet on the tracheal wall, and of the necessity for establishing a patent airway above the jet so that exhalation can occur.

Extensive studies of side-effects of jet ventilation have not been made. Mention has been made of minimal hemodynamic effect (Carlon *et al.*, 1981) in one clinical study, and Carlon *et al.* (1983) have shown that blood pressure is inversely related to mean airway pressure. Keszler *et al.* (1982) have examined the lungs of dogs ventilated with either conventional or jet ventilation and shown no difference in gross or microscopic evidence of barotrauma. Lungs ventilated with the jet ventilator showed less hyperaeration. The infants treated by Pokora *et al.* (1983), on the other hand, showed major evidence of tracheal damage.

Despite the successful application of jet ventilation in both animal and human studies, good means of choosing appropriate settings have not been established. Variables include bias flow, driving pressure behind the jet, frequency, duration of the jet pulse, and the size and location of the cannula. Each of these may affect gas exchange, pressure and volume delivered to the respiratory system, and lung volume.

Choice of bias flow rate is relatively simple, since all that is necessary is a flow great enough to prevent rebreathing from the circuit and to maintain the desired level of continuous distending pressure. The correct flow may thus be determined on the same basis as for continuous distending airway pressure.

There is less basis for the choice of some of the other settings. This is in part because the respiratory system has not been fully characterized in terms of oscillation mechanics, and in part because the jet ventilators themselves have not been well characterized. Oscillation mechanics are further discussed later in this chapter. The characteristic of the jet ventilator that most needs definition is the tidal volume delivered to the respiratory system. Factors that determine the tidal volume are the jet driving pressure, duration of the jet, the size of the cannula, the position of the cannula and the characteristics of the respiratory system. The volume of the gas jet itself is obviously determined by the driving pressure and duration of the jet as well as the cannula size. Additional gas that may be entrained from the bias flow is affected by the above factors as well as the location of the jet tip and the characteristics of the venturi. Location of the jet tip will also affect the composition of the entrained gas, since if the tip is at the end of the endotracheal tube near the carina rebreathing must occur, whereas if it is in the bias gas flow more of the entrained gas will be fresh.

In addition to tidal volume, lung volume is also of concern during jet ventilation. Lung volume is determined in part by the continuous distending pressure applied. It is also affected by the relationship of expiratory duration to the time constant of the respiratory system and attachments. There have been anecdotal reports of increasing end-expiratory volume during jet ventilation, and this has been documented by Rouby *et al.* (1983). We have seen this in our own laboratory when certain combinations of tidal volume and expiratory duration were used. For example, in a rabbit ventilated at 125 min^{-1} (*Figure 3.2*), as the percentage of inspiratory time was increased from 10 to 30–50%, there was a marked increase in lung volume from relaxation volume to near total lung capacity. This could

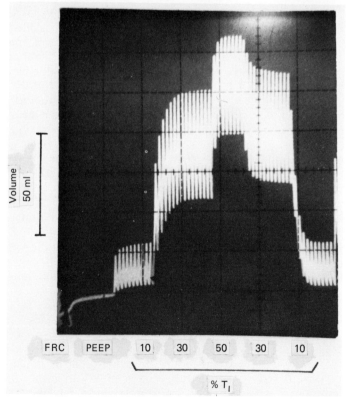

Figure 3.2 Tracing of lung volume during jet ventilation of a rabbit at 125 min^{-1}. There is a marked increase in lung volume as inspiratory time becomes a greater fraction of total cycle time. Tidal volume is maximal at 30% inspiratory time. (From data of Frantz and Close, 1985a)

obviously have deleterious cardiovascular effects as well as place the subject at risk for pneumothorax.

At present there is no rational basis for choosing settings, and it must be done by trial and error. This situation should improve as experience is gained, and the ventilators themselves are better characterized.

As mentioned previously, most use of jet ventilators to date has been at rates of $250 \, \text{min}^{-1}$ or less, where tidal volume is greater than dead space volume. Preliminary data from our laboratory (Close and Manchester, 1983) suggest that at much higher rates ($600-1000 \, \text{min}^{-1}$), tidal volume becomes much smaller. At these rates jet ventilation may become similar to oscillatory ventilation (HFO).

HIGH FREQUENCY OSCILLATION

High frequency oscillation is the most interesting of the new techniques since it represents the biggest departure from conventional methods. The single feature that differentiates HFO from other techniques is the use of tidal volume less than dead space volume. This feature requires that gas exchange must occur by mechanisms different from conventional ventilation. The frequency range for HFO has not been defined, but rates of $180-3000 \, \text{min}^{-1}$ have been reported.

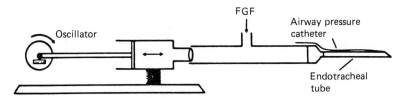

Figure 3.3 Diagram of piston pump high frequency oscillator. Oscillations are created by the piston driven by a motor and flywheel. The stroke volume can be varied by changing the point of attachment of the connecting rod to the flywheel. Fresh gas is supplied through a high impedance side port labelled FGF in the diagram. (Reproduced from Marchak *et al.*, 1981, by courtesy of the Editors and Publisher, *Journal of Pediatrics*)

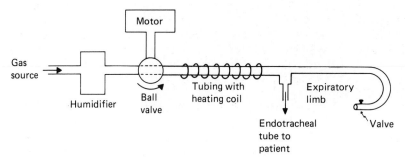

Figure 3.4 Schematic diagram of Emerson airflow interrupter as used in our studies (Frantz *et al.*, 1982; Frantz, Werthammer and Stark, 1983; Frantz and Close, 1985b). A bias flow of gas is interrupted by the ball valve turned on a motor shaft. A high impedance expiratory limb is used to direct oscillations to the subject. Mean pressure can be varied using the distal valve.

The first description of HFO appears to have been in Germany by Lunkenheimer and associates (Lunkenheimer *et al.*, 1972, 1978). These investigators were originally trying to excite the heart using pressure oscillations of up to 40 Hz through the airway, and noted that the technique enhanced pulmonary gas exchange.

Several methodologies have been used to create high frequency oscillations, including loudspeakers, piston pumps (*Figure 3.3*), vibrating diaphragms and airflow interrupters (*Figure 3.4*). Physiologically it may not be too important how the oscillations are created as long as they can be characterized. For research purposes it is useful to have sinusoidal oscillations of known volume amplitude; thus most experimental studies have utilized loudspeakers (Lehr, Barkyoumb and Drazen, 1981; Lehr *et al.*, 1982) or piston pumps (Bohn *et al.*, 1980; Slutsky, 1980, 1981; Lehr *et al.*, 1981) as flow generators. From a clinical point of view these devices may be too complicated, and some sort of flow interrupter (Fletcher and Epstein, 1982; Frantz, Werthammer and Stark, 1983; Frantz and Close, 1985b) may be more desirable. Most HFO devices have incorporated some type of low pass filter, usually a long tube, into the expiratory portion of the circuit. The purpose of this filter is to allow passage of the bias flow, and direct oscillations to the patient's airway. Ngeow and Mitzner (1982) have described a closed-circuit system that contains a CO_2 absorber and oxygen supply that eliminates some humidification and oscillatory flow loss problems.

The mechanisms of gas exchange during HFO are not yet fully understood. Since tidal volume is less than dead space volume, convection alone cannot account for gas exchange. Nonetheless, there is some movement of gas by convection. It appears that three basic processes may be involved in gas exchange, but their relative contributions are not established (Slutsky *et al.*, 1981). These include: bulk flow by convection, convective mixing between lung units and augmented diffusion.

The tidal volumes moved with HFO are less than 2 ml/kg body weight, or less than dead space volume (Slutsky *et al.*, 1981a). While such volumes are obviously insufficient to ventilate peripheral alveoli, they will provide gas exchange in the trachea and perhaps even in the nearest alveoli. Thus bulk flow will provide some exchange of fresh gas during HFO.

Lehr *et al.* (Lehr, Barkyoumb and Drazen, 1981; Lehr *et al.*, 1982), Fredberg *et al.* (1984) and Allen *et al.* (1983) have provided evidence that peripheral alveoli ventilate asynchronously during HFO. The magnitude of this asynchrony is sufficient that individual lung units may exchange gas with one another three times for each time the entire lung is cleared. This inter-regional gas mixing, often referred to as 'Pendelluft', may result in homogenization of alveolar gas concentration and is a second convective mechanism that may contribute to gas exchange during HFO.

Finally, Fredberg (1980) has postulated that augmented diffusion may contribute substantially to gas exchange during HFO. Simple molecular diffusion plays a part in gas exchange in the distal airspaces during conventional ventilation. When diffusion is enhanced by the rapid to-and-fro movement of the high frequency oscillations, gas transport by diffusion may occur over a longer portion of the airway. Augmented diffusion is theoretically sufficient to account for gas exchange during HFO, and empiric evidence is compatible with this mechanism (Slutsky *et al.*, 1980).

In all probability, gas exchange during HFO may be accounted for by some combination of convection in central airways, convective mixing between lung units and augmented diffusion. Their relative proportions may vary depending on experimental circumstance, the species being studied and the type of generator used for the oscillations.

High frequency oscillation has been studied in several animal models, both with normal and diseased lungs. Bohn *et al.* (1980) demonstrated adequate gas exchange in normal dogs using oscillatory volumes approximately equal to dead space volume, and rates of 5–30 Hz. Wright *et al.* (1981) successfully ventilated rabbits treated with oleic acid. They found that carbon dioxide elimination was improved with increasing oscillatory volume from 2.6 to 8.9 ml, increasing frequency from 5 to 30 Hz and increasing bias flow of fresh gas. Oxygenation improved as mean airway pressure was increased. Thompson *et al.* (1982), on the other hand, were unable to show differences in oxygenation or cardiac output in oleic acid-treated dogs during conventional or high frequency ventilation. They did also show that oxygenation increased with increasing mean airway pressure. Oxygenation during HFO and conventional ventilation in rabbits with lung injury due to lavage or oleic acid injection were compared by Kolton *et al.* (1982). In both forms of lung injury, oxygenation was superior during HFO provided that adequate lung volume was established by inflation to a pressure exceeding opening pressure and then maintained with mean airway pressure above opening pressure. Presumably the improved oxygenation during HFO is a result of maintaining lung units open during the entire respiratory cycle by means of the relatively high mean airway pressure and small pressure oscillations. Breen, Ali and Wood (1984) studied gas exchange and perfusion in lungs of open chest dogs with unilobar pulmonary edema created by selective injection of oleic acid. When mean airway pressure was matched during conventional ventilation and high frequency oscillatory ventilation, the lobar venous admixture increased and the relative perfusion decreased in the edematous lobe. When mean airway pressure was increased slightly during HFO, edematous lobar venous admixture decreased and relative perfusion increased compared to conventional ventilation. Lobar venous P_{CO_2} also decreased. The authors conclude that increasing mean airway pressure may open collapsed, flooded regions resulting in increased oxygen transfer, perfusion, and ventilation, and that HFO *per se* does not necessarily account for the changes seen.

The effect of HFO on lung morphology, surfactant and lymph flow has been examined by several groups. Frank *et al.* (1975) ventilated dogs at 20–24 Hz for 2–5 h without effect on light or electron microscopic morphology. We (Frantz *et al.*, 1982) found no change in surfactant, light and electron microscopic morphology, wet-to-dry weight ratios or pressure–volume curves in normal cats ventilated for 4 h on either conventional or high frequency ventilation. Hamilton *et al.* (1983) examined morphology in rabbits ventilated either conventionally or with HFO after injury caused by lung lavage. They found better oxygenation and better survival in the HFO-treated animals. All of the conventionally treated animals developed hyaline membranes, but those treated with HFO did not. Surfactant and pressure–volume curves were examined in monkeys treated with HFO by Truog *et al.* (1983). They found no differences from conventionally treated animals.

There have been few studies of long-term effects of HFO in animals. Rehder, Schmid and Knopp (1983) have treated dogs with HFO for 36 h. The dogs all maintained adequate gas exchange and cardiovascular function. No effect on lung pressure–volume relationships was noted; however, all dogs treated with HFV had small pleural effusions, whereas these were not present in conventionally ventilated dogs.

Lung lymph flow has been examined in two studies. Lymph flow was less and lymph-to-plasma protein ratio greater in lambs ventilated at 25 Hz by Bland *et al.* (1982). Examination of the lungs after sacrifice showed no edema or extravascular water. These investigators concluded that HFO had no adverse effect on lymph flow and may be beneficial in decreasing net lung fluid filtration. Lymph flow was unchanged in the adult sheep studied by Jefferies, Hamilton and O'Brodovich (1983). The sheep responded with a normal increase in lymph flow when air microemboli were injected into the pulmonary vasculature. Our observation of unchanged lung wet-to-dry ratios also suggests no effect of HFO on net lung water (Frantz *et al.*, 1982).

The vibratory nature of HFO has suggested that HFO might affect mucus clearance. Two dog studies have been carried out to date with conflicting results. When high frequency compressions were applied to the chest wall, movement of a carbon particle placed on the tracheal surface was observed to be increased by as much as 340% (King *et al.*, 1983). On the other hand, clearance of an aerosol of radiolabelled sulfur colloid was greatly diminished during HFO via the airway (McEvoy *et al.*, 1982a). In addition, large amounts of mucus were observed in the tracheas of the dogs after HFO, and a bolus of radiolabel placed in the trachea was observed to disperse and move rapidly to distal airways during HFO. Tracheal mucus velocity during conventional ventilation after HFO was normal. The reasons for these disparate results are not clear, but may relate to the differing techniques used for ventilation.

Gas exchange during HFV has been examined using a number of approaches. The group at the Harvard School of Public Health have studied CO_2 elimination in normal dogs as well as adults with normal and diseased lungs (Goldstein *et al.*, 1981; Slutsky *et al.*, 1981; Rossing *et al.*, 1981, 1982). In general they have found that CO_2 elimination is proportional to oscillatory flow, i.e. frequency times tidal volume. They found no significant effect of increasing lung volume (Slutsky *et al.*, 1981). In humans with lung disease the relationship to oscillatory flow was no longer obtained above a critical frequency, and CO_2 elimination was related to tidal volume alone (Rossing *et al.*, 1981). The investigators concluded that gas transport to the lung periphery was limited by the mechanical characteristics of the lung above the critical frequency. Carbon dioxide elimination in dogs given intravenous histamine infusion was also proportional to oscillatory flow, but the amount of CO_2 elimination was lower than in controls (Rossing *et al.*, 1982). The investigators concluded that the mechanical properties of the lung accounted for decreased delivery of oscillatory flow to the gas-exchanging units of the lung during histamine infusion.

Investigators at the Mayo Clinic have examined gas transport and pulmonary perfusion during HFO by studying distribution and clearance of inspired and injected radio-isotopes (Schmid, Knopp and Rehder, 1981; Brusasco, Knopp and Rehder, 1983). Clearance of labelled xenon was uniform in dogs during HFO at 16 and 30 Hz with a stroke volume of $2.6 \, \text{ml} \cdot \text{kg}^{-1}$. Vertical gradients in pulmonary perfusion were demonstrated when labelled xenon was injected into the right atrium during HFO or apnea. After the injections, xenon concentrations in dependent regions decreased and those in independent regions increased, indicating inter-regional mixing. After concentrations became similar in all regions, the lung continued to clear uniformly. Brusasco, Knopp and Rehder (1983) have partitioned gas transport during HFO into that due to regional conductance along airways, and inter-regional conductance. They found regional conductance to be nearly uniform when stroke volume was less than two-thirds of the dead space volume. When stroke volume was greater than this and the frequency 5 Hz, regional conductance to dependent regions was larger than that to independent regions. The average regional conductance for the whole lung increased with stroke volume at all frequencies, but was greatest when stroke volume was high and frequency was low for any given product of the two.

To test the importance of diffusion in gas transport during HFO, Knopp *et al.* (1983) examined washout of gases of different diffusivity. They found no differences in washout of mixtures of He and SF_6 or He and Ar, and concluded that diffusion was not rate limiting in either transient-state washout of inert gases or steady-state transport of respiratory gases. Robertson *et al.* (1982) have examined the exchange of respiratory and inert gases in dogs ventilated at 10 Hz. They concluded that augmented diffusion accounted for the primary transport of gas from alveolus to airway opening, and that substantial inter-regional mixing of gas occurred as well. The multiple inert gas technique was also used by McEvoy *et al.* (1982). Like Robertson *et al.* (1982), these investigators found that elimination of the most soluble gas was increased over those less soluble. They propose that this increased elimination is due to absorption and desorption from the liquid lining layer of the airway and hypothesize that CO_2 transfer may be facilitated by this mechanism.

An interesting observation during HFO of both animals and man is that, in many cases, spontaneous respiration ceases. This may in part be due to effects on blood gas tensions, but appears also to be related to stimulation of pulmonary mechanoreceptors. Man, Man and Kappagoda (1983) recorded electrical activity from the vagus and phrenic nerves in dogs ventilated conventionally or with HFO at 25 Hz. They found that vagal fibers were stimulated continuously and to a greater extent during HFO than with static lung inflation. HFO diminished phrenic nerve activity, and this diminution was abolished by functional vagotomy. The investigators concluded that increased vagal activity during HFO probably accounts for the cessation of spontaneous respiration. Banzett, Lehr and Geffroy (1983) came to a similar conclusion based on their measurements of lung volume, airway pressure and respiratory muscle electromyograms in dogs. They found that during HFO at 15 Hz, expiratory time was prolonged to the point of apnea without effect on inspiratory time or peak diaphragmatic electrical activity. The effect was blocked by vagotomy.

Although most experimental work to date has involved application of forced oscillations at the airway opening, gas exchange may also be accomplished with high frequency oscillations at the chest wall. Ward, Power and Nicholas (1983) oscillated isolated perfused rat lungs in a plethysmograph. They found normal oxygen uptake when frequency was varied from 5 to 40 Hz. Although tidal volume decreased with increasing frequency, expired minute ventilation was relatively constant. Zidulka *et al.* (1983) demonstrated that oxygenation and carbon dioxide elimination could be maintained in dogs when a blood pressure cuff wrapped around the thorax was oscillated with a piston pump. Harf, Bertrand and Chang (1984) ventilated rats with a piston pump at 20 Hz via the trachea or via the body surface while they were in a whole body plethysmograph. They found identical oxygenation and CO_2 elimination using the two techniques. Oscillation at the body surface may thus prove to be a desirable method for providing gas exchange in unintubated patients.

Although HFO has been more thoroughly studied from a physiological point of view than other techniques, it has had less clinical application. Goldstein *et al.* (1981) and Rossing *et al.* (1981) have used the technique for short periods in adults, more to examine gas exchange than to test for therapeutic effects. Butler *et al.* (1980) and Marchak *et al.* (1981) have successfully applied the technique to patients ranging in age from infancy to adulthood. Although the patients achieved adequate gas exchange, the studies were not designed to show therapeutic benefit. Use of HFO did result in improved oxygenation. Since the endotracheal tube represents a major source of resistance to transport of gas during HFO, Rossing *et al.* (1984) have examined the effect of changing the bias flow of fresh gas from the distal to the proximal end of the endotracheal tube in adults with lung disease. They found a 50% improvement of CO_2 elimination when the bias flow was located at the end of the endotracheal tube near the carina.

We have used a flow interrupter technique to ventilate a group of infants with respiratory distress syndrome or pulmonary interstitial emphysema (Frantz, Werthammer and Stark, 1983). As in the above studies, adequate gas exchange was achieved with tracheal pressure swings lower than those on conventional ventilation. There appeared to be clinical improvement in the patients with interstitial emphysema; the study was not, however, controlled.

The optimal frequency for HFO is not yet clear. There are two approaches to choice of frequency: observation of effects on gas exchange and theoretical considerations based on oscillation mechanics of the respiratory system. Studies of the effects of changing frequency on gas exchange are confounded by the fact that with many systems used for HFO, frequency and tidal volume changes are difficult to make independently, and no study has resulted in evidence of the superiority of a given frequency.

The oscillatory mechanical behavior of the lung is consistent with a model made up of an elastance, resistance and inertance in series (Allen *et al.*, 1983; Dorkin *et al.*, 1983; Keefe *et al.*, 1983; Fredberg *et al.*, 1984). From such a model one predicts that for a given oscillatory flow tracheal pressure swings will be minimized at the resonant frequency of the respiratory system. Alveolar pressure swings will, however, be minimized at the highest possible frequency, and may exceed tracheal pressure swings at resonance. We have observed such amplification of tracheal pressures in both excised dog and rabbit lungs (Allen *et al.*, 1983; Keefe *et al.*, 1983; Fredberg *et al.*, 1984). The clinician is left with the conflict of deciding whether he wishes to minimize tracheal pressure swings by ventilating at the resonant frequency, or minimize alveolar pressure swings by ventilating at the highest frequency at which adequate gas exchange is obtained.

There have not been many studies of oscillation mechanics in human infants. We have used a loudspeaker plethysmograph to measure frequency dependence of impedance of the respiratory systems in six intubated infants with respiratory distress syndrome or pulmonary interstitial emphysema (Dorkin *et al.*, 1983). Their resonant frequences were from 13–23 Hz, with fairly broad ranges of minimal impedance. The data fit well with the resistance–inertance–compliance model referred to above, and thus the considerations for choice of ventilatory frequency based on this model should be applicable.

Thus far, no adverse side-effects have been attributed to HFO. The animal studies referred to above showed no effect on lung morphology, lymph flow or surfactant. In hemodynamic studies of human infants we have seen no effect on cardiac output, pulmonary artery pressure and resistance or systemic artery pressure and resistance (Vincent *et al.*, 1984). Todd, Toutant and Shapiro (1981) demonstrated that ventilation at $60-200\,min^{-1}$ had no effect on hemodynamics in cats. They also noted that ventilation at these rates effectively eliminated respiration-associated effects on intracranial pressure and brain surface movement.

PRESSURE MEASUREMENTS DURING HIGH FREQUENCY VENTILATION

A major attraction of high frequency ventilation is the claim that lower mean and dynamic pressures within the airway may be required for adequate gas exchange. Pressures measured at the airway opening, in the ventilator circuit, or even in the trachea may not be adequate estimates of pressures in the alveoli. There are several possible sources of error. First, the pressure measuring system may not have adequate frequency response. Typically those transducers designed for blood pressure measurement or for measurement of pressures at conventional ventilatory rates fall into this category. The problem may be confounded when catheters or stub adapters are used in conjunction with tracheal pressure measurements. Jackson and Vinegar (1979) have described a system for testing of frequency response of transducer–catheter systems. Comparison with a reference transducer of known frequency response may also be done. Before pressure measurements made during high frequency ventilation are to be believed, some assessment of frequency response of the measuring system must be made.

Given an adequate measuring system, the location where measurements are made is also of importance. We have compared pressure swings measured in the

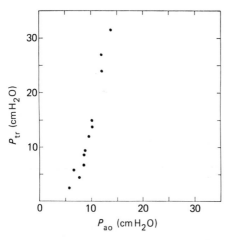

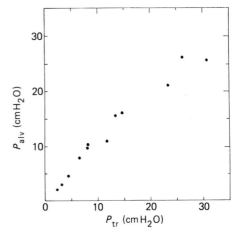

Figure 3.5 Pressure swings in the trachea plotted versus pressure swings at the airway opening during jet ventilation of rabbits. Pressure swings at the airway opening grossly underestimate those in the trachea. (From data of Frantz and Close, 1985a)

Figure 3.6 Pressure swings in the alveoli plotted versus those in the trachea during jet ventilation of a rabbit. Tracheal pressure swings are reasonably good estimates of alveolar pressure swings. (From data of Frantz and Close, 1985a)

ventilator circuit with those measured in the trachea during jet ventilation (*Figure 3.5*). It is evident from the figure that pressure at the airway opening does not even closely approximate that in the trachea. Tracheal pressure swings, on the other hand, are reasonable approximations of those in the alveoli during jet ventilation (*Figure 3.6*). During high frequency oscillation tracheal pressure swings may underestimate those in the alveoli near the resonant frequency of the respiratory system (*Figure 3.7*). Thus barotrauma to the lung periphery may occur despite small pressure swings in the trachea.

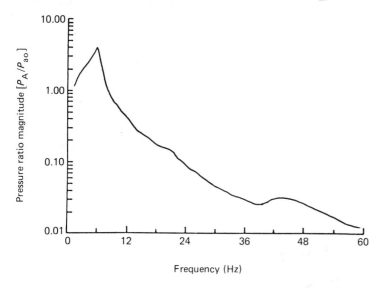

Figure 3.7 Ratio of pressure in the alveoli to that at the airway opening during high frequency oscillation of excised dog lungs at a distending pressure of 10 cm H_2O. Alveolar pressure is four times that at the airway opening near the resonant frequency, and falls as frequency increases. (From data of Keefe *et al.*, 1983)

Estimates of mean pressures during high frequency ventilation may also be affected by many factors. Simon, Weinmann and Mitzner (1982) estimated mean alveolar pressure by occluding the airway at end-expiration and measuring the relaxation pressure. They found that mean alveolar pressure exceeded mean pressure measured at the airway opening during HFO. Similar results were obtained when this technique was used by Breen, Ali and Wood (1984). We, on the other hand, found no difference between mean pressures at the airway opening, trachea or alveoli when these were measured directly in closed chest rabbits (Frantz and Close, 1985b). The changes in end-expiratory volume observed by Rouby *et al.* (1983) and us (Close and Manchester, 1983; Frantz and Close, 1985a) during jet ventilation, as well as the increase in mean alveolar pressure observed in our study, emphasize the magnitude of changes in mean airway pressure during jet ventilation as well as the inadequacy of attempting to assess mean alveolar pressure based on measurements made at the airway opening.

In conclusion, high frequency ventilation of any form has not yet been proven a superior means of ventilation for patients with lung disease. While it has potential benefits, there are real dangers. Better means of assessing pressures, or a further understanding of the relationships between pressures at the airway opening, trachea and alveoli, are needed. In addition, the relationship between lung volume and jet ventilator settings must be further defined. Finally, controlled clinical studies of safety and efficacy must be carried out before the techniques can be accepted for routine clinical use.

References

ALLEN, J. L., KEEFE, D. H., FREDBERG, J. J., GLASS, G. M. and FRANTZ, I. D. (1983) Alveolar pressures and pulmonary impedance during high frequency oscillation in excised rabbit lungs. *Pediatric Research*, **17**, 370A

BANZETT, R., LEHR, J. and GEFFROY, B. (1983) High-frequency ventilation lengthens expiration in the anesthetized dog. *Journal of Applied Physiology: Respiratory, Environmental and Exercise Physiology*, **55**, 329–334

BLAND, R. D., KIM, M. H., LIGHT, M. J. and WOODSON, J. L. (1980) High frequency mechanical ventilation in severe hyaline membrane disease: an alternative treatment? *Critical Care Medicine*, **8**, 275

BLAND, R. D., RAJ, J. U., HAZINSKI, T. A., SEDIN, G. E. and GOLDBERG, R. B. (1982) Lung fluid balance during vibratory ventilation in lambs. *Pediatric Research*, **16**, 280A

BOHN, D., MIYASAKA, K., MARCHAK, B., THOMPSON, W., FROESE, A. and BRYAN, A. (1980) Ventilation by high frequency oscillation. *Journal of Applied Physiology: Respiratory, Environmental and Exercise Physiology*, **48**, 710–716

BORG, U., ERIKSSON, I., LYTTKENS, L., NILSSON, L-G. and SJOSTRAND, U. (1977) High-frequency positive-pressure ventilation (HFPPV) applied in bronchoscopy under general anaesthesia. *Acta Anaesthesiologica Scandinavica Supplement*, 69–81

BREEN, P. H., ALI, J. and WOOD, L. D. H. (1984) High-frequency ventilation in lung edema: effects on gas exchange and perfusion. *Journal of Applied Physiology: Respiratory, Environmental and Exercise Physiology*, **56**, 187–195

BRUSASCO, V., KNOPP, T. J. and REHDER, K. (1983) Gas transport during high-frequency ventilation. *Journal of Applied Physiology: Respiratory, Environmental and Exercise Physiology*, **55**, 472–478

BUTLER, W., BOHN, M., BRYAN, A. and FROESE, A. (1980) Ventilation by high frequency oscillation in humans. *Anesthesia and Analgesia; Current Researches*, **59**, 577–584

CARLO, W. A., CHATBURN, R. L., MARTIN, R. J., LOUGH, M. D., SHIVPURI, C. R., ANDERSON, J. V. *et al.* (1984) Decrease in airway pressure during high-frequency jet ventilation in infants with respiratory distress syndrome. *Journal of Pediatrics*, **104**, 101–107

CARLON, G. C., HOWLAND, W. S., RAY, C., MIODOWNIK, S., GRIFFIN, J. P. L. and GROEGER, J. S. (1983) High-frequency jet ventilation: a prospective randomized evaluation. *Chest*, **84**, 551–559

CARLON, G. C., KAHN, R. C., HOWLAND, W. S., RAY, C. and TURNBULL, A. (1981) Clinical experience with high frequency jet ventilation. *Critical Care Medicine*, **9**, 1–6

CARLON, G. C., MIODOWNIK, S., RAY, C. and KAHN, R. C. (1981a) Technical aspects and clinical implications of high frequency jet ventilation with a solenoid valve. *Critical Care Medicine*, **9**, 47–50

CARLON, G. C., RAY, C., GRIFFIN, J., MIODOWNIK, S. and GROEGER, J. S. (1983a) Tidal volume and airway pressure on high frequency jet ventilation. *Critical Care Medicine*, **11**, 83–86

CARLON, G. C., RAY, C. JR, KLAIN, M. and MCCORMACK, P. M. (1980) High-frequency positive-pressure ventilation in management of a patient with bronchopleural fistula. *Anesthesiology*, **52**, 160–162

CARLON, G. C., RAY, C. JR, PIERRI, M. K., GROEGER, J. and HOWLAND, W. S. (1982) High-frequency jet ventilation: theoretical considerations and clinical observations. *Chest*, **81**, 350–353

CHATBURN, R. L. and MCCLELLAN, L. D. (1982) A heat and humidification system for high frequency jet ventilation. *Respiratory Care*, **27**, 1386–1391

CLOSE, R. H. and MANCHESTER, P. (1983) Alveolar pressure swings and tidal volume measurement during high frequency jet ventilation. *Respiratory Care*, **28**, 1327

DAVEY, A. J., LAY, G. R. and LEIGH, J. M. (1982) High frequency venturi jet ventilation: comparison of a proximal central jet with a distal wall jet. *Anaesthesia*, **37**, 947–950

DORKIN, H. L., STARK, A. R., WERTHAMMER, J. W., STRIEDER, D. J., FREDBERG, J. J. and FRANTZ III, I. D. (1983) Respiratory system impedance from 4 to 40 Hz in paralyzed intubated infants with respiratory disease. *Journal of Clinical Investigation*, **72**, 903–910

EL-BAZ, N. M., KITTLE, C. F., FABER, L. P. and WELSHER, W. (1982) High-frequency ventilation with an uncuffed endobronchial tube: a new technique for one-lung anesthesia. *Journal of Thoracic and Cardiovascular Surgery*, **84**, 823–828

ERIKSSON, I. and SJOSTRAND, U. (1977) Experimental and clinical evaluation of high-frequency positive-pressure ventilation (HFPPV) and the pneumatic valve principle in bronchoscopy under general anaesthesia. *Acta Anaesthesiologica Scandinavica*, **64**, 83–100

FLETCHER, P. R., EPSTEIN, M. A. and EPSTEIN, R. A. (1982) A new ventilator for physiologic studies during high-frequency ventilation. *Respiration Physiology*, **47**, 21–37

FLETCHER, P. R. and EPSTEIN, R. A. (1982) Constancy of physiological dead space during high-frequency ventilation. *Respiration Physiology*, **47**, 39–49

FRANK, I., NOACK, W., LUNKENHEIMER, P. P., ISING, H., KELLER, H., DICKHUTH, H. H. *et al.* (1975) Light and electron microscopic investigations of pulmonary tissue after high frequency positive pressure ventilation (HFPPV). *Anaesthetist*, **24**, 171–176

FRANTZ, I. D. and CLOSE, R. H. (1985a) Elevated lung volume and alveolar pressure during jet ventilation of rabbits. *American Review of Respiratory Disease*, **131**, 134–138

FRANTZ, I. D. and CLOSE, R. H. (1985b) Alveolar pressure swings during high frequency ventilation in rabbits. *Pediatric Research*, **19**, 162–166

FRANTZ, I. D., STARK, A., DAVIS, J. M., DAVIES, P. and KITZMILLER, T. J. (1982) High frequency ventilation does not affect pulmonary surfactant, liquid, or morphologic features in normal cats. *American Review of Respiratory Disease*, **126**, 909–913

FRANTZ, I. D., WERTHAMMER, J. and STARK, A. R. (1983) High-frequency ventilation in premature infants with lung disease: adequate gas exchange at low tracheal pressure. *Pediatrics*, **71**, 483–488

FREDBERG, J. J. (1980) Augmented diffusion in the airways can support pulmonary gas exchange. *Journal of Applied Physiology: Respiratory, Environmental and Exercise Physiology*, **49**, 232–238

FREDBERG, J. J., KEEFE, D. H., GLASS, G. M., CASTILE, R. G. and FRANTZ, I. D. (1984) Alveolar pressure inhomogeneity during small amplitude high frequency oscillation. *Journal of Applied Physiology: Respiratory, Environmental and Exercise Physiology*, **57**, 788–800

GALLAGHER, T. J. (1983) High-frequency ventilation. *Medical Clinics of North America*, **67**, 633–643

GILLESPIE, D. J. (1983) High-frequency ventilation: a new concept in mechanical ventilation. *Mayo Clinic Proceedings*, **58**, 187–196

GOLDSTEIN, D., SLUTSKY, A. S., INGRAM, R. H., WESTERMAN, P., VENEGAS, J. and DRAZEN, J. (1981) CO_2 elimination by high frequency ventilation (4 to 10 Hz) in normal subjects. *American Review of Respiratory Disease*, **123**, 251–255

HAMILTON, P. P., ONAYEMI, A., SMYTH, J. A., GILLAN, J. E., CUTZ, E., FROESE, A. B. *et al.* (1983) Comparison of conventional and high-frequency ventilation: oxygenation and lung pathology. *Journal of Applied Physiology: Respiratory, Environmental and Exercise Physiology*, **55**, 131–138

HARF, A., BERTRAND, C. and CHANG, H. K. (1984) Ventilation by high-frequency oscillation of thorax or at trachea in rats. *Journal of Applied Physiology: Respiratory, Environmental and Exercise Physiology*, **56**, 155–160

HEIJMAN, K., HEIJMAN, L., JONZON, A. *et al.* (1972) High-frequency positive-pressure ventilation during anaesthesia and routine surgery in man. *Acta Anaesthesiologica Scandinavica*, **16**, 176

JACKSON, A. C. and VINEGAR, A. (1979) A technique for measuring frequency response of pressure, volume and flow transducers. *Journal of Applied Physiology*, **47**, 462–467

JEFFERIES, A. L., HAMILTON, P. and O'BRODOVICH, H. M. (1983) Effect of high-frequency oscillation on lung lymph flow. *Journal of Applied Physiology: Respiratory, Environmental and Exercise Physiology*, **55**, 1373–1378

JONZON, A., OBERG, P. A., SEDIN, G. *et al.* (1970) High frequency low tidal volume positive pressure ventilation. (Abstract) *Acta Physiologica Scandinavica*, **80**, 21A

JONZON, A., OBERG, P. A., SEDIN, G. *et al.* (1971) High-frequency positive-pressure ventilation by endotracheal insufflation. *Acta Anaesthesiologica Scandinavica Supplement*, **43**

KEEFE, D., GLASS, G., CASTILE, R., FRANTZ, I. D., STARK, A. R. and FREDBERG, J. (1983) Alveolar pressure during high frequency oscillations in excised dog lungs. *Federation Proceedings*, **42**, 763

KESZLER, M., KLEIN, R., MCCLELLAN, L., NELSON, D. and PLATT, M. (1982) Effects of conventional and high frequency jet ventilation on lung parenchyma. *Critical Care Medicine*, **10**, 514–516

KING, M., PHILIPS, D. M., GROSS, D., VARTIAN, V., CHANG, H. K. and ZIDULKA, A. (1983) Enhanced tracheal mucus clearance with high frequency chest wall compression. *American Review of Respiratory Diseases*, **128**, 511–515

KLAIN, M. and SMITH, B. (1977) High frequency percutaneous transtracheal jet ventilation. *Critical Care Medicine*, **5**, 280–287

KNOPP, T. J., KAETHNER, T., MEYER, M., REHDER, K. and SCHEID, P. (1983) Gas mixing in the airways of dog lungs during high-frequency ventilation. *Journal of Applied Physiology: Respiratory, Environmental and Exercise Physiology*, **55**, 1141–1146

KOLTON, M., CATTRAN, C. B., KENT, G., VOLGYESI, G., FROESE, A. B and BRYAN, A. C. (1982) Oxygenation during high-frequency ventilation compared with conventional mechanical ventilation in two models of lung injury. *Anesthesia and Analgesia; Current Researches*, **61**, 323–332

LEHR, J. L., BARKYOUMB, J. and DRAZEN, J. M. (1981) Gas transport during high frequency ventilation. *Federation Proceedings*, **40**, 384

LEHR, J. L., DRAZEN, J. M., WESTERMAN, P. A. and ZATZ, S. L. (1982) Regional expansion of excised dog lungs during high frequency ventilation. *Federation Proceedings*, **41**, 1747

LUNKENHEIMER, P. P., ISING, H., FRANK, I., SCHARSICH, M., WELHAM, K. and DITTRICH, H. (1978) Enhancement of carbon dioxide elimination by intrapulmonary high frequency pressure alternation during 'apnoeic oxygenation'. *Advances in Experimental Medicine and Biology*, **94**, 599–603

LUNKENHEIMER, P. P., RAFFFLENBEUL, W., KELLER, H., FRANK, I., DICKHUTH, H. H. and FUHRMANN, C. (1972) Application of transtracheal pressure oscillations as a modification of 'diffusion respiration'. *British Journal of Anaesthesia*, **44**, 627

McEVOY, R. D., DAVIES, N. J., HEDENSTIERNA, G., HARTMAN, M. T., SPRAGG, R. G. and WAGNER, P. D. (1982) Lung mucociliary transport during high frequency ventilation. *American Review of Respiratory Disease*, **126**, 452–456

McEVOY, R. D., DAVIES, N. J. H., MANNINO, F. L., PRUTOW, R. J., SCHUMACKER, P. T. *et al.* (1982a) Pulmonary gas exchange during high-frequency ventilation. *Journal of Applied Physiology*, **52**, 1278–1287

MAN, G. C. W., MAN, S. F. P. and KAPPAGODA, C. T. (1983) Effects of high-frequency oscillatory ventilation on vagal and phrenic nerve activities. *Journal of Applied Physiology: Respiratory, Environmental and Exercise Physiology*, **54**, 502–507

MARCHAK, B., THOMPSON, W., DUFFTY, P., MIYAKI, T., BRYAN, M., BRYAN, A. *et al.* (1981) Treatment of RDS by high frequency oscillatory ventilation: A preliminary report. *Journal of Pediatrics*, **99**, 287–292

NGEOW, Y. K. and MITZNER, W. (1982) A new system for ventilating with high-frequency oscillation. *Journal of Applied Physiology*, **53**, 1638–1642

POKORA, T., BING, D., MAMMEL, M. and BOROS, S. (1983) Neonatal high-frequency jet ventilation. *Pediatrics*, **72**, 27–32

REHDER, K., SCHMID, E. R. and KNOPP, T. J. (1983) Long-term high frequency ventilation in dogs. *American Review of Respiratory Disease*, **128**, 476–480

ROBERTSON, H. T., COFFEY, R. L., STANDAERT, T. A. and TRUOG, W. E. (1982) Respiratory and inert gas exchange during high-frequency ventilation. *Journal of Applied Physiology*, **52**, 683–689

ROSSING, T. H., SLUTSKY, A. S., INGRAM, R. H., KAMM, R. D. and SHAPIRO, A. H. (1982) CO_2 elimination by high frequency oscillation in dogs – effects of histamine infusion. *Journal of Applied Physiology*, **53**, 1256–1262

ROSSING, T. H., SLUTSKY, A. S., LEHR, J. L., DRINKER, P. A., KAMM, R. and DRAZEN, J. M. (1981) Tidal volume and frequency dependence of carbon dioxide elimination by high-frequency ventilation. *New England Journal of Medicine*, **305**, 1375–1379

ROSSING, T. H., SOLWAY, J., SAARI, A. F., GAVRIELY, N., SLUTSKY, A. S., LEHR, J. L. *et al.* (1984) Influence of the endotracheal tube on CO_2 transport during high-frequency ventilation. *American Review of Respiratory Disease*, **129**, 54–57

ROUBY, J. J., FUSCIARDI, J., BOURGAIN, J. L. and VIARS, P. (1983) High-frequency jet ventilation in postoperative respiratory failure: determinants of oxygenation. *Anesthesiology*, **59**, 281–287

SANDERS, R. D. (1967) Two ventilating attachments for bronchoscopes. *Delaware Medical Journal*, **39**, 170–175

SCHMID, E. R., KNOPP, T. J. and REHDER, K. (1981) Intrapulmonary gas transport and perfusion during high-frequency oscillation. *Journal of Applied Physiology*, **51**, 1507–1514

SCHUSTER, D. P., KLAIN, M. and SNYDER, J. V. (1982) Comparison of high frequency jet ventilation to conventional ventilation during severe acute respiratory failure in humans. *Critical Care Medicine*, **10**, 625–630

SCHUSTER, D. P., SNYDER, J. V., KLAIN, M. and GRENVIK, A. (1981) High-frequency jet ventilation during the treatment of acute fulminant pulmonary edema. *Chest*, **80**, 682–685

SIMON, B., WEINMANN, G. and MITZNER, W. (1982) Significance of mean airway pressure during high frequency ventilation (HFV). *Physiologist*, **25**, 282

SJOSTRAND, U. (1977) Review of the physiological rationale for and development of high-frequency positive-pressure ventilation – HFPPV. *Acta Anaesthesiologica Scandinavica Supplement*, **64**, 7–27

SJOSTRAND, U. (1980) High-frequency positive-pressure ventilation (HFPPV): a review. *Critical Care Medicine*, **8**, 345–364

SJOSTRAND, U., JONZON, A., SEDIN, G. *et al.* (1973) High-frequency positive-pressure ventilation. *Opuscula Medica* (Abstract), **18**, 74

SLUTSKY, A. S., BROWN, R., LEHR, J. *et al.* (1981) High frequency ventilation: a promising new approach to mechanical ventilation. *Medical Instrumentation*, **15**, 228–233

SLUTSKY, A., DRAZEN, J., INGRAM, R., KAMM, R., SHAPIRO, A., FREDBERG, J. *et al.* (1980) Effective pulmonary ventilation with small-volume oscillations at high frequency. *Science,* **209,** 609–611

SLUTSKY, A. S., KAMM, R. D., ROSSING, T. H., LORING, S. H., LEHR, J., SHAPIRO, A. H. *et al.* (1981a). Effects of frequency, tidal volume, and lung volume on CO_2 elimination in dogs by high frequency (2–30 Hz), low tidal volume ventilation. *Journal of Clinical Investigation,* **68,** 1475–1484

SMITH, R. B. (1982) Ventilation at high respiratory frequencies: high frequency positive pressure ventilation, high frequency jet ventilation and high frequency oscillation. *Anaesthesia,* **37,** 1011–1018

THOMPSON, W. K., MARCHAK, B. E., FROESE, A. B. and BRYAN, A. C. (1982) High-frequency oscillation compared with standard ventilation in pulmonary injury model. *Journal of Applied Physiology,* **52,** 543–548

TODD, M., TOUTANT, S. M. and SHAPIRO, H. M. (1981) The effects of high-frequency positive pressure ventilation on intracranial pressure and brain surface movement in cats. *Anesthesiology,* **54,** 496–504

TRUOG, W. E., STANDAERT, T. A., MURPHY, J., PALMER, S., WOODRUM, D. E. and HODSON, W. A. (1983) Effect of high-frequency oscillation on gas exchange and pulmonary phospholipids in experimental hyaline membrane disease. *American Review of Respiratory Disease,* **127,** 585–589

TURNBULL, A. D., CARLON, G., HOWLAND, W. S. and BEATTIE, E. J. (1980) High-frequency jet ventilation in major airway or pulmonary disruption. *Annals of Thoracic Surgery,* **5,** 468–474

VINCENT, R. N., STARK, A. R., LANG, P., CLOSE, R. H., NORWOOD, W. I., CASTANEDA, A. R. *et al.* (1984) Hemodynamic response to high frequency ventilation in infants following cardiac surgery. *Pediatrics,* in press

WARD, H. E., POWER, J. H. T. and NICHOLAS, T. E. (1983) High-frequency oscillations via the pleural surface: an alternative mode of ventilation? *Journal of Applied Physiology: Respiratory, Environmental and Exercise Physiology,* **54,** 427–433

WOO, P. and EURENIUS, S. (1982) Dynamics of venturi jet ventilation through the operating laryngoscope. *Annals of Otology, Rhinology and Laryngology,* **91,** 615–621

WRIGHT, K., LYRENE, R. K., TRUOG, W. E., STANDAERT, T. A., MURPHY, J. and WOODRUM, D. E. (1981) Ventilation by high-frequency oscillation in rabbits with oleic acid lung disease. *Journal of Applied Physiology: Respiratory, Environmental and Exercise Physiology,* **50,** 1056–1060

ZIDULKA, A., GROSS, D., MINAMI, H., VARTIAN, V. and CHANG, H. K. (1983) Ventilation by high-frequency chest wall compression in dogs with normal lungs. *American Review of Respiratory Disease,* **127,** 709–713

4

Bronchopulmonary dysplasia

Eduardo Bancalari

The term 'bronchopulmonary dysplasia' (BPD) was introduced in 1967, by Northway, Rosan and Porter (1967) to describe a series of pulmonary changes that developed in a group of infants with respiratory distress syndrome (RDS) following prolonged intermittent positive pressure ventilation (IPPV). After this original description, there have been many reports describing similar patients and this problem has become the most common pulmonary sequelae in newborns who survive mechanical ventilation.

In their first report, Northway et al. (1967) described four stages of the disease according to the clinical, radiographic and pathological findings. The first stage is essentially indistinguishable from the acute phases of RDS. In the second stage between the fourth and tenth day, there is radiographic opacification of both lung fields and the main pathological findings are necrosis and repair of bronchial and alveolar epithelium. In the third stage, between 10 to 20 days, the chest radiograph shows small areas of radiolucency alternating with areas of increased density giving a spongy appearance to the lung. Pathology shows increased proliferation, edema and metaplasia of the bronchial epithelium. In stage IV, the areas of overdistension become more marked, especially in the bases with bands of increased density. Frequently, there is cardiomegaly. Pathological findings include emphysema, alternating with areas of collapse and fibrosis, and hyperplasia of smooth muscle in small airway, and pulmonary vessels. There is also metaplasia of bronchial epithelium with obstruction of the lumen in some areas. This stage usually occurs after the fourth week of life and is characterized clinically by severe respiratory failure, with hypoxemia and hypercapnia. The manifestations of the first three stages are not specific and are difficult to differentiate from a complicated course of RDS. Because of this we prefer to limit the term BPD to the more chronic stages of the disease which correspond to the stage IV of Northway et al. (1967).

INCIDENCE

The incidence of BPD varies widely in different reports (Mayes, Perkett and Stahlman, 1983; Harrod et al., 1974). Although part of this variation may be real and due to differences in patient susceptibility and management, most of the

54

discrepancies lie in the way the figures are obtained and in the criteria used to diagnose BPD. While some authors include only patients with a clinical and radiographic evolution that fits the original description by Northway *et al.* (1967), most centers including ourselves have adopted a more liberal definition and include all patients that, after requiring mechanical ventilation during the first week of life, remain oxygen dependent for more than 28 days and have persistent increased densities with or without hyperinflation on chest radiographs. We prefer to call this entity chronic lung disease rather than BPD. There are also differences in the base population in which the incidence of BPD is calculated. While some reports include all infants who require mechanical ventilation, others consider only those infants with RDS. The incidence is obviously higher in the latter group. The indications for IPPV and the survival rate of ventilated infants also influences the incidence of BPD. With increasing survival of very small prematures the number of infants at risk of developing chronic lung disease also increases.

The incidence of BPD in infants with RDS who receive IPPV and survive varies between 10 and 20% (Edwards, Dyer and Northway, 1977; Brown *et al.*, 1978; Bancalari *et al.*, 1979). Assuming the incidence of RDS in newborns weighing less than 2.5 kg to be approximately 14% (Farrell and Avery, 1975), it can be estimated that 35 000 infants will develop RDS each year in the USA. If one-third of these infants require mechanical ventilation, with 70–80% survival and 15% of these infants developing BPD, approximately 1300 infants will survive with this condition each year in this country. The number of infants surviving with milder forms of chronic lung damage may be much higher. BPD is, therefore, a problem of great medical and social importance.

CLINICAL PRESENTATION

The diagnosis of BPD is based on clinical and radiographic characteristics, but there are no specific clinical signs or laboratory alterations that confirm the diagnosis. The majority of infants who develop BPD are born prematurely, although there are also cases reported in infants born at term (Barnes *et al.*, 1969; Rhodes, Hall and Leonidas, 1975). With rare exceptions, all of them require mechanical ventilation with intermittent positive pressure during the first days of life. The indication for ventilation is usually respiratory failure due to RDS, but it can also occur in infants who require mechanical ventilation for other causes of respiratory failure such as pneumonia, meconium aspiration, patent ductus arteriosus (PDA) and apnea of prematurity (Philip, 1975; Rhodes, Hall and Leonidas, 1975; Friis-Hansen *et al.*, 1976; Moylan and Shannon, 1979; Mayes, Perkett and Stahlman, 1983). While the infants with BPD described by Northway and colleagues had severe respiratory failure during the initial course of their disease, infants who have only mild or moderate forms of pulmonary disease may also develop BPD (Philip, 1975; Bancalari *et al.*, 1979). Once BPD has occurred, infants usually require mechanical ventilation and oxygen therapy for long periods of time varying from weeks to several months. In many cases, this prolonged need for respiratory assistance is caused by complications that occur during the acute stages of the respiratory failure such as intracranial hemorrhage, pulmonary interstitial emphysema or pneumothorax, and pulmonary infection. The persistence of a patent ductus arteriosus with left heart failure is another condition that frequently compromises pulmonary function and prolongs the need for IPPV in prematures with RDS. By aggravating the pulmonary failure these complications also make the use of higher inspired oxygen concentrations and airway pressures more likely. This may establish a vicious cycle in which the required therapy produces further aggravation of the pulmonary damage. It is common, therefore, that these patients require ventilation with high airway pressures and inspired oxygen concentrations for many weeks or months, although this is not always related to their initial respiratory disease. A large number of very small infants have mild respiratory disease initially requiring ventilation with low pressures and oxygen concentration, but, after a few days or weeks of ventilation, show progressive deterioration in their lung function and develop chronic lung disease. The cause of this deterioration is not always clear but, in many cases, is produced by bacterial or viral infection or heart failure secondary to a PDA (*Figure 4.1*).

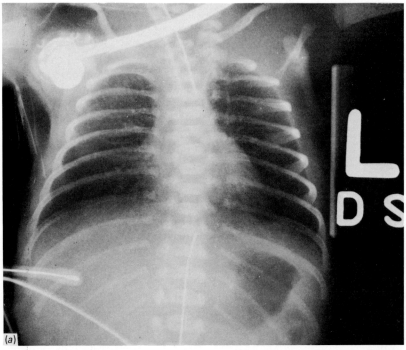

Figure 4.1 (*a*) Chest radiograph obtained on the first day of life in an infant with RDS, showing a characteristic reticulogranular pattern

Some infants with BPD die because of progressive respiratory failure while others die of acute complications. Most show a slow but steady improvement in their lung function and, after variable periods of time, can be weaned from the ventilator. This is usually a very tedious and difficult process, during which time higher oxygen concentrations may be required to maintain adequate oxygenation. The $PaCO_2$ may also rise to levels over 60–70 mmHg as the ventilator settings are lowered. After extubation some infants may persist with chest retractions and tachypnea and frequently have rales and bronchial sounds on auscultation. Because of the respiratory failure, they take oral feeds with difficulty and may require tube

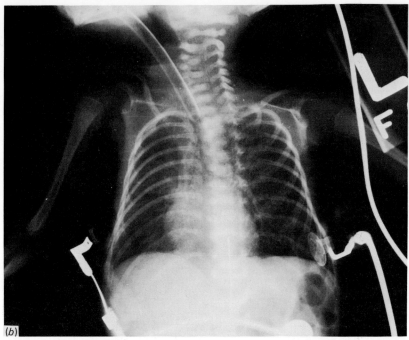

Figure 4.1 (b) Same infant 15 days later, showing a reduction in the densities and better aeration of both lungs

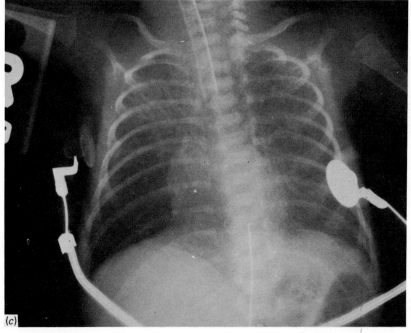

Figure 4.1 (c) At 19 days of age there is opacification of the left lung and right upper lobe, compatible with pneumonia

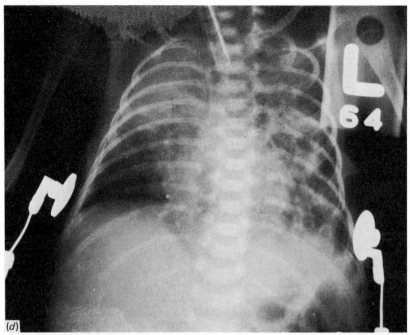

Figure 4.1 (*d*) At 24 days the increased densities persist, but there are cystic areas evolving, especially in the left lung

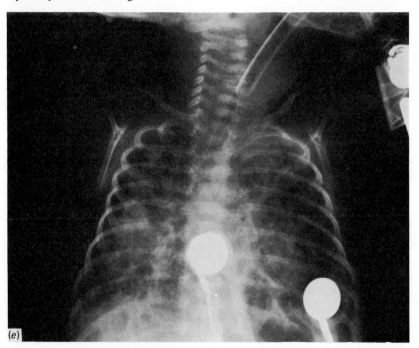

Figure 4.1 (*e*) At 48 days the infant is still intubated and there are bilateral radiolucent areas surrounded by radiodense strands that may correspond to collapse and/or fibrosis

feeding. Weight gain is usually below normal even when the number of calories is appropriate for their age. This may be due to the higher energy expenditure produced by the increased work of breathing (Weinstein and Oh, 1981).

With prolonged respiratory failure, some infants may develop signs of right heart failure with cardiomegaly, hepatomegaly and fluid retention, secondary to pulmonary hypertension. In these cases the need for fluid restriction further limits the number of calories that can be given. Right ventricular failure was a frequent complication of BPD some years ago, but is seen less commonly now (Fouron *et al.*, 1980; Melnick *et al.*, 1980). This is probably related to the milder forms of BPD seen today, and to the fact that their PaO_2 is maintained at a normal level. Echocardiographic evaluation of infants with BPD has shown relatively normal pulmonary artery pressures as long as the PaO_2 is maintained above 55 mmHg (Halliday, Dumpit and Brady, 1980; Melnick *et al.*, 1980). Acute pulmonary infection, either bacterial or viral, is a frequent complication that further disrupts the unstable equilibrium in which these patients survive, worsening their respiratory failure.

Radiographic manifestations

The four stages of BPD reported by Northway and his colleagues (1967) were based primarily on the radiographic evolution described earlier in this chapter. Although this process is present in some infants who develop BPD, many patients do not follow this course, but still reach a final chronic picture similar to the stage IV described by Northway (Opperman *et al.*, 1977; Edwards, 1979; Wung *et al.*, 1979). As mentioned earlier, infants with conditions other than RDS may also develop BPD and, therefore, their initial films may be different from those of stage I. The radiographic characteristics of stage II are also non-specific and may reflect deterioration of RDS, but also may be produced by pulmonary edema, hemorrhage or infection. Not only are the changes of stage II absent in many infants who develop the advanced form of BPD, but they may be present in a large number of infants who recover without pulmonary sequelae.

The radiographic changes of stage III are somewhat more specific and usually convey more chronicity to the picture. Yet, on some occasions, the cysts correspond to severe pulmonary interstitial emphysema and may clear within a few days. This stage can also be absent in patients who ultimately develop stage IV BPD.

Thus, the only changes that are required to make the diagnosis of BPD as originally described are those seen in the more advanced stages of the disease, characterized by an X-ray picture with hyperlucent areas alternating with strands of radiodensity (*Figure 4.2*). The radiographic course before this stage is extremely variable and is influenced by the many complications that may occur in preterm neonates who require mechanical ventilation for extended periods of time.

Recently, an increasing number of very small infants who require IPPV for long periods of time develop chronic lung disease, but their chest radiographs do not show the typical changes of stage IV BPD. Instead, they may show mild hyperexpansion with fine diffuse bilateral lung densities, and sometimes cardiomegaly (Edwards, 1979) (*Figure 4.3*). It is likely that these patients have a similar disease, but of a lesser severity than those described originally.

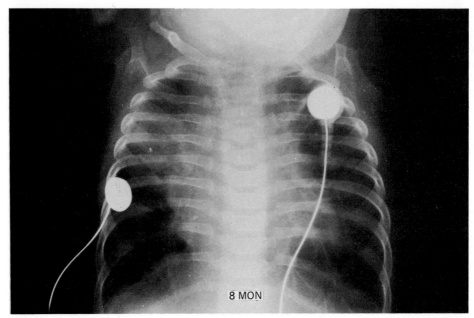

Figure 4.2 Chest radiograph of an 8-month-old infant showing marked hyperlucency in both bases with strands of radiodensity more prominent on the upper lung fields. The cardiac silhouette is enlarged. This picture is compatible with BPD stage IV. (Reproduced from Bancalari and Goldman, 1982, by courtesy of the Editor and Publishers, *Advances in Perinatal Medicine*)

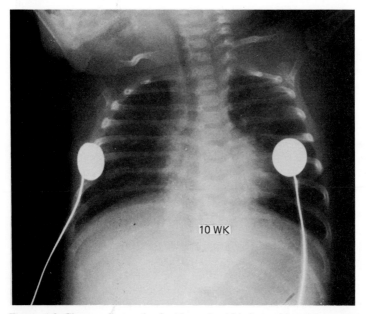

Figure 4.3 Chest radiograph of a 10-week-old infant with mild strands of increased density in both lungs and some hyperinflation of the left lower lobe. This corresponds to a milder form of chronic lung disease

In conclusion, the radiographic progression through the four classical stages of BPD is now uncommon, so that absence of stages I–III does not rule out the diagnosis of BPD. Since stages I, II and III are not specific, one cannot base the diagnosis of BPD on these changes alone. Only a radiographic picture showing chronic pulmonary involvement plus a clinical course that is compatible with BPD allows one to make this diagnosis with some degree of consistency.

Pulmonary function

Patients with BPD have respiratory failure with varying degrees of hypoxemia and hypercapnia. The disruption of pulmonary function is secondary to airway obstruction, fibrosis, emphysema and areas of collapse characteristic of BPD. Minute volume is usually normal, but this is accomplished with a smaller tidal volume and a higher respiratory rate than normal (Watts, Ariagno and Brady, 1977). Thus, there is an increase in dead space ventilation partially explaining the alveolar hypoventilation and CO_2 retention seen in these patients.

Infants with BPD characteristically have a marked increase in airway resistance (Barnes *et al.*, 1969; Stocks, Godfrey and Reynolds, 1978; Morray *et al.*, 1982; Gerhardt *et al.*, 1983). This results in a decreased dynamic compliance and a large increase in the work of breathing. Static compliance has been found to be normal or increased (Barnes *et al.*, 1969) indicating that the decrease in dynamic compliance is mainly due to the increased airway resistance. In the face of airway obstruction, dynamic compliance becomes frequency dependent and decreases at higher respiratory rates.

Functional residual capacity (FRC) may be decreased, normal or increased, depending on the severity and stage of the pulmonary involvement (Bryan *et al.*, 1973; Gerhardt *et al.*, 1983). Because of the maldistribution of inspired gas in infants with BPD, measurements of FRC by nitrogen washout or helium dilution must be interpreted with caution.

The distribution of ventilation is abnormal in infants with advanced BPD. Watts, Ariagno and Brady (1977) found a significant delay in the nitrogen washout in infants with BPD when compared with infants who received IPPV, but did not develop BPD. The alteration in the distribution of ventilation reflects the involvement of the small airway in these patients. Ventilation studies on infants with BPD using xenon-133, have shown that the hyperinflated areas in the bases of the lungs are ventilated less than the upper lobes (Moylan and Shannon, 1979). This indicates that the hyperinflation is not due to compensatory hyperventilation, but is due to emphysema. In infants with milder forms of chronic lung disease, the distribution of gas is usually normal as measured by nitrogen clearance delay (Goldman *et al.*, 1983).

In contrast, the increased airway resistance is observed in most infants who receive IPPV, even when they do not have clinical or radiographic evidence of residual pulmonary disease (Ahlstrom, 1975; Stocks and Godfrey, 1976; Stocks, Godfrey and Reynolds, 1978). This increased airway resistance may last for several months or years and is not observed in infants with RDS who received oxygen therapy, but not IPPV.

Most infants with severe BPD have marked hypoxemia and hypercapnia and require supplemental oxygen to maintain a PaO_2 above 50 mmHg. The amount and duration of oxygen therapy varies according to the severity of the pulmonary damage. In most cases when given 100% O_2, the PaO_2 increases over 100 mmHg, indicating that the hypoxemia is due to a combination of abnormal ventilation/ perfusion ratios and some degree of hypoventilation, rather than anatomical right-to-left shunting. The oxygen requirement decreases gradually as the disease process improves, but increases during feeding, physical activity or during episodes of pulmonary infection or edema.

The increased $PaCO_2$ is secondary to alveolar hypoventilation and to an increased alveolar–arterial CO_2 gradient produced by a mismatch of ventilation and perfusion (Watts, Ariagno and Brady, 1977). The chronic hypercapnia results in an increased blood bicarbonate that tends to compensate for the respiratory acidosis. This increase in base can be exaggerated by the use of diuretics that are frequently indicated in infants with BPD. *Table 4.1* shows the results of serial pulmonary function tests performed in our laboratory on infants with chronic lung disease who have been followed up to 18 months of age (Gerhardt *et al.*, 1983). The results during the first 6 months of life show a decreased FRC with marked increase in pulmonary resistance and decreased lung compliance. With increasing age, FRC and compliance tend to normalize suggesting that alveolar growth is not significantly altered. In contrast, specific pulmonary conductance (SGL) remains decreased during the second year of life indicating that the airway obstruction persists in spite of the lung growth. It is not known whether this alteration disappears later in life or whether the increased airway resistance is irreversible and may persist through into adult life.

Cardiovascular manifestations

Many of the patients with BPD reported earlier in the literature had evidence of pulmonary hypertension with signs of right ventricular failure. The chest radiograph and the electrocardiogram frequently showed evidence of right ventricular hypertrophy. Harrod *et al.* (1974) and Berman *et al.* (1982), performed cardiac catheterization in infants with BPD ranging from 2 to 28 months of age, and found an elevated mean pulmonary artery pressure, that in some infants even persisted after increasing the inspired oxygen concentration (FiO_2) up to 0.8. The ratio of right ventricular pre-ejection period to ejection time (RPEP/RVET) measured echocardiographically has been utilized as a non-invasive method to indirectly evaluate pulmonary artery pressure. Using this method, Fouron *et al.* (1980) showed that the presence of pulmonary hypertension is a poor prognostic sign in infants with BPD. Infants with a normal ratio had a good outcome despite persistence of abnormalities in the chest radiograph. On the other hand, all infants who later expired had a ratio over 0.3 indicating some degree of pulmonary hypertension. Using the same technique, Halliday, Dumpit and Brady (1980) and Melnick *et al.* (1980) found evidence of normal or mildly increased pulmonary artery pressure in infants with BPD. The ratio RPEP/RVET was not modified by a higher inspired oxygen concentration, but increased when the oxygen was lowered. It appears, therefore, that pulmonary hypertension is present only in the more severe cases of BPD and signals a poor prognosis. It is likely that with milder forms of BPD, better monitoring of PaO_2 and avoidance of long periods of hypoxemia may reduce the development of cor pulmonale.

Table 4.1 Pulmonary function in infants with chronic lung disease

Age (months)	Weight (g)	C_L (ml/cm H_2O per kg)	R_L (cm $H_2O \cdot l^{-1} \cdot s^{-1}$)	FRC (ml · kg^{-1})	SC_L (ml/cm H_2O per ℓ FRC)	SG_L (l·s^{-1}·cm H_2O^{-1} per ℓ FRC)
1 (n = 4)	1300 ± 390	0.81 ± 0.20	149 ± 65	14.6 ± 1.9	54.2 ± 14.7	0.47 ± 0.28
6 (n = 14)	5650 ± 1160	0.72 ± 0.22	119 ± 44	15.5 ± 2.9	48.4 ± 16.5	0.31 ± 0.25
12 (n = 14)	8430 ± 1460	1.01 ± 0.25	70 ± 16	17.8 ± 4.5	57.6 ± 15.0	0.11 ± 0.04
18 (n = 7)	9780 ± 1340	1.18 ± 0.27	53 ± 18	20.7 ± 5.0	58.0 ± 9.0	0.12 ± 0.03

C_L = Lung compliance.
FRC = Functional residual capacity.
SC_L = Specific lung compliance (expressed per liter FRC).

R_L = Pulmonary resistance.
SG_L = Specific pulmonary conductance (expressed per liter FRC).

Differential diagnosis

The diagnosis of BPD is based mainly on the clinical course and radiographic findings. As mentioned before, it is impossible to make a clinical diagnosis of BPD during the early stages because the clinical and radiographic findings are non-specific. In addition, it is difficult to predict which of the patients who have changes compatible with early stages of BPD will progress to stage IV and which infants will improve without developing chronic lung disease. For these reasons, the diagnosis of BPD can only be made with some degree of certainty in the more advanced stages of the disease. Even in this stage, the changes are not specific and, therefore, it is likely that one may include patients with chronic lung changes secondary to a variety of etiologies. In an attempt to reduce this problem, we prefer making the diagnosis of BPD only in infants who develop chronic respiratory failure with hypoxemia and hypercapnia lasting more than 28 days. In addition, the diagnosis of BPD should be made only in those infants who have received mechanical ventilation and who have demonstrated persistent radiographic changes characterized by hyperinflation and/or strands of increased density. Using these criteria one limits the diagnosis of BPD to the more severe cases and eliminates other forms of chronic lung disease that may occur during the newborn period. The following are some of the chronic lung problems that should be differentiated from BPD.

Wilson–Mikity

The advanced stages of this disease have clinical and radiographic similarities to BPD and, therefore, the differential diagnosis is based mainly on the initial clinical course. While BPD occurs in infants who require IPPV, the chronic lung changes described by Wilson and Mikity occurred in preterm infants who did not initially have significant pulmonary disease and, therefore, were not treated with IPPV (Wilson and Mikity, 1960; Swyer *et al.*, 1965). There are many very-low-birth-weight infants who require IPPV after the first days or weeks of life because of apnea or heart failure secondary to a PDA, and subsequently also develop chronic lung changes. In these cases it is not clear whether the pulmonary changes are secondary to the mechanical ventilation or whether they would have occurred even without the use of IPPV, thus better fitting the diagnostic criteria of the Wilson–Mikity syndrome. In these patients it is preferable to use the term chronic lung disease rather than BPD or Wilson–Mikity. It is possible that BPD and Wilson–Mikity have a similar pathogenesis, and that the differentiation based on prior use of IPPV is artificial. Although some pathological differences between these two conditions have been described, many of these appear to be more quantitative than qualitative.

Pulmonary interstitial emphysema

This is a complication that occurs frequently in prematures requiring IPPV and is primarily a radiographic diagnosis of air rupturing from alveoli into the perivascular lung tissues. There exist both diffuse and localized varieties, although their causes do not appear to differ. In the more severe cases the gas can coalesce into cystic areas that simulate focal emphysema as seen in BPD (Bauer *et al.,* 1978). These areas are more localized, occur early during the course of the disease and usually disappear within a few days. When they persist for a longer time they commonly precede the development of BPD (Stocker and Madewell, 1977).

Congenital heart disease

Obstruction of the pulmonary venous drainage can produce a radiographic picture similar to BPD. This occurs, however, during the first days of life and is usually accompanied by other evidence of cardiovascular abnormality. Infants with left-to-right shunting and increased pulmonary blood flow frequently develop respiratory failure that must also be differentiated from BPD. The clinical signs of heart disease and echocardiography or cardiac catheterization help in the differential diagnosis.

Pneumonia

Viral pneumonia such as that produced by cytomegalovirus can have radiographic findings similar to those of BPD. Most of these cases have changes present at birth if the infection is congenital, but if the infection occurs later it may be difficult to differentiate from BPD (Whitley *et al.,* 1976; Edwards, 1979). In fact, the pulmonary infection may produce severe respiratory failure requiring the use of mechanical ventilation and predispose the infant to develop BPD. Viral cultures and serial antibody titers must be obtained to confirm the diagnosis of cytomegalovirus pneumonia. Recurrent aspiration of gastric contents secondary to gastroesophageal reflux can also result in chronic pulmonary changes similar to BPD (Danus, Casar and Larrain, 1976).

Cystic fibrosis may also present early in life. However, like most of the conditions mentioned above, the respiratory failure and radiographic changes will precede the use of IPPV rather than follow its use as in BPD.

In summary, while there are many conditions that can produce chronic pulmonary disease in the neonate, the diagnosis of BPD is usually made in cases where the pulmonary changes follow the use of prolonged mechanical ventilation. Although in most infants with BPD the initial indication for IPPV is RDS, there are many cases in which the ventilator is used for respiratory failure due to other causes.

PATHOGENESIS

The exact mechanisms that lead to the morphological and functional disruption of the lungs seen in patients with BPD have not been clearly established. Because the disease occurs almost exclusively in infants who receive mechanical ventilation with positive pressure, this mode of therapy has been considered one of the most likely causes of BPD. Other factors that may be involved in the pathogenesis of this problem include oxygen toxicity, prematurity, lung damage produced by severe RDS and pulmonary edema due to a patent ductus arteriosus or excessive fluid administration.

Intermittent positive pressure

Most cases of BPD occur in infants who require IPPV. Only a few cases of BPD have been described in infants who were ventilated with intermittent negative pressure (Stern *et al.*, 1970; Monin *et al.*, 1976). This low incidence might be partially due to the lower survival of very small infants ventilated with negative pressure alone. In a long-term follow-up of infants who survived after being ventilated with negative pressure, Shepard *et al.* (1968) described residual pulmonary changes similar to those of BPD in six out of 19 infants. These authors attributed those changes to the reparative process of the initial lung insult, but, in fact, those changes may correspond to a milder form of BPD. The strongest advocates for the role of IPPV in the development of BPD are Reynolds and Taghizadeh (1974). They reported an increased survival and decreased incidence of BPD in their nursery after introducing a modality of IPPV with longer inspiration, lower peak airway pressure and lower rate. This was a retrospective study and the diagnosis of BPD was based on postmortem examinations. Subsequently, the same authors (Taghizadeh and Reynolds, 1976) reported results from a second pathological study in which they examined lungs of 112 infants dying from RDS. From this analysis they confirmed their impression that the more severe lesions of BPD correlated best with the use of high airway pressures. In another retrospective analysis, Moylan *et al.* (1978) also observed a decrease in the incidence of alveolar rupture and BPD coincident with the use of lower peak airway pressures during IPPV. Similar results were published by Berg *et al.* (1975) who reported a decreased incidence of BPD from 36.2 to 17.2% after introducing positive end-expiratory pressure and lower peak inspiratory pressures in their nursery. Additional evidence for the long-term detrimental effect of positive pressure on lung function was provided by Stocks (Stocks and Godfrey, 1976; Stocks, Godfrey and Reynolds, 1978) who found that infants who were mechanically ventilated with intermittent positive pressure have an increase in airway resistance that persists at least up to one year of age. Airway resistance was normal in infants with RDS treated only with oxygen or continuous positive pressure, suggesting that the intermittent positive pressure, and not the oxygen or end-expiratory pressure, was responsible for the airway damage.

Most of this information is from retrospective data and, therefore, it is difficult to determine whether the high pressures had a casual effect on the chronic lung damage or whether these high settings were required after the lung damage was already established. No prospective study controlling for other variables that may influence the development of BPD has shown a relationship between positive pressure and BPD. In fact, there are studies demonstrating the opposite. In one of them, 110 infants with RDS were ventilated with different peak airway pressures and inspiratory durations. No significant differences were found in the incidence of chronic lung disease between infants ventilated with low pressures and prolonged inspiration and those ventilated with higher pressures and shorter inspiration (Bancalari *et al.*, 1980). Additional evidence that high peak airway pressure may not be the critical factor in the pathogenesis of BPD was presented by Brown *et al.* (1978) who described seven cases of BPD, only one of whom received pressures above 30 cmH$_2$O. In two subsequent prospective studies using different inspiratory to expiratory ratios during the acute phase of RDS no differences were found in the incidence of BPD between the two treatment groups (Spahr *et al.*, 1980; Heicher, Kasting and Harrod, 1981).

De Lemos *et al.* (1969) tried to establish the role of positive pressure and oxygen in the production of pulmonary damage in lambs. While animals exposed to 100% O_2 died within 2–4 days of severe lung damage, those that were ventilated with air did not demonstrate any significant pulmonary changes. The relevance of these results in relation to the pathogenesis of BPD is limited because IPPV was used for a relatively short period of time and because the lungs in these animals were initially normal. Nilsson (1979) showed that positive pressure ventilation with air produced widespread necrosis of bronchiolar epithelium in premature rabbits while no lesions occurred in mature animals. The same authors (Nilsson, Grossmann and Robertson, 1978) were able to prevent the development of the bronchiolar lesions by depositing a surfactant solution in the upper airway before the animals were ventilated. These results suggest that the decreased compliance secondary to the increased surface tension can be an important factor in the development of bronchiolar lesions secondary to IPPV in the preterm animal.

In infants with RDS, it is difficult to separate the effect of pressure from all the other factors that may influence the development of BPD. Most of these patients require aggressive respiratory support, including high pressures and oxygen concentrations and frequently have complications such as PDA and pulmonary interstitial emphysema that may predispose them to BPD. Although it is likely that positive pressure contributes to the damage of the small airway and to the maldistribution of the inspired gas, there is not enough clinical or experimental evidence to single out one aspect of ventilation as the critical factor in the pathogenesis of BPD.

Oxygen toxicity

In their original report of BPD, Northway and colleagues postulated that the pulmonary lesions were due to the effects of high oxygen concentrations on a lung that was healing from severe RDS. This conclusion was based on the fact that all infants who developed BPD had received high oxygen concentrations for more than 150 hours. This hypothesis was reinforced later by Edwards, Dyer and Northway (1977) who found that the occurrence of BPD in 62 infants was related to the duration of exposure to oxygen concentrations above 40% and not to the duration of mechanical ventilation or endotracheal intubation. Similar results and conclusions have been reported by Banerjee, Girling and Wigglesworth (1972) and Rhodes, Hall and Leonidas (1975), but most infants in these studies received both oxygen and positive pressure ventilation, making interpretation of the results difficult.

Clinically and experimentally, it is well established that a high inspired oxygen concentration can produce severe functional and morphological changes in the lungs, some of which are similar to those observed in BPD (Winter and Smith, 1972). During the first days of exposure to 100% O_2, the pulmonary changes are characterized by interstitial edema and swelling of endothelial cells followed by destruction of type I alveolar cells. After a week of exposure to 100% O_2 there is hyperplasia of type II alveolar epithelial cells with further destruction of type I cells and marked interstitial edema with increased cellularity composed mainly of macrophages and fibroblasts. Bronchiolar changes are particularly striking, and consist of mucosal necrosis with metaplasia and proliferation of bronchiolar epithelium and peribronchiolar edema and obstruction (Nash, Blennerhassett and Pontoppidan, 1967; Northway *et al.*, 1969; Lum *et al.*, 1978). These changes in the bronchioles are probably responsible for the uneven aeration and areas of emphysema that are observed in newborn mice after several days of oxygen exposure (Hellstrom and Nergardh, 1965). These changes are similar to those observed in the advanced stages of BPD. If the animals are allowed to recover in room air, most of these changes will regress, but there may be residual thickening of the interstitium with fibrous tissue.

Because of the evidence that oxygen may play an important role in the pathogenesis of BPD, interest has been focused on the susceptibility of the newborn to the toxic effects of oxygen. The cytotoxicity of oxygen seems to be related to the formation of highly reactive free radicals such as superoxide anion, hydroxyl radical, singlet oxygen and peroxide. The effects of these oxygen metabolites are neutralized by endogenous enzyme systems, such as superoxide dismutase (SOD), glutathione peroxidase and catalase. The neonatal animal's lung is able to respond with a larger increase in pulmonary SOD activity when exposed to high oxygen than the adult animal. This may explain the increased tolerance of the neonatal animal to hyperoxia compared to the mature animal (Yam, Frank and Roberts, 1978).

Little information is available regarding these antioxidant systems in human neonatal lung. Frank, Autor and Roberts (1977) showed that plasma of premature infants with RDS did not stimulate an increase in SOD activity in premature rat's lungs when exposed to oxygen, whereas plasma of most premature infants without RDS did support this enzyme activity. This deficiency in infants with RDS may increase their susceptibility to the toxic effects of oxygen. In addition, Bonta, Gawron and Warshaw (1977) were able to show decreasing SOD levels over several days in three infants with RDS who developed BPD.

Continued exposure to high oxygen concentrations is accompanied by an influx of polymorphonuclear leukocytes containing proteolytic enzymes such as elastase. The anti-proteinase defense system has been observed to be significantly impaired in human infants exposed to greater than 60% inspired oxygen for 6 or more days (Bruce *et al.*, 1982). Consistent with these findings, Merritt *et al.* (1981b) showed elevation in pulmonary effluent neutrophils, macrophages, and elastase activity in infants with RDS who eventually developed BPD. Therefore, proteolytic damage of structural elements in alveolar walls may be an important etiological factor in the development of BPD. Administration of an anti-elastase or other proteinase inhibitor may offer a future preventive approach in the care of these infants.

Another factor that may protect against the effects of high oxygen is vitamin E. In rabbit pups, the administration of vitamin E significantly reduced the lung changes produced by exposure to 100% oxygen (Wender *et al.*, 1980). Although, in a preliminary report, it was suggested that vitamin E could also reduce the incidence of BPD in infants with RDS treated with IPPV (Ehrenkranz *et al.*, 1978), these results were not confirmed in a larger number of infants (Ehrenkranz, Ablow and Warshaw, 1979; Saldanha, Cepeda and Poland, 1982).

While some of the previous data tends to support the possibility that oxygen may play a role in the pathogenesis of BPD, there are some findings that do not support its importance as a single factor. The first one is the very low incidence of BPD in infants who receive high oxygen concentrations for long periods of time, but are not ventilated with positive pressure. Second, there is an increasing number of patients reported in the literature who develop BPD after receiving only low oxygen concentrations or high concentrations for only short periods of time (Philip, 1975; Edwards, Dyer and Northway, 1977; Bancalari *et al.*, 1979).

In conclusion, exposure to high oxygen concentrations for extended periods of time may play a role in the pathogenesis of BPD, but other concomitant factors are required for the development of the chronic pulmonary changes characteristic of this disease.

Pulmonary edema

Most infants with BPD have evidence of a PDA at some point during their clinical course (Brown *et al.*, 1978; Bancalari *et al.*, 1979; Mayes, Perkett and Stahlman, 1983) or at postmortem examination (Northway, Rosan and Porter, 1967; Taghizadeh and Reynolds, 1976). In addition, Brown *et al.* (1978) found that infants who developed BPD had received greater fluid intake during the first five days of life when compared with infants who did not develop BPD. Spitzer, Fox and Delivoria-Papadopoulos (1981) published data suggesting that infants who do not increase their diuresis during the first days of life may be at higher risk for developing BPD than those who have a large diuresis. These findings suggest that an increased pulmonary blood flow and/or interstitial fluid in the lung is another factor that increases the risk of BPD in preterm infants. Increased pulmonary blood flow due to a PDA and the resulting increase in interstitial fluid cause a decrease in pulmonary compliance and increase in airway resistance (Bancalari *et al.*, 1977). These two changes may prolong the need for mechanical ventilation with higher ventilatory pressures and oxygen concentrations increasing the risk for BPD (Cotton *et al.*, 1978; Merritt *et al.*, 1978; Obeyesekere, Pankhurst and Yu, 1980; Merritt *et al.*, 1981a). The increased resistance can also alter the time constant of different segments of the lung and impair the distribution of the inspired gas favoring uneven lung expansion. In a recent study pulmonary function was evaluated in a group of infants early during the course of RDS to define risk factors for BPD (Goldman *et al.*, 1983). Infants who subsequently developed chronic lung disease (CLD) had increased pulmonary resistance from the first week of life, while infants who did not develop CLD had lower resistance values. This observation raises the possibility that increased airway resistance may play a significant role in the pathogenesis of BPD, and this measurement could be used to predict which infants are at higher risk during the first days of life. This may also open the possibility for early intervention in order to lower airway resistance and possibly reduce the incidence of chronic lung disease.

Primary pulmonary disease

Although prematurity and the underlying pulmonary disease may be important factors in the development of BPD, it is very difficult to analyse their independent role because they usually coexist with many other variables implicated in the pathogenesis of BPD. The vast majority of patients with BPD are premature and have RDS, but the problem can also occur in full-term infants (Northway, Rosan and Porter, 1967; Rhodes, Hall and Leonidas, 1975) and in newborns with diseases other than RDS (Philip, 1975; Friis-Hansen *et al.*, 1976).

In a recent report, the possibility of a genetic predisposition to abnormal airway reactivity in infants with BPD has been raised. Nickerson and Taussig (1980) found a stronger family history of asthma in infants with BPD than in controls. *Figure 4.4* shows the interaction of some of the factors that may play an important role in the pathogenesis of neonatal chronic lung disease.

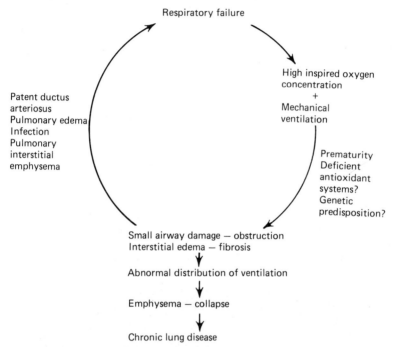

Figure 4.4 Factors that may participate in the pathogenesis of neonatal chronic lung disease

PATHOLOGICAL CHANGES

The pathological changes seen in the early stages of BPD are similar to those present in patients dying during the first days of life with severe RDS. In the more chronic forms of the disease, the changes become more characteristic. Macroscopically, the lungs have a grossly abnormal appearance; they are firm, heavy and have a darker color than normal. The surface is irregular, many times showing emphysematous areas alternating with areas of collapse (*Figures 4.5* and *4.6*).

On histological examination, these lungs are characterized by areas of emphysema, sometimes coalescent into larger cystic areas, surrounded by areas of atelectasis (*Figure 4.7*). There is widespread bronchial and bronchiolar mucosal hyperplasia and metaplasia that reduces the lumen in many of the small airways (*Figure 4.8*). In some cases, there may be excessive mucus secretion with exudation of alveolar macrophages. Except for the hypertrophy of the peribronchiolar smooth muscle that persists throughout the course of the disease, the involvement

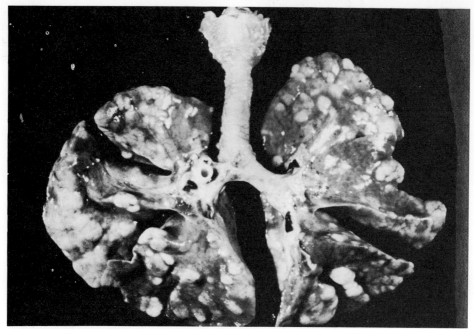

Figure 4.5 Macroscopic appearance of lungs with severe BPD showing uneven expansion. (Reproduced from Bancalari and Goldman, 1982, by courtesy of the Editor and Publishers, *Advances in Perinatal Medicine*)

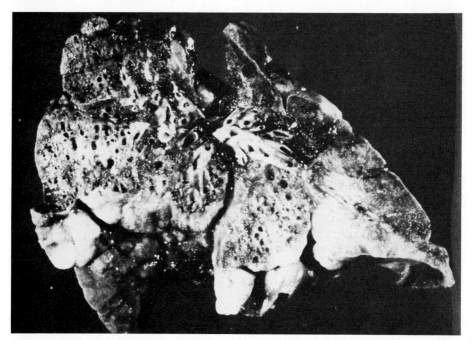

Figure 4.6 Macroscopic section of lungs with severe BPD showing areas of emphysema and collapse

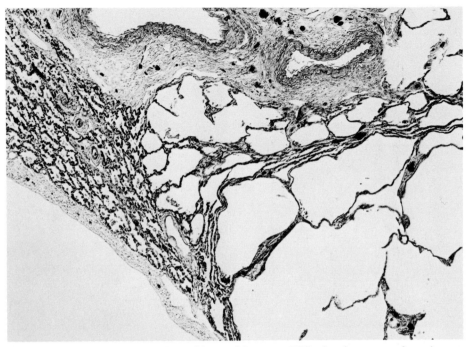

Figure 4.7 Low magnification view of lung with severe BPD showing areas of emphysema alternating with areas of partial collapse. (Reproduced from Bancalari and Goldman, 1982, by courtesy of the Editor and Publishers, *Advances in Perinatal Medicine*)

of the small airway is more prominent during the early stages becoming less marked after the first month of evolution (Reynolds and Taghizadeh, 1974). In addition, there is interstitial edema and an increase in fibrous tissue with focal thickening of the basal membrane separating capillaries from alveolar spaces (*Figure 4.9*). Lymphatics are frequently dilated and tortuous. In many cases there are vascular changes of pulmonary hypertension, such as medial muscle hypertrophy and elastic degeneration. There may also be evidence of right ventricular hypertrophy, and in some cases left ventricular hypertrophy as well (Melnick *et al.,* 1980).

Tracheal aspirate cytology

In recent years, the cytopathological examination of tracheobronchial aspirate has been proposed as a tool to diagnose BPD while the infant is receiving mechanical ventilation (Merritt *et al.,* 1981a). Infants who develop BPD have a large number of bronchial epithelial exfoliated cells. These cells have prominent chromocenters and an increased nuclear/cytoplasm ratio, suggestive of cell regeneration.

PREVENTION

It is likely that BPD results from the interaction of multiple contributing factors. Therefore, the prevention of BPD must be attempted by minimizing all these factors, especially in the small premature infants most susceptible to development

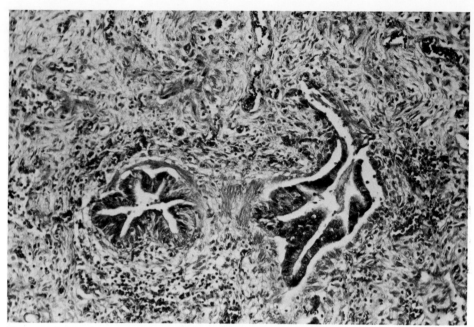

Figure 4.8 Small airways showing hyperplasia of the epithelium partially obstructing the lumen. Peribronchial muscle is hypertrophied, most alveoli are collapsed, and there is an increase in interstitial fibrous tissue. (Reproduced from Bancalari and Goldman, 1982, by courtesy of the Editor and Publishers, *Advances in Perinatal Medicine*)

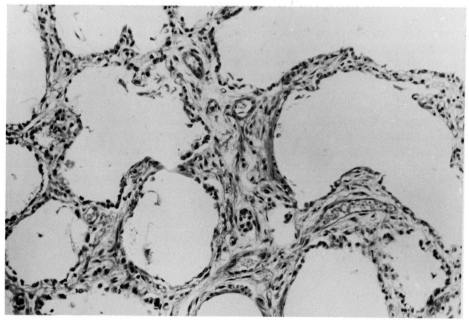

Figure 4.9 Alveolar septa thickened by edema and fibroblastic proliferation. (Reproduced from Bancalari and Goldman, 1982, by courtesy of the Editor and Publishers, *Advances in Perinatal Medicine*)

of this condition. When these infants require mechanical ventilation, one must use the lowest peak airway pressure required to obtain adequate ventilation and this pressure must be lowered rapidly as the mechanical characteristics of the lungs improve. Inspiratory times between 0.3 and 0.5 s are usually adequate with flow rates between 5 and 10 $\ell \cdot min^{-1}$. Shorter inspiratory times and higher flow rates are not recommended because they may exaggerate the maldistribution of the inspired gas. Longer inspiratory times may increase the risk of alveolar rupture and cardiovascular side-effects. The end-expiratory pressure must be adjusted so that the minimum oxygen concentration necessary to keep the PaO_2 above 50 mmHg is used. Fluid administration must be carefully controlled and restricted, especially if there is evidence of a PDA. In this case, the use of diuretics and early intervention with drugs or surgery in order to close the ductus will improve lung function and reduce the exposure to prolonged IPPV and high oxygen concentrations (Cotton *et al.*, 1978; Merritt *et al.*, 1978; Gerhardt and Bancalari, 1980). This may result in a lower incidence of BPD (Merritt *et al.*, 1981b).

Various collaborative studies are currently examining newer innovative approaches to the management of the preterm infant with RDS requiring assisted ventilation. The current status of high frequency ventilation is discussed in Chapter 3, while the potential usefulness of surfactant therapy has recently been extensively reviewed (Taeusch, Clements and Benson, 1983). A major objective of these lines of investigation remains to reduce the incidence of BPD.

MANAGEMENT

The management of infants with BPD should be directed at maintaining adequate arterial blood gases and, at the same time, avoiding progression of the pulmonary lesions. Weaning these patients from the ventilator is difficult and has to be accomplished gradually. When the patient is able to maintain an acceptable PaO_2 and $PaCO_2$ with peak pressures under 25 cm H_2O and an FiO_2 lower than 0.5, the ventilator rate is gradually reduced allowing the infant to increase spontaneous ventilation. During this process it is common for the inspired oxygen concentration to be increased and the $PaCO_2$ to rise into the 50s or 60s. As long as the pH is within acceptable limits, this degree of hypercapnia may need to be accepted in order to wean the patient from the ventilator. In some infants, theophylline can be used as a respiratory stimulant during the weaning. When the patient is able to maintain acceptable blood gas levels on a continuous positive airway pressure of 2–4 cm H_2O, and without the ventilator cycling, extubation can be attempted. During the days following extubation, it is important to do chest physiotherapy and, if necessary, direct endotracheal suctioning to prevent airway obstruction and lung collapse due to retained secretions.

Oxygen therapy

Although it is necessary to reduce the FiO_2 as soon as possible to avoid its toxic effects, nonetheless, it is important to maintain the PaO_2 at a level sufficient to assure adequate tissue oxygenation and avoid the pulmonary hypertension and cor pulmonale that can result from chronic hypoxemia. Furthermore, oxygen therapy does not produce respiratory depression in infants with chronic lung disease

(Hazinski *et al.*, 1981). Thus, the PaO_2 should be maintained above 50–55 mmHg at all times. Oxygen can be administered through a hood, tent, face mask or nasal catheter. During feeds, oxygen consumption increases and PaO_2 may decrease, so it may be necessary to provide a higher FiO_2 to avoid hypoxemia. In many cases, oxygen therapy is required for several months or even years. Some of these patients can be sent home receiving oxygen therapy. This may offer significant advantages in terms of a better environment for the patient and cost savings for the family (Pinney and Cotton, 1976).

The determination of the necessary FiO_2 must be based on a combination of arterial blood gas and transcutaneous measurements. The former is difficult because each time that an arterial or capillary blood sample is being obtained these infants react with vigorous crying which may result in hypoxemia. This problem may be avoided by the use of local anesthesia prior to arterial puncture. The use of the transcutaneous oxygen monitor is helpful, although transcutaneous PO_2 frequently underestimates arterial PO_2 when these infants are beyond 10 weeks postnatal age (Rome *et al.*, 1984).

Fluid management

Infants with BPD tolerate excessive or even normal fluid intake poorly and have a marked tendency to accumulate an excessive amount of interstitial fluid in the lung. This leads to a deterioration of their pulmonary function with exaggeration of the hypoxemia and hypercapnia. The tendency to increase extravascular lung water may be due to increased capillary pressure, increased capillary permeability or decreased lymphatic drainage. The increased capillary pressure can be secondary to the left ventricular dysfunction that has been described in patients with chronic respiratory failure (Kachel, 1978; Melnick *et al.*, 1980). The increased capillary permeability may be secondary to the effects of high oxygen concentration in the inspired gas on the capillary endothelium. Decreased lymphatic drainage may result from the compression of lymphatics by interstitial fluid and fibrous tissue and also from the increased central venous pressure due to cor pulmonale.

In order to reduce lung fluid, water intake should be limited in infants with BPD to the minimum required to provide the necessary calories for their metabolic needs and growth. When increased lung water persists despite fluid restriction, chronic diuretic administration can be used successfully especially in patients with evidence of cor pulmonale (Noble, Trenchard and Guz, 1966; Sniderman *et al.*, 1978). The use of diuretics in these infants is associated with a rapid improvement in lung compliance and decrease in resistance, but the blood gases may not show significant improvement (Kao *et al.*, 1983b; Tapia *et al.*, 1983). The reduction in pulmonary capillary pressure observed after furosemide administration is not entirely due to the increased elimination of sodium and water, but seems to be, in part, secondary to an increase in venous capacitance and reduced venous return (Dikshit *et al.*, 1979). Complications of chronic diuretic therapy include hypokalemia, hyponatremia, metabolic alkalosis and hypercalciuria.

The use of theophylline has also been recommended in infants with BPD (Rooklin *et al.*, 1979). This drug may have several beneficial effects, including diuresis, bronchodilation and respiratory center stimulation, but there is limited controlled experience with its use in these type of patients. The inconsistent results from bronchodilator therapy in patients with BPD warrant their routine use only in the presence of bronchospasm (Tal, Bar-Yishay and Godfrey, 1982; Kao *et al.*, 1983a).

Recently, steroids were given to a group of infants with BPD with improvement in lung function during the administration of dexamethasone for a period of 10 days (Sobel *et al.*, 1983). It is not clear whether this transient improvement in lung function justifies the use of a drug that may increase the risk of serious infection.

Nutritional needs are difficult to meet in these patients because of poor feeding tolerance, the need to restrict fluids and the increased caloric needs due to the excessive work of breathing (Weinstein and Oh, 1981). Thus, the use of parenteral hyperalimentation and nasogastric feeding using concentrated diets for extended periods of time is frequently necessary.

A special emphasis on psychosensory stimulation is important to compensate for the lack of family influence and the abnormal environment in which these infants spend such a large portion of a critical period of their development.

OUTCOME

The survival of infants with BPD has markedly improved in recent years. While 70% of the infants described by Northway, Rosan and Porter (1967) died, in more recent series the mortality has been markedly reduced (Rhodes, Hall and Leonidas, 1975; Edwards, Dyer and Northway, 1977; Bancalari *et al.*, 1979; Mayes, Perkett and Stahlman, 1983). A significant proportion of the deaths of infants with BPD occur after discharge from the hospital (Edwards, Dyer and Northway, 1977) and are usually due to acute respiratory infections. The reduction in mortality over the recent years is not due to one specific modality of treatment, but is a consequence of the overall improvement in the care these patients are receiving. Because most of the originally described infants died with right heart failure, the improved outcome may be related to closer monitoring of arterial blood gases and avoidance of chronic hypoxemia. This reduces the risk of pulmonary hypertension and cor pulmonale. The lower mortality is also due to the milder form of BPD increasingly seen over recent years.

The hospital stay of infants with severe BPD is frequently very long. This is primarily because of the need for supplemental inspired oxygen and can, therefore, be reduced considerably if the patients are given oxygen at home (Pinney and Cotton, 1976). Growth and development may be delayed in some infants with BPD (Mayes, Perkett and Stahlman, 1983). This is partly due to the difficulties in providing adequate nutrition and partly because of the lack of normal sensory stimulation received by these infants in an oxygen tent, isolated from their environment. Major developmental deficits are usually associated with preceding perinatal and neonatal events rather than the presence of BPD (Markestad and Fitzhardinge, 1981).

Little is known regarding the long-term evolution of the pulmonary lesions in BPD. While most infants show progressive improvement of their respiratory status, they frequently have episodes of deterioration due to respiratory tract infection with airway obstruction and increasing hypoxemia that require readmission to the hospital. Radiographic changes also show improvement, but in some cases they may persist for several years (Harrod *et al.*, 1974; Johnson *et al.*, 1974).

There are few long-term sequential studies of pulmonary function in infants with BPD. This is partially because of the difficulty in performing these studies in children before 5 or 6 years of age. Evidence of airway obstruction with air trapping and bronchial hyper-reactivity was recently reported in nine survivors with BPD at 7–9 years of age (Smyth *et al.*, 1981). Follow-up data from our institution (Gerhardt *et al.*, 1983) also suggests that the increased airway resistance persists for at least two years, raising the possibility that infants with BPD may have persistently abnormal pulmonary function for extended periods of time.

Acknowledgement

The author thanks Drs Rita Fojaco and Bill Buck for providing the pathological illustrations.

References

AHLSTROM, H. (1975) Pulmonary mechanics in infants surviving severe neonatal respiratory insufficiency. *Acta Paediatrica Scandinavica*, **64**, 69

BANCALARI, E., ABDENOUR, G. E., FELLER, R. *et al.* (1979) Bronchopulmonary dysplasia: clinical presentation. *Journal of Pediatrics*, **95**, 819

BANCALARI, E., FELLER, R., GERHARDT, T., ABDENOUR, G., GANNON, J. and MELNICK, G. (1980) Prospective evaluation of different IPPV settings in infants with RDS. *Clinical Research*, **28**, 870A

BANCALARI, E. and GOLDMAN, S. L. (1982) Bronchopulmonary dysplasia. In *Advances in Perinatal Medicine*. Eds A. Milunsky, E. A. Friedman and L. Gluck. pp. 162–182. New York: Plenum Medical Book Company

BANCALARI, E., JESSE, M. J., GELBRAND, H. *et al.* (1977) Lung mechanics in congenital heart disease with increased and decreased pulmonary blood flow. *Journal of Pediatrics*, **90**, 192

BANERJEE, C. K., GIRLING, D. J. and WIGGLESWORTH, J. S. (1972) Pulmonary fibroplasia in newborn babies treated with oxygen and artificial ventilation. *Archives of Disease in Childhood*, **47**, 509

BARNES, N. D., HULL, D., GLOVER, W. J. *et al.* (1969) Effects of prolonged positive-pressure ventilation in infancy. *Lancet*, **2**, 1096

BAUER, C. R., BRENNAN, M. J., DOYLE, C. *et al.* (1978) Surgical resection for pulmonary interstitial emphysema in the newborn infant. *Journal of Pediatrics*, **93**, 656

BERG, T. J., PAGTAKHAN, R. D., REED, M. H. *et al.* (1975) Bronchopulmonary dysplasia and lung rupture in hyaline membrane disease: influence of continuous distending pressure. *Pediatrics*, **55**, 51

BERMAN, W. JR, YABEK, S. M., DILLON, T., BURSTEIN, R. and CORLEW, S. (1982) Evaluation of infants with bronchopulmonary dysplasia using cardiac catheterization. *Pediatrics*, **70**, 708

BONTA, B. W., GAWRON, E. R. and WARSHAW, J. B. (1977) Neonatal red cell superoxide dismutase enzyme levels: possible role as a cellular defense mechanism against pulmonary oxygen toxicity. *Pediatric Research*, **11**, 754

BRYAN, M. H., HARDIE, M. J., REILLY, B. J. *et al.* (1973) Pulmonary function studies during the first year of life in infants recovering from the respiratory distress syndrome. *Pediatrics*, **52**, 169

BROWN, E. R., STARK, A., SOSENKO, I. *et al.* (1978) Bronchopulmonary dysplasia: possible relationship to pulmonary edema. *Journal of Pediatrics*, **92**, 982

BRUCE, M., BOAT, T., MARTIN, R., DEARBORN, D. and FANAROFF, A. (1982) Proteinase inhibitors and inhibitor inactivation in neonatal airways secretions. *Chest*, **81** (Supplement), 44

COTTON, R. B., STAHLMAN, M. T., BENDER, H. W. *et al.* (1978) Randomized trial of early closure of symptomatic patent ductus arteriosus in small preterm infants. *Journal of Pediatrics*, **93**, 647

DANUS, O., CASAR, C. and LARRAIN, A. (1976) Esophageal reflux: an unrecognized cause of recurrent obstructive bronchitis in children. *Journal of Pediatrics*, **89**, 220

DE LEMOS, R., WOLFSDOR, J., NACHMAN, R. *et al.* (1969) Lung injury from oxygen in lambs: the role of artificial ventilation. *Anesthesiology*, **30**, 609

DIKSHIT, K., VYDEN, J. K., FORRESTER, J. S. *et al.* (1979) Renal and extrarenal hemodynamic effects of furosemide in congestive heart failure after acute myocardial infarction. *New England Journal of Medicine*, **288**, 1087

EDWARDS, D. K. (1979) Radiographic aspects of bronchopulmonary dysplasia. *Journal of Pediatrics*, **85**, 823

EDWARDS, D. K., DYER, W. M. and NORTHWAY, W. H. JR (1977) Twelve years' experience with bronchopulmonary dysplasia. *Pediatrics*, **59**, 839

EHRENKRANZ, R., ABLOW, R. C. and WARSHAW, J. B. (1979) Prevention of bronchopulmonary dysplasia with vitamin E administration during the acute stages of respiratory distress syndrome. *Journal of Pediatrics*, **95**, 873

EHRENKRANZ, R. A., BONTA, B. W., ABLOW, R. C. *et al.* (1978) Amelioration of bronchopulmonary dysplasia after vitamin E administration. *New England Journal of Medicine*, **299**, 564

FARRELL, P. M. and AVERY, M. E. (1975) Hyaline membrane disease. *American Review of Respiratory Disease*, **111**, 657

FOURON, J. C., LE GUENNEC, J. C., VILLEMANT, D. *et al.* (1980) Value of echocardiography in assessing the outcome of bronchopulmonary dysplasia of the newborn. *Pediatrics*, **65**, 529

FRANK, L., AUTOR, A. P. and ROBERTS, R. J. (1977) Oxygen therapy and hyaline membrane disease: the effect of hyperoxia on pulmonary superoxide dismutase activity and the mediating role of plasma or serum. *Journal of Pediatrics*, **90**, 105

FRIIS-HANSEN, B., KAMPER, J., BOISON-MOLLER, J. *et al.* (1976) The incidence of pulmonary fibroplasia among 263 infants treated with intermittent positive pressure ventilation. In *Neonatal Intensive Care*. Eds J. B. Stetson and P. R. Swyer. p. 445. St Louis, Missouri: W. H. Greene Inc.

GERHARDT, T. and BANCALARI, E. (1980) Lung compliance in neonates with patent ductus arteriosus before and after surgical ligation. *Biology of the Neonate*, **38**, 96

GERHARDT, T., TAPIA, J. L., GOLDMAN, S. L., HEHRE, D., FELLER, R. and BANCALARI, E. (1983) Serial lung function measurements in infants with chronic lung disease (CLD). *Pediatric Research*, **17**, 376A

GOLDMAN, S. L., GERHARDT, T., SONNI, R. *et al.* (1983) Early prediction of chronic lung disease by pulmonary function testing. *Journal of Pediatrics*, **102**, 613

HALLIDAY, H. L., DUMPIT, F. M. and BRADY, J. P. (1980) Effects of inspired oxygen on echocardiographic assessment of pulmonary vascular resistance and myocardial contractility in bronchopulmonary dysplasia. *Pediatrics*, **65**, 536

HARROD, J. R., L'HEUREUX, P., WANGENSTEEN, O. D. *et al.* (1974) Long-term follow-up of severe respiratory distress syndrome treated with IPPB. *Journal of Pediatrics*, **84**, 277

HAZINSKI, T. A., HANSEN, T. N., SIMON, J. A. and TOOLEY, W. H. (1981) Effect of oxygen administration during sleep on skin surface oxygen and carbon dioxide tensions in patients with chronic lung disease. *Pediatrics*, **67**, 626

HEICHER, D. A., KASTING, D. S. and HARROD, J. R. (1981) Prospective clinical comparison of two methods for mechanical ventilation of neonates: rapid rate and short inspiratory time versus slow rate and long inspiratory time. *Journal of Pediatrics*, **98**, 957

HELLSTROM, B. and NERGARDH, A. (1965) The effect of high oxygen concentrations and hypothermia on the lung of the newborn mouse. *Acta Paediatrica Scandinavica*, **54**, 457

JOHNSON, J. D., MALACHOWSKI, N. C., GROBSTEIN, R. *et al.* (1974) Prognosis of children surviving with the aid of mechanical ventilation in the newborn period. *Journal of Pediatrics*, **84**, 272

KACHEL, R. (1978) Left ventricular function in chronic obstructive pulmonary disease. *Chest*, **74**, 286

KAO, L. C., KEENS, T. G., SARGENT, C. W. and WARBURTON, D. (1983a) Bronchodilators decrease airway resistance in bronchopulmonary dysplasia. *American Review of Respiratory Disease*, **127**, 212

KAO, L. C., WARBURTON, D., SARGENT, C. W., PLATZKER, A. C. G. and KEENS, T. G. (1983b) Furosemide acutely decreases airways resistance in chronic bronchopulmonary dysplasia. *Journal of Pediatrics*, **103**, 624

LUM, H., SCHWARTZ, L. W., DUNGWORTH, D. L. *et al.* (1978) A comparative study of cell renewal after exposure to ozone or oxygen. *American Review of Respiratory Disease*, **118**, 335

MARKESTAD, T. and FITZHARDINGE, P. M. (1981) Growth and development in children recovering from bronchopulmonary dysplasia. *Journal of Pediatrics*, **98**, 597

MAYES, L., PERKETT, E. and STAHLMAN, M. T. (1983) Severe bronchopulmonary dysplasia: a retrospective review. *Acta Paediatrica Scandinavica*, **72**, 225

MELNICK, G., PICKOFF, A. S., FERRER, P. L., PEYSER, J., BANCALARI, E. and GELBAND, H. (1980) Normal pulmonary vascular resistance and left ventricular hypertrophy in young infants with bronchopulmonary dysplasia: An echocardiographic and pathologic study. *Pediatrics*, **66**, 589

MERRITT, T. A., COCHRANE, C. G., HOLCOMB, K. *et al.* (1983) Elastase and α_1-proteinase inhibitor activity in tracheal aspirates during respiratory distress syndrome. *Journal of Clinical Investigation*, **72**, 656

MERRITT, T. A., DISESSA, T. G., FELDMAN, B. H. *et al.* (1978) Closure of the patent ductus arteriosus with ligation and indomethacin: a consecutive experience. *Journal of Pediatrics*, **93**, 639

MERRITT, T. A., HARRIS, J. P., ROGHMANN, K. *et al.* (1981a) Early closure of the patent ductus arteriosus in very-low-birth-weight infants: a controlled trial. *Journal of Pediatrics*, **99**, 281

MERRITT, T. A., STUARD, I. D., PUCCIA, J. *et al.* (1981b) Newborn tracheal aspirate cytology: classification during respiratory distress syndrome and bronchopulmonary dysplasia. *Journal of Pediatrics,* **98,** 949

MONIN, P., CASHORE, W. J., HAKANSON, D. O. *et al.* (1976) Assisted ventilation in the neonate: comparison between positive and negative respirators. *Pediatric Research,* **10,** 464

MORRAY, J. P., FOX, W. W., KETTRICK, R. G. and DOWNES, J. J. (1982) Improvement in lung mechanics as a function of age in the infant with severe bronchopulmonary dysplasia. *Pediatric Research,* **16,** 290

MOYLAN, F. M. B. and SHANNON, D. C. (1979) Preferential distribution of lobar emphysema and atelectasis in bronchopulmonary dysplasia. *Pediatrics,* **63,** 130

MOYLAN, F. M. B., WALKER, A. M., KRAMER, S. S. *et al.* (1978) The relationship of bronchopulmonary dysplasia to the occurrence of alveolar rupture during positive pressure ventilation. *Critical Care Medicine,* **6,** 140

NASH, G., BLENNERHASSETT, J. B. and PONTOPPIDAN, H. (1967) Pulmonary lesions associated with oxygen therapy and artificial ventilation. *New England Journal of Medicine,* **276,** 368

NICKERSON, B. G. and TAUSSIG, L. M. (1980) Family history of asthma in infants with bronchopulmonary dysplasia. *Pediatrics,* **65,** 1140

NILSSON, R. (1979) Lung compliance and lung morphology following artificial ventilation in the premature and full-term rabbit neonate. *Scandinavian Journal of Respiratory Diseases,* **60,** 206

NILSSON, R., GROSSMANN, G. and ROBERTSON, B. (1978) Lung surfactant and the pathogenesis of neonatal bronchiolar lesions induced by artificial ventilation. *Pediatric Research,* **12,** 249

NOBLE, M. I. M., TRENCHARD, D. and GUZ, A. (1966) The value of diuretics in respiratory failure. *Lancet,* **2,** 257

NORTHWAY, W. H. Jr, ROSAN, R. C. and PORTER, D. Y. (1967) Pulmonary disease following respirator therapy of hyaline membrane disease. *New England Journal of Medicine,* **276,** 357

NORTHWAY, W. H. Jr, ROSAN, R. C., SHAHINIAN, L. *et al.* (1969) Radiologic and histologic investigation of pulmonary oxygen toxicity in newborn guinea pigs. *Investigative Radiology,* **4,** 148

OBEYESEKERE, H. I., PANKHURST, S. and YU, V. Y. H. (1980) Pharmacological closure of ductus arteriosus in preterm infants using indomethacin. *Archives of Disease in Childhood,* **55,** 271

OPPERMANN, H. C., WILLE, L., BLEYL, U. *et al.* (1977) Bronchopulmonary dysplasia in premature infants: a radiological and pathological correlation. *Pediatric Radiology,* **5,** 137

PHILIP, A. G. (1975) Oxygen plus pressure plus time: the etiology of bronchopulmonary dysplasia. *Pediatrics,* **55,** 44

PINNEY, M. A. and COTTON, E. K. (1976) Home management of bronchopulmonary dysplasia. *Pediatrics,* **58,** 856

REYNOLDS, E. O. R. and TAGHIZADEH, A. (1974) Improved prognosis of infants mechanically ventilated for hyaline membrane disease. *Archives of Disease in Childhood,* **49,** 505

RHODES, P. G., HALL, R. T. and LEONIDAS, J. C. (1975) Chronic pulmonary disease in neonates with assisted ventilation. *Pediatrics,* **55,** 788

ROME, E. S., STORK, E. K., CARLO, W. A. and MARTIN, R. J. (1984) Limitations of transcutaneous PO_2 and PCO_2 monitoring in infants with bronchopulmonary dysplasia. *Pediatrics,* **74,** 217

ROOKLIN, A. R., MOOMJIAN, A. S., SHUTACK, J. G. *et al.* (1979) Theophylline therapy in bronchopulmonary dysplasia. *Journal of Pediatrics,* **95,** 882

SALDANHA, R. L., CEPEDA, E. E. and POLAND, R. L. (1982) The effect of vitamin E prophylaxis on the incidence and severity of bronchopulmonary dysplasia. *Journal of Pediatrics,* **101,** 89

SHEPARD, F. M., JOHNTSON, R. B. JR, KLATTE, E. C. *et al.* (1968) Residual pulmonary findings in clinical hyaline membrane disease. *New England Journal of Medicine,* **279,** 1063

SMYTH, J. A., TABACHNIK, E., DUNCAN, W. J., REILLY, B. J. and LEVISON, H. (1981) Pulmonary function and bronchial hyperreactivity in long-term survivors of bronchopulmonary dysplasia. *Pediatrics,* **68,** 336

SNIDERMAN, S., CHUNG, M., ROTH, R. *et al.* (1978) Treatment of neonatal chronic lung disease with furosemide. *Clinical Research,* **26,** 201A

SOBEL, D. B., LEWIS, K., DEMING, D. D. and MCCANN, E. M. (1983) Dexamethasone improves lung function in infants with chronic lung disease. *Pediatric Research,* **17,** 390A

SPAHR, R. C., KLEIN, A. M., BROWN, D. R. *et al.* (1980) Hyaline membrane disease. *American Journal of Diseases of Children,* **134,** 373

SPITZER, A. R., FOX, W. W. and DELIVORIA-PAPADOPOULOS, M. (1981) Maximum diuresis – a factor in predicting recovery from respiratory distress syndrome and the development of bronchopulmonary dysplasia. *Journal of Pediatrics,* **98,** 476

STERN, L., RAMOS, A. D., OUTERBRIDGE, E. W. *et al.* (1970) Negative pressure artificial respiration: use in treatment of respiratory failure of the newborn. *Canadian Medical Association Journal,* **102,** 595

STOCKER, J. T. and MADEWELL, J. E. (1977) Persistent interstitial emphysema: another complication of the respiratory distress syndrome. *Pediatrics,* **59,** 847

STOCKS, J. and GODFREY, S. (1976) The role of artificial ventilation, oxygen, and CPAP in the pathogenesis of lung damage in neonates: assessment by serial measurement of lung function. *Pediatrics,* **57,** 352

STOCKS, J., GODFREY, S. and REYNOLDS, E. O. R. (1978) Airway resistance in infants after various treatments for hyaline membrane disease: special emphasis on prolonged high levels of inspired oxygen. *Pediatrics,* **61,** 178

SWYER, P. R., DELIVORIA-PAPADOPOULOS, M., LEVISON, H. *et al.* (1965) Pulmonary syndrome of Wilson and Mikity. *Pediatrics,* **36,** 374

TAEUSCH, H. W., CLEMENTS, J. and BENSON, B. (1983) Exogenous surfactant for human lung disease. *American Review of Respiratory Disease,* **128,** 791

TAGHIZADEH, A. and REYNOLDS, E. O. R. (1976) Pathogenesis of bronchopulmonary dysplasia following hyaline membrane disease. *American Journal of Pathology,* **82,** 241

TAL, A., BAR-YISHAY, E., EYAL, F. and GODFREY, S. (1982) Lack of response to bronchodilator of airway obstruction after mechanical ventilation in the newborn. *Critical Care Medicine,* **10,** 361

TAPIA, J. L., GERHARDT, T., GOLDBERG, R. N., GOMEZ-DEL-RIO, M., HEHRE, D. and BANCALARI, E. (1983) Furosemide and lung function in neonates with chronic lung disease (CLD). *Pediatric Research,* **17,** 338A

WATTS, J. L., ARIAGNO, R. L. and BRADY, J. P. (1977) Chronic pulmonary disease in neonates after artificial ventilation: distribution of ventilation and pulmonary interstitial emphysema. *Pediatrics,* **60,** 273

WEINSTEIN, M. R. and OH, W. (1981) Oxygen consumption in infants with bronchopulmonary dysplasia. *Journal of Pediatrics,* **99,** 958

WENDER, D. F., THULIN, G. E., SMITH, G. J. W. *et al.* (1980) Vitamin E affects lung morphologic response to hyperoxia. *Pediatric Research,* **14,** 653

WHITLEY, R. J., BRASFIELD, D., REYNOLDS, D. W. *et al.* (1976) Protracted pneumonitis in young infants associated with perinatally acquired cytomegaloviral infection. *Journal of Pediatrics,* **89,** 16

WILSON, M. G. and MIKITY, V. G. (1960) A new form of respiratory disease in premature infants. *American Journal of Diseases in Children,* **99,** 119

WINTER, P. M. and SMITH, G. (1972) The toxicity of oxygen. *Anesthesiology,* **37,** 210

WUNG, J. T., KOONS, A. H., DRISCOLL, J. M. *et al.* (1979) Changing incidence of bronchopulmonary dysplasia. *Journal of Pediatrics,* **85,** 845

YAM, J., FRANK, L. and ROBERTS, R. J. (1978) Oxygen toxicity: comparison of lung biochemical responses in neonatal and adult rats. *Pediatric Research,* **12,** 115

5
Cardiorespiratory monitoring for sudden infant death syndrome

Joan Hodgman

Cardiorespiratory monitoring is carried out under three circumstances in connection with the sudden infant death syndrome (SIDS). The first of these is for research investigation into the etiology of the syndrome. Because most of the infants succumbing to SIDS do so while sleeping, this type of monitoring usually takes place in a laboratory where sleep and cardiorespiratory variables can be monitored during sleep and waking. The second reason for monitoring is to evaluate an individual infant who is believed to be at increased risk for SIDS. This is usually done in a sleep laboratory connected to a clinical service as part of a diagnostic work-up. The third reason is to detect life-threatening events in an infant at increased risk and involves continuous monitoring at home for periods of weeks or months. Controversy surrounds all of these and especially the last.

Since SIDS is the unexpected death of an infant not perceived to be seriously ill, selection of appropriate infants for monitoring has posed serious problems. Certain epidemiological factors can identify groups of infants at increased risk for SIDS. An infant who has experienced a life-threatening apnea for which no explanation can be found on diagnostic study has been designated a 'near-miss' for SIDS, or an aborted SIDS (Gunteroth, 1977). These infants are at increased risk of subsequently dying of SIDS. The actual risk of subsequent death is not great, varying from 1.4 to 2.5% in large series (Bergman, Beckwith and Ray, 1975; Southall, 1983). Infants who required vigorous positive pressure resuscitation have been reported to be at greatest risk in one series (Kelly, Shannon and O'Connell, 1978), but this has not been the experience of others (Duffty and Bryan, 1982; Hodgman et al., 1982a). The exclusion nature of the diagnosis of unexplained apnea contributes to this being a somewhat heterogeneous group of infants for study.

Infants born to a family with a previous SIDS death are also at increased risk. The rate of SIDS in subsequent siblings has been reported to be 4–5 times that of the general population (Froggatt, Lynas and MacKenzie, 1971; Peterson, Chinn and Fisher, 1980). Here again, although this increase is highly significant statistically, the actual rate of approximately 1% means that the risk for an individual infant is small.

The third identifiable risk group is the premature infant. These infants are also more likely to die of SIDS than are infants born at term and the risk appears to increase with decreasing gestational age (Kulkani *et al.*, 1978; Teberg *et al.*, 1982). There were two deaths from SIDS in 178 infants weighing less than 1500 g at birth discharged from our nursery, for a rate of 1.1%.

Although the risk of SIDS is increased for these three types of infants as a group, the individual infant within the group who will actually die of SIDS cannot be identified ahead of time.

Other statistical determinators have been associated with an increased incidence of SIDS. For example, young multiparous mothers who necessarily have a short intergestational period are significantly more likely to have their second infant die (Bergman *et al.*, 1972; Kraus and Borhani, 1972; Peterson, van Belle and Chinn, 1979). These factors have not been used to define risk groups for study, even though they are consistently reported.

INVESTIGATIONAL LABORATORY MONITORING

Monitoring for SIDS began in the sleep laboratory in the 1970s. Study of sleep was revealing its complexity, and also delineating sleep pathology such as sleep apnea. At the same time serious attention was being focused on the near-miss infant and the idea that SIDS was a consequence of sleep apnea seemed a logical conclusion (Steinschneider, 1972; Guilleminault *et al.*, 1975). A concept of pre-existing autonomic instability predisposing to SIDS began to replace the more traditional belief that these infants were entirely normal before death. Isolated findings in tracings from newborn infants who later died of SIDS were reported as showing abnormal cardiac habituation (Salk, Grellong and Dietrich, 1974), increased respiratory rate (Thoman, Miano and Freese, 1977), and cardiac arrhythmia (Lipsitt, Starner and Oh, 1979). A differentiation was made between predisposing factors which placed an infant at risk and precipitating factors which immediately preceded death. A research strategy was developed where infants at increased risk for SIDS were studied in order to determine abnormalities in cardiorespiratory behaviors that could predispose to death. The early reports were seriously flawed by lack of appropriate control data. Findings in infants with unexplained apnea were reported without realizing that much of the reported behaviors was within normal limits for young infants.

Data on normal infants beyond the neonatal period are in short supply especially during early infancy. Perhaps the most lasting contribution of our own work will be the consistent study of a group of 25 normal term infants from the first week to the sixth month of life. These infants were selected for gestational age, intrauterine growth and socioeconomic class as well as birth weight. Cardiorespiratory and sleep variables were monitored for 12 hours overnight at 1 week and 1, 2, 3, 4 and 6 months. The most important message arising from the study of these infants is the non-monotonic nature of infant development during the first 3 months. Changes do not necessarily proceed in a linear fashion over time as the infant matures. For example, while respiratory rates drop from birth to 6 months, the rate of fall is more rapid during early infancy (Hoppenbrouwers *et al.*, 1978b). Heart rates during this time are following a different pattern, first rising after birth, peaking at 1–2 months, falling rapidly until 3 months and then stabilizing (Harper *et al.*, 1976). The patterns for these and other variables are shown in *Figure 5.1*. Periodic breathing in normal term infants is surprisingly common appearing between 5 and 8% of the time when the infant is in active sleep. Density of periodic breathing

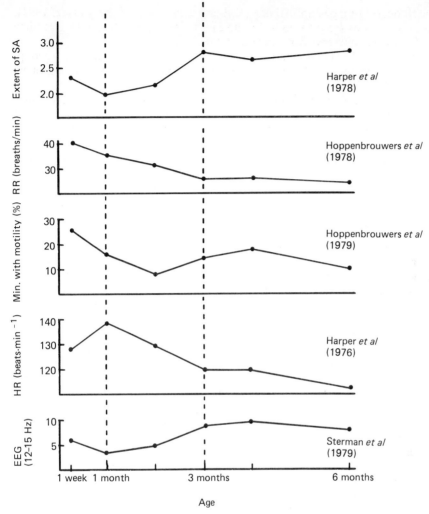

Figure 5.1 Schematic representation of a number of physiological variables during QS. Note the non-monotonic rate and direction of changes. (Reproduced from Hoppenbrouwers and Hodgman, 1982, by courtesy of the Editor and Publishers, *Neuropediatrics*)

follows a non-linear pattern, increasing at 1 and 2 months, at the same time that the density of central apnea longer than 6 s decreases rapidly (*Figure 5.2*). The first 3 months constitute a time of rapid change as contrasted to relative stability thereafter. The first year should be considered as comprising two developmental periods with the first 3 months characterized by rapid and non-monotonic changes in the maturing organism. The importance of accurate age matched controls is obvious, especially in the first 3 months of life. Controls for preterm infants present a particular problem. Although the practice of using post-conceptional rather than postnatal ages for comparisons decreases some of the variance caused by different gestational ages at birth, the preterm infant does not necessarily develop along the

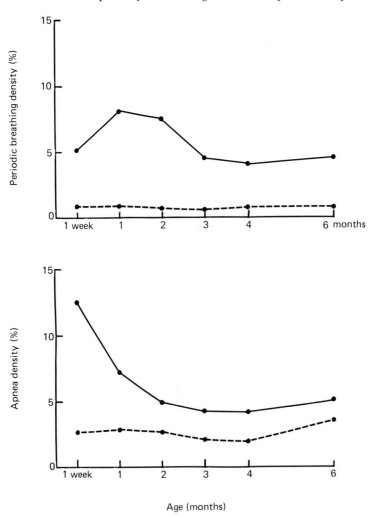

Figure 5.2 Top: periodic breathing density in AS (●——●) and QS (●---●) as a function of age. Note the non-monotonic pattern in AS and the low density in QS. Bottom: approximately 2.5 out of every 100 min in QS contain an apnea, while apnea in AS decreases rapidly from 1 every 8 min at 1 week to 1 every 20 min at 2 months. (Reproduced from Hoppenbrouwers *et al.*, 1977, by courtesy of the Editor and Publishers; copyright of the American Academy of Pediatrics, 1977)

identical path of the full-term infant. This becomes a practical consideration in SIDS research because preterm infants either comprise or are over-represented in two of the groups at increased risk.

   All of the studies of normal infants during early infancy also demonstrate marked individual variation in cardiorespiratory variables (Stein *et al.*, 1979; Flores-Guevara *et al.*, 1982). Standard deviations exceeding the mean in incidence of apnea are not unusual in active sleep (AS), and even in quiet sleep (QS) the s.d. is regularly at least 50% of the mean (Hoppenbrouwers *et al.*, 1977). This variability exemplifies the relative instability characteristic of the normal young infant. Almost all investigators find significant gender differences in the incidence of apnea (Thoman *et al.*, 1978; Hoppenbrouwers *et al.*, 1980b; Steinschneider and Weinstein, 1983). Another factor influencing results is the socioeconomic status of the family. Infants of low income families are known to have both increased morbidity and mortality during infancy and this is manifested by increased numbers of minor abnormalities in cardiorespiratory function (Hoppenbrouwers, Zanini and Hodgman, 1979b). Risk infants are more likely to be from lower socioeconomic class, while control infants are more likely to be from the middle class, yet this factor is frequently not considered in matching risk and control infants.

The near-miss infant

The majority of studies using cardiorespiratory monitoring have been performed in the near-miss infant. The diagnosis in all cases has been based on the history of an apneic event considered life threatening by the caretakers. The majority of these have occurred at home, but some have been observed in the hospital. Additional criteria include the presence of color change, of pallor or cyanosis, neuromuscular change (usually hypotonia but occasionally stiffening), and the need for vigorous resuscitation by the caretakers. Some investigators have required that the infants be asleep at the time of the attack. In all cases, no cause for the apnea was uncovered by clinical study. Reported studies where near-miss infants have been compared with controls are listed chronologically in *Table 5.1*. The most striking finding for the total group is the similarity of near-miss and normal infants. Few significant differences have been found in cardiorespiratory behavior when near-miss infants are compared with appropriate controls.

The next most striking finding is the variation of results among investigators. For example, an increase in periodic breathing was reported by Kelly and Shannon (1979), a decrease in periodic breathing by Navelet, Benoit and Lacombe (1979) and no difference from normals by Guilleminault *et al.* (1979) and Hodgman *et al.* (1982a). A similar lack of consistency exists in the reporting of apnea. In the 2 reports where apnea duration exceeded 6 s, both study groups were selected by the presence of prolonged apnea during sleep in preliminary recordings and compared to infants without recorded sleep apnea (Steinschneider, 1977; Haidmayer *et al.*, 1982). Only Kahn *et al.* (1982a) found prolonged apnea longer than 10 s which was limited to the near-miss infant. Increases in short apnea of 2–5 s were found by some but not all investigators (Monod *et al.*, 1976; Nogues and Sampson-Dollfus, 1979). Guilleminault *et al.* (1979) reported more short obstructive apnea in both normal and risk infants at 6 weeks of age, another example of non-monotonic development. They also reported an increase in short obstructive apnea in the near-miss infants as compared to controls between 3 weeks and 4.5 months during total sleep time, a finding confirmed by Kahn *et al.* (1982), but not by others.

Studies of response to hypercarbic stimuli have also produced conflicting results. A decrease in ventilatory response to CO_2 was reported by Shannon, Kelly and O'Connell (1977), not confirmed by either Brady *et al.* (1978) or Ariagno, Nagel and Guilleminault (1980), while Haddad *et al.* (1981) actually found an increase in CO_2 response in the near-miss infant. Responses to a mild hypoxic challenge have differed from normal in all the near-miss infants studied, but, again, the specific response has varied. Brady *et al.* (1978) found a decrease in respiratory rate and an

Table 5.1 Cardiac and respiratory findings in near miss for SIDS

Author	Year	Study infants	Control infants	Age monitored	Recording methods	RR	Apnea	HR	Other
Monod et al.	1976	6 (term) 5 SIDS (4 preterm)	12 NB (term) 15 infants	NB 3 months	Laboratory nap Sleep state Thoraco-abdominal strain gauge Nasal thermistor		↑ ≥2 s nm and SIDS ↑ ≥5 s nm and SIDS None >10 s Obstructive rare		↑ apnea: male infants in all groups
Steinschneider	1977	28 sleep apnea >20 s (50% LBW)	25 no sleep apnea (32% LBW)	4–223 days m̄ 31 days	Laboratory nap Hyperthermia (90%) Thoracic strain gauge		↑ ≥2 s sleep apnea ↑ ≥5 s sleep apnea		↑ PB: sleep apnea group
Shannon, Kelly and O'Connell	1977	11 (resuscitated × 2) m̄ 14 weeks	12 sex matched m̄ 11.5 weeks	Up to 37 weeks	Laboratory – short observations QS only CO_2 response	No diff.			↑ end-tidal CO_2: nm ↓ CO_2 response: nm
Brady et al.	1978	5 (1 preterm) 3 preterm apnea	8 preterm	2 weeks 6 months	Laboratory – 20 min observations QS only Hypoxic challenge (17% O_2)	No diff. with hypoxic challenge ↓	No diff. ↑ ≥6 s none >12 s	No diff. No change	No diff: PB or end-tidal CO_2 ↑ PB No change: end-tidal CO_2
Hoppenbrouwers et al.	1978a	7	9 age matched	3 months	Laboratory – 12 h overnight Sleep state Thoraco-abdominal strain gauge Nasal thermistor	RR, HR, and motility with each apnea ≥6 s			↑ motility preceding apnea ↓ RR following apnea ↓ drop in HR following apnea

Authors	Year	n (study)	n (control)	Age	Conditions				
Nogues and Sampson-Dollfus	1979	10	27	2–12 months	Laboratory nap or early night Sleep state	↑	↑ 2–5 s		
Kelly and Shannon	1979	32 (term)	32 age and sex matched	2–45 weeks	Home 8 h overnight impedance		No diff. >10 s ↓ $\bar{m}$ duration	↑ PB (total time, av. and longest duration)	No diff.: PB
Guilleminault et al.	1979	29 (term)	30 age matched	3 weeks–6 months	Laboratory – 24 h Sleep state Thoraco-abdominal strain gauge Nasal and oral thermistors		No diff.: central No diff. >10 s ↑ mixed and obstructive at 3 and 4.5 months		
Ariagno, Nagel and Guilleminault	1980	9	5 term	1–4 months	Laboratory sleep state CO_2 and hypoxic response	No diff.		No diff.	No diff.: CO_2 response ↑ PB both groups with hypoxia: ? less in nm ↓ arousal with hypoxia
Leistner et al.	1980	12 (1 preterm) 2 weeks–4 months	18 term	1, 2, 3, 4 months	Laboratory Nap Sleep state			↑ AS ↑ QS	↓ short and overall R–R variability
Haddad et al.	1981	12 (same as above)	19 (2–37 weeks GA)	1, 2, 3, 4 months	Laboratory Nap Sleep state Barometric CO_2 response	↑			No diff.: V_O ↓ V_T ↑ CO_2 response
Hodgman et al.	1982	17 (3 preterm)	17 age and sex matched	3–28 weeks	Laboratory 12 h – overnight Sleep state Thoracic and abdominal strain gauge Nasal thermistor	↑ trend	↓ trend: 2–5 s No diff.: obstructive Long central rare Obstructive rare	↑ trend	No diff.: PB

Table 5.1 continued over

Table 5.1 (continued)

Author	Year	Study infants	Control infants	Age monitored	Recording methods	RR	Apnea	HR	Other
Haidmayer et al.	1982	6 / 48 sleep apnea or anesthesia related	233 pediatric surgery admissions	4–197 days	Laboratory – 1 h / Impedance		↑ ≥6 s sleep apnea		No diff.: Q–T_c
McCulloch et al.	1982	11 mean = 7.3 weeks	22 term mean = 29.3 weeks	1–3 months	Laboratory / Nap / Sleep state / Thoraco-abdominal strain gauge / Nasal thermistor / CO_2 response / Hypoxic response	No diff.: baseline in QS	No diff.: ≥3 s response to hypoxia in QS		No diff.: PB response to hypoxia in QS / ↓ hypoxic and hypercarbic arousal
Kahn et al. / Kahn et al.	1982a / 1982b	25	25 age matched	4–28 weeks	Laboratory – 12 h overnight / Sleep state / Thoracoabdominal strain gauge / Nasal and oral thermistors / $P_{TC}O_2$		>10 s nm only / No diff. <10 s / Short obstructive apnea uncommon but more common in nm		No diff.: $P_{TC}O_2$ / Drop in O_2 related to apnea duration / ↑ O_2 drop: obstructive apnea
Scott et al.	1982	10	10 age matched	2–8 months	Esophageal and gastric catheters				Normal to ↑ Transdiaphragm pressure

nm = near miss; NB = newborn; SIDS = sudden infant death syndrome; RR = respiratory rate; HR = heart rate; Diff. = difference; PB = periodic breathing; QS = quiet sleep; AS = active sleep; GA = gestational age; Q–T_c = corrected Q–T interval; $\overline{m}$ = mean; $\dot{V}_O$ = minute ventilation; V_T = tidal volume.

increase in periodic breathing and longer apnea, while Ariagno, Nagel and Guilleminault (1980) and McCulloch *et al.* (1982) did not confirm these findings but reported a decreased arousal in response to hypoxia.

In spite of this variation in reported findings, some consistency has emerged. One of the most consistent findings has been an increase in respiratory rates in the risk infants. Either a significant change or a trend towards more rapid rates has been found by all investigators reporting the results of daytime or overnight sleep recordings (Nogues and Samson-Dollfus, 1979; Haddad *et al.*, 1981; Hodgman *et al.*, 1982a). Heart rates have been increased in those few sleep studies where they have been reported (Leistner *et al.*, 1980; Hodgman and Hoppenbrouwers, 1984). The results from our study of near-miss infants are presented in *Figure 5.3*. These findings are particularly interesting because similar findings have been reported for subsequent siblings and for infants who subsequently died of SIDS (*see below* and Thoman, Miano and Freese, 1977).

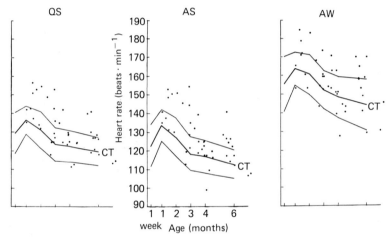

Figure 5.3 Median heart rate for each near-miss infant at each age is plotted against the median and one standard deviation for the control (CT) infants. Heart rates for near-miss infants were within the expected normal range but with a tendency to be above the normal median. QS = quiet sleep; AS = active sleep; AW = awake

One-fifth of our near-miss infants had some peculiarity in cardiorespiratory behavior such as excessive apnea, or fixed or abnormally variable heart rate, but no two infants showed the same findings (Hodgman *et al.*, 1984). The significance of these findings is unknown and care should be exercised in attributing clinical importance to them as the same findings occur in normal infants.

Sources of the variation among investigators include differences in monitoring technique. Length of the monitoring sessions will influence the results, with long sessions accentuating numbers of apnea (Hoppenbrouwers *et al.*, 1980c). Time of night will make a difference, particularly as the infant develops diurnal rhythms in cardiorespiratory behavior (Hoppenbrouwers *et al.*, 1979a). While not consistently studied, there is a strong suggestion that results of monitoring in the home will differ considerably from that carried out in a laboratory. All of these factors added to the uncertain nature of an exclusion diagnosis, the inherent variability of the

Table 5.2 Cardiac and respiratory findings in subsequent siblings of SIDS

Author	Year	Study infants	Control infants	Age	Monitor procedures	RR	Apnea	HR	Other
Nogues and Sampson-Dollfus	1979	10	27	2–12 months	Laboratory nap Sleep state	↑	↑ 2–5 s SSS		
Hoppenbrouwers et al.	1978a	9	9 age matched	3 months	Laboratory – 12 h overnight Sleep state Thoraco-abdominal strain gauges Nasal thermistor				No diff.: motility preceding apnea, cardiac deceleration or respiratory rate following apnea
Harper et al.	1978b	10	10 age matched	1 week and 1,2,3,4,6 months	Laboratory – 12 h overnight Sleep state Thoraco-abdominal strain gauges Nasal thermistor			↑ at 3 months	↓ HR variability
Hoppenbrouwers et al.	1980b	26	25 age matched	1 week and 1,2,3,4,6 months	Laboratory – 12 h overnight Sleep state Thoraco-abdominal strain gauges Nasal thermistor	↑ SSS	↓ 2–5 s / No diff. ≥6 s / Obstructive rare but ↓ SSS		↑ respiratory variability

Author	Year	N	Controls	Age	Recording	Apnea	Findings
Kelly et al.	1980	48	48 age and sex matched	2 days–25 weeks	Home pneumogram		↑ PB
Hoppenbrouwers et al.	1981	15 (term)	16 age matched	32–33 weeks GA 35–37 weeks GA	Laboratory – 12 h overnight Maternal sleep state Fetal heart rate		↓ mat. stage IV sleep No diff.: FHR ↑ FHR variability ↑ bradycardia
Kahn et al.	1982a	25	25 age matched	5–18 weeks	Laboratory – 12 h overnight Sleep state Thoraco-abdominal strain gauge Nasal and oral thermistors $P_{TC}O_2$	No diff.: central none ≥10 s	No diff.: $P_{TC}O_2$ in O_2 ↓ in O_2 related to apnea duration
Kahn et al.	1982b					No diff.: obstructive (rare)	

SSS = subsequent siblings of SIDS; GA = gestational age; diff. = difference; HR = heart rate; RR = respiratory rate; FHR = fetal heart rate.

young infant and the need for careful age and sex matching of controls probably explains the heterogeneity of the findings in the near-miss infant.

Subsequent siblings of SIDS

Although fewer studies have been reported involving the subsequent siblings of infants who have died of SIDS, these infants have the advantages as a study group that they can be identified ahead of time, studied on a prearranged and consistent schedule, and matched concurrently with normal infants. The information available is presented in *Table 5.2*. Again, the most striking finding in the risk infants is their close similarity to normal controls. However, subtle changes between these infants and normals have been found in most of the studied parameters. Respiratory rates have been consistently higher, short apnea fewer, and heart rates faster (*Figures 5.4–5.6*). It is of particular interest that these same findings have been reported in the near-miss infant.

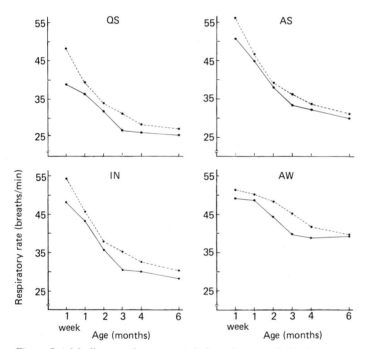

Figure 5.4 Median respiratory rate in breaths per min for 25 subsequent siblings (- - - -) and 25 control (—) infants. Subsequent siblings breathed significantly faster than controls in all states at 3 months. QS = quite sleep; AS = active sleep; IN = indeterminate sleep; AW = awake. (Reproduced from Hoppenbrouwers *et al.*, 1980b, by courtesy of the Editor and Publishers; copyright of the American Academy of Pediatrics, 1980)

The ability to identify the subsequent sibling during gestation has made it possible to study this group as fetuses. Increased variability and an increase in bradycardia was found in the fetal heart rate at 32 and 36 weeks gestation (Hoppenbrouwers *et al.*, 1981). This is of particular interest in light of the increasing data suggesting that SIDS infants are abnormal from before birth

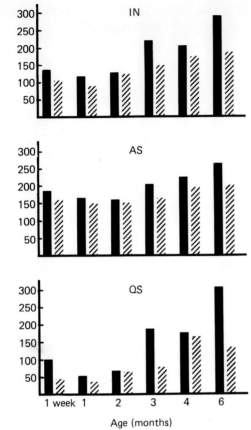

Figure 5.5 Sleep state related density of breathing pauses between 2 to 5 s. Note the reduced incidence in subsequent siblings particularly at 3 and 6 months in QS. ■ Controls; ☒ siblings. (Reproduced from Hoppenbrouwers *et al.*, 1980b, by courtesy of the Editor and Publishers, copyright of the American Academy of Pediatrics, 1980)

(Naeye, Ladis and Drage, 1976; Naeye, 1977; Hoppenbrouwers and Hodgman, 1982).

Maternal anxiety during pregnancy and early infancy is understandably increased with subsequent siblings. One of the manifestations of this anxiety is reflected in earlier feeding of solids to the subsequent sibling, resulting in more rapid early weight gain when compared to control infants (Hodgman and Hoppenbrouwers, 1984). Increased heart rates have been associated with caloric intake in the young infant (Chessex *et al.*, 1981). How much of the differences in cardiorespiratory behavior observed in the subsequent siblings can be attributed to differences in caretaking cannot be answered at the present time.

Premature infants

Rather surprisingly, similar data from laboratory recordings of premature infants are not available. Considerable information is available for the neonatal period, but almost none concerning the cardiorespiratory behavior of the preterm infant

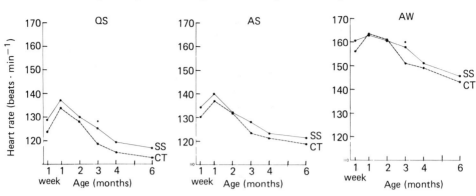

Figure 5.6 Heart rates of subsequent siblings (SS) and control (CT) infants. Note the delayed decrease in heart rate between 2 and 3 months for the subsequent siblings. $P<0.06$. Reproduced from Harper *et al.*, 1982, by courtesy of the Editor and Publishers, *Sleep*)

during infancy beyond the neonatal period. Apnea of prematurity occurring after the first week is relatively uncommon. In our large center with over 1000 term infants delivered monthly, we find approximately one case of unexplained apnea a month persisting beyond the first week (Hodgman *et al.*, 1982b). Although relationship, if any, between apnea in the nursery and SIDS following discharge has not been consistently explored, the available evidence suggests that the infant with apnea in the nursery is not at increased risk (Southall *et al.*, 1982).

DIAGNOSTIC MONITORING

A work-up for a near-miss infant should include cardiorespiratory monitoring. Ideally, the monitoring session should be carried out overnight as abnormalities are more likely to occur during the early morning hours. Excessive central apnea and cardiac abnormalities can be readily detected on standard impedance and ECG monitors. Detection of obstructive apnea is more difficult, requiring at least a nasal thermistor preferably associated with an esophageal catheter. Even with these precautions, it is difficult to clearly differentiate obstructive apnea from normal behavior. For example, when the glottis is closed, movements which are normal and perhaps advantageous for the preterm infant cannot be separated from obstructive apnea with chest motion but no airflow (Van Someren and Stothers, 1983). Although sleep state has not been reported as grossly abnormal in risk infants, proper interpretation of cardiorespiratory variables requires that sleep state be known (Gould *et al.*, 1977). Since the majority of infants will have normal findings, this overnight recording will be disappointing most of the time except in a negative sense. Detailed study of responses to inhaled gases and other more complex techniques do not seem indicated in the usual clinical setting. These are still investigational in nature and should be employed only if some special indication exists.

Appropriate management when cardiorespiratory changes are found raises other questions. Whether treatment is indicated for the occasional infant with apnea beyond the norm is unknown. Even less information is available concerning the proper care for infants with cardiac findings of too little or too much variability in heart rate. Much is made of the association of 'bradycardia' with apnea as a risk factor; however, the phenomenon referred to is really cardiac deceleration rather than a persistent slowing of the heart rate. These drops in heart rate are a normal response to many exogenous and endogenous stimuli. In our studies of normal infants, we have recorded as many as 741 cardiac decelerations to below 100 beats · min^{-1} in a 12-h recording (Hodgman *et al.,* 1984). These decelerations are frequently, but not exclusively, associated with apnea. Onset of the deceleration occurs shortly after the onset of apnea and before any significant decrease has occurred in O_2 levels; consequently, hypoxia is not the cause of the drop in heart rate (Kahn *et al.,* 1982a). Consistent damping of this normal response is seen in seriously ill infants, but whether transient loss of variability carries any risk is unknown. Whether excess reactivity poses any disadvantage to an infant is also unknown at the present time. I believe the finding of brief drops in heart rate should be equated with the V-shaped dips seen in the fetal heart tracings which are known to be benign (Hon, 1968). The limits of normality need to be defined in this area of cardiac behavior in the same way that normal and abnormal respiratory pauses are being defined.

Cardiorespiratory monitoring of the asymptomatic subsequent sibling for clinical diagnosis is not warranted. It is not helpful to monitor these infants in the nursery in an effort to identify those few who will have future difficulty because early findings have not predicted later behavior in risk infants (Gould *et al.,* 1977; Hoppenbrouwers *et al.,* 1980c).

HOME MONITORING

Long-term monitoring at home has been recommended for infants perceived to be at risk for SIDS in an effort to interrupt life-threatening events. The popularity of the treatment is presumably based on the seriousness of the condition for which it is recommended in spite of the fact that no studies have been performed to demonstrate its effectiveness. Although the risk even in identifiable risk groups is small, it is risk of death and is frightening to parents and physicians.

The selection of infants for home monitoring has been based primarily on the epidemiology of SIDS. The infants for whom monitoring at home is recommended are most frequently those in the risk groups described above. Further refinements based on the infant's performance during cardiorespiratory monitoring such as prolonged sleep apnea, increased incidence of periodic breathing, and cardiac decelerations or other abnormalities may be added to the indications. This approach is not very logical, as all investigators agree that the infant at risk of dying cannot be differentiated from the remaining group by cardiorespiratory parameters. The use of pneumogram criteria developed on term infants in order to identify which premature infant to monitor seems particularly ill advised. In studies of healthy preterm infants we have found apnea from 20 to 30 s duration in 4.5% of the 66 infants studied (Hodgman *et al.,* 1982b). Periodic breathing that has been used to justify monitoring occurred in 85% of these healthy infants and was present during at least 20% of an 8-h overnight recording in 14% of the group. Cardiac decelerations were also common, being recorded in 68% of the infants. A recent report by Southall *et al.* (1982) throws further doubt on the wisdom of using findings such as these to identify risk as they find no correlation with apnea or cardiac irregularity in the neonatal period and subsequent death from SIDS.

Which monitor to use has been the subject of some controversy as well. Impedance monitors which are most available for home use have significant disadvantages. The most serious of these is the inability to differentiate chest movement without airflow (Warburton, Stark and Taeusch, 1977). Cardiac pulsations may also be picked up by the monitor and interpreted as breathing movements. For these reasons, adding a cardiac monitor to the impedance monitor has been recommended. Obstructive apnea is regularly associated with cardiac deceleration which begins early in the episode before significant hypoxia has appeared (Kahn *et al.*, 1982b). Consequently, a cardiac monitor should protect against missing a significant obstructive apnea. Frequent false alarms are also a problem with the available cardiac monitors which alarm when the heart rate drops below the set rate for a few seconds during a normal cardiac deceleration. Monitors should be modified to alarm only after the heart rate drop has persisted for a significant period or, in other words, when true bradycardia is present. Our data derived from healthy preterm infants would suggest an interval of no less than 30 s (Hodgman *et al.*, 1982b). A new monitor based on the acoustic detection of airflow has recently been developed (Werthammer *et al.*, 1983). Although it has not as yet had extensive clinical trials, it bears promise of avoiding several of the objections to impedance monitoring.

Monitoring has been justified on the basis of the number of alarms recorded and resuscitation given by parents to their infants on the assumption that such efforts represent life-saving interventions in spite of the problems with false alarms. Recurrence rates for the near-miss infant have varied between 43 and 67% (Ariagno *et al.*, 1983; Duffty and Bryan, 1982; Hodgman *et al.*, 1982a; Rosen, Frost and Harrison, 1983). Interestingly, the rates are not different between series where home monitoring was regularly employed and those where it was not. Which infant will experience a recurrence cannot be accurately predicted. Multiple episodes of recurrent apnea have been associated with a significant increase in need for resuscitation (Kelly, Shannon and O'Connell, 1978). Deaths have occurred on the monitors apparently due to respiratory obstruction or cardiac arrhythmia (Lewak, 1975; Kelly, Shannon and O'Connell, 1978; Duffty and Bryan, 1982; Rosen, Frost and Harrison, 1983). Whether the incidence is less than would occur under natural circumstances is impossible to evaluate properly without controlled studies. Experience with home monitors has been reported by a number of investigators (Kelly, Shannon and O'Connell, 1978; Duffty and Bryan, 1982; Kahn and Blum, 1982; Ariagno *et al.*, 1983) and summarized by Southall (1983) in a recent publication. The available data does not suggest a marked effect from monitoring. The mortality rate of 3.98% for monitored infants, is not different from the 2.5% reported for mortality before monitoring was in use (Bergman, Beckwith and Ray, 1975).

Evaluation of the effect of prolonged monitoring on the family has been reported by two groups both of whom enthusiastically espouse home monitoring (Black, Hersher and Steinschneider, 1978; Cain, Kelly and Shannon, 1980). The reports document responses varying from relief of anxiety to severe stress on the family constellation. Both groups emphasize the need for a knowledgable and readily available support system. A report detailing the normal development up to 9 months of the involved infants was reassuring (Black, Steinschneider and Sheehe, 1979), but long-term results are not as yet available.

SUMMARY

Home monitoring has not made much difference in the mortality from SIDS. This would be expected since most infants cannot be identified by epidemiological risk. Pre-existing apnea is not a common finding in infants who have died (Froggatt, Lynas and MacKenzie, 1971; Southall *et al.*, 1982). Home monitoring is accepted in spite of the lack of confirming studies because the condition is so frightening and there is no better alternative at the present time. Whoever recommends or employs this type of management must not lose sight of the fact that it is fraught with problems and the efficacy is questionable.

There are no reliable cardiorespiratory findings on which to base recommendations for home monitoring. Interestingly, one of the more consistent findings in studies of risk groups, namely increased respiratory rate, has not been used in this regard. Perceived risk based on history of the infant and epidemiology of SIDS remains the major criterion. In any clinical situation, level of parental anxiety must be given strong consideration.

Investigative monitoring has added greatly to our understanding of the development of cardiorespiratory behaviors in the young infant. Study of groups of infants known to be at increased risk for SIDS has demonstrated minor differences between these infants and controls. Increases in respiratory rate and heart rate, and decreases in the incidence of short apnea have been consistent findings in both near-miss infants and subsequent siblings. These studies have not uncovered the etiology of SIDS. Sleep monitoring in spite of its early promise has been disappointing in this regard. New directions are required at this point. Further investigation into arousal mechanisms which have been shown to be deranged in the near-miss infant seems one particularly appealing approach.

Acknowledgements

The studies referred to in this chapter were carried out with funds from NIHCHD Contracts number NO1-HD-2-2777 and HD4-2810 and Grant number HD 13689-03; the National Foundation for SIDS (Los Angeles Chapter); the Guild for Infant Survival (San Gabriel Valley Chapter and Orange County Chapter); Arthur B. Zimtbaum Foundation of New York. We express our deep appreciation for this support.

References

ARIAGNO, R. L., GUILLEMINAULT, C., KOROBKIN, R., BOEDDIKER, M. and BALDWIN, R. (1983) 'Near-miss' for sudden infant death syndrome infants: a clinical problem. *Pediatrics,* **71,** 726–730

ARIAGNO, R., NAGEL, L. and GUILLEMINAULT, C. (1980) Waking and ventilatory responses during sleep in infants near-miss for sudden infant death syndrome. *Sleep,* **3,** 351–359

BERGMAN, A. B., BECKWITH, J. B. and RAY, C. G. (1975) The apnea monitor business. *Pediatrics,* **56,** 1–3

BERGMAN, A. B., RAY, C. G., POMEROY, M. A., WAHL, P. W. and BECKWITH, J. B. (1972) Studies of the sudden death syndrome in King County, Washington, III. Epidemiology. *Pediatrics,* **49,** 860–870

BLACK, L., HERSHER, L. and STEINSCHNEIDER, A. (1978) Impact of the apnea monitor on family life. *Pediatrics,* **62,** 681–685

BLACK, L., STEINSCHNEIDER, A. and SHEEHE, P. R. (1979) Neonatal respiratory instability and infant development. *Child Development,* **50,** 561–564

BRADY, J. P., ARIAGNO, R. L., WATTS, J. L., GOLDMAN, S. L. and DUMPIT, F. M. (1978) Apnea, hypoxemia, and aborted sudden infant death syndrome. *Pediatrics,* **62,** 686–691

CAIN, L. P., KELLY, D. H. and SHANNON, D. C. (1980) Parents' perceptions of the psychological and social impact of home monitoring. *Pediatrics,* **66,** 37–41

CHESSEX, P., REICHMAN, B. L., VERELLEN, G. J. E. *et al.* (1981) Relation between heart rate and energy expenditure in the newborn. *Pediatric Research,,* **15,** 1077–1082

DUFFTY, P. and BRYAN, M. H. (1982) Home apnea monitoring in 'near-miss' sudden infant death syndrome (SIDS) and in siblings of SIDS victims. *Pediatrics,* **70,** 69–74

FLORES-GUEVARA, R., PLOUIN, P., CURZI-DASCALOVA, L. *et al.* (1982) Sleep apneas in normal neonates and infants during the first 3 months of life. *Neuropediatrics,* **13,** 21–28

FROGGATT, P., LYNAS, M. A. and MACKENZIE, G. (1971) Epidemiology of sudden unexpected death in infants ('cot death') in Northern Ireland. *British Journal of Preventive and Social Medicine,* **25,** 119–134

GOULD, J. B., LEE, A. F. S., JAMES, O., SANDER, L., TEAGER, H. and FINEBERG, N. (1977) The sleep state characteristics of apnea during infancy. *Pediatrics,* **59,** 182–194

GUILLEMINAULT, C., ARIAGNO, R., KOROBKIN, R. *et al.* (1979) Mixed and obstructive sleep apnea and near miss for sudden infant death syndrome. 2. Comparison of near miss and normal control infants by age. *Pediatrics,* **64,** 882–891

GUILLEMINAULT, C., PERAITA, R., SOUQUET, M. and DEMENT, W. C. (1975) Apneas during sleep in infants: possible relationship with sudden infant death syndrome. *Science,* **190,** 677–679

GUNTEROTH, W. G. (1977) Sudden infant death syndrome (crib death). *American Heart Journal,* **93,** 784–787

HADDAD, G. G., LEISTNER, H. L., LAI, T. L. and MELLINS, R. B. (1981) Ventilation and ventilatory pattern during sleep in aborted sudden infant death. *Pediatric Research,* **15,** 879–833

HAIDMAYER, R., PFEIFFER, K. P., KENNER, T. and KURZ, R. (1982) Statistical evaluation of respiratory control in infants to assess possible risk for the sudden infant death syndrome (SIDS). *European Journal of Pediatrics,* **138,** 145–150

HARPER, R. M., HOPPENBROUWERS, T., STERMAN, M. B., MCGINTY, D. J. and HODGMAN, J. E. (1976) Polygraphic studies of normal infants during the first months of life: I. Heart rate and variability as a function of state. *Pediatric Research,* **10,** 945–951

HARPER, R. M., LEAKE, B., HODGMAN, J. G. and HOPPENBROUWERS, T. (1982) Developmental patterns heart rate and heart rate variability during sleep and waking in normal infants and infants at risk for SIDS. *Sleep,* **5,** 28–38

HARPER, R. M., LEAKE, B., HOPPENBROUWERS, T., STERMAN, M. B., MCGINTY, D. J. and HODGMAN, J. (1978b) Polygraphic studies of normal infants and infants at risk for the sudden infant death syndrome: Heart rate and variability as a function of state. *Pediatric Research,* **12,** 778–785

HARPER, R. M., WALTER, D. O., LEAKE, B. *et al.* (1978a) Development of sinus arrhythmia during sleeping and waking states in normal infants. *Sleep,* **1,** 33–48

HODGMAN, J. E. and HOPPENBROUWERS, T. (1984) Clinical characteristics of subsequent siblings of SIDS. In *Ontogeny of Sleep and Cardiopulmonary Regulation: Factors Related to Risk for the Sudden Infant Death Syndrome.* Eds M. B. Sterman, J. E. Hodgman, C. R. Stark and H. J. Hoffman. Section III. Part A. Washington, DC: National Institute for Child Health and Development

HODGMAN, J. E., HOPPENBROUWERS, T., CABAL, L., RUIZ, M. E. and CHAVEZ, A. (1982b) Respiratory and cardiac patterns in healthy premature infants after the first week. *Clinical Research* (Abstract), **30,** 143A

HODGMAN, J. E., HOPPENBROUWERS, T., GEIDEL, S. *et al.* (1982a) Respiratory behavior in near-miss sudden infant death syndrome. *Pediatrics,* **69,** 785–792

HODGMAN, J. E., HOPPENBROUWERS, T., HARPER, R. M. and STERMAN, M. B. (1984) The infant with unexplained apnea; near miss for SIDS. In *Ontogeny of Sleep and Cardiopulmonary Regulation: Factors Related to Risk for the Sudden Infant Death Syndrome.* Eds M. B. Sterman, J. E. Hodgman, C. R. Stark and H. J. Hoffman. Section III. Part B. Washington, DC: NICHD

HON, E. H. (1968) *An Atlas of Fetal Heart Rate Patterns.* New Haven, Connecticutt: Harty Press, Inc.

HOPPENBROUWERS, T., HARPER, R. M., HODGMAN, J. E., STERMAN, M. B. and MCGINTY, D. J. (1978b) Polygraphic studies of normal infants during the first six months of life: II. Respiratory rate and variability as a function of state. *Pediatric Research,* **12,** 120–125

HOPPENBROUWERS, T. and HODGMAN, J. E. (1982) Sudden infant death syndrome (SIDS): an integration of ontogenetic pathologic, physiologic and epidemiologic factors. *Neuropediatrics,* **13,** 36–51

HOPPENBROUWERS, T., HODGMAN, J. E., ARAKAWA, K., HARPER, R. and STERMAN, M. B. (1980c) Respiration during the first six months of life in normal infants: III. Computer identification of breathing pauses. *Pediatric Research,* **14,** 1230

HOPPENBROUWERS, T., HODGMAN, J. E., ARAKAWA, K. *et al.* (1978a) Sleep apnea as part of a sequence of events: a comparison of three months old infants at low and increased risk for sudden infant death syndrome (SIDS). *Neuropadiatrie*, **9**, 320–337

HOPPENBROUWERS, T., HODGMAN, J. E., HARPER, R. M., HOFFMAN, E., STERMAN, M. B. and MCGINTY, D. J. (1977) Polygraphic studies of normal infants during the first six months of life: III. Incidence of apnea and periodic breathing. *Pediatrics*, **60**, 418–425

HOPPENBROUWERS, T., HODGMAN, J. E., HARPER, R. M. and STERMAN, M. B. (1979b) Motility patterns as a function of state and time of night. *Sleep Research*, **8**, 124

HOPPENBROUWERS, T., HODGMAN, J. E., HARPER, R. M. and STERMAN, M. B. (1980a) Respiration during the first six months of life in normal infants: IV. Gender differences. *Early Human Development*, **4**, 167–177

HOPPENBROUWERS, T., HODGMAN, J. E., HARPER, R. M. and STERMAN, M. B. (1981) Fetal heart rates in siblings of infants with sudden infant death syndrome. *Obstetrics and Gynecology*, **58**, 319–326

HOPPENBROUWERS, T., JENSEN, D., HODGMAN, J., HARPER, R. and STERMAN, M. (1979a) Respiration during the first six months of life in normal infants: II. The emergence of a circadian pattern. *Neuropadiatrie*, **10**, 264–280

HOPPENBROUWERS, T., HODGMAN, J. E., McGINTY, D., HARPER, R. M. and STERMAN, M. B. (1980b) Sudden infant death syndrome: sleep apnea and respiration in subsequent siblings. *Pediatrics*, **66**, 205–214

HOPPENBROUWERS, T., ZANINI, B. and HODGMAN, J. E. (1979) Intrapartum fetal heart rate and sudden infant death syndrome. *American Journal of Obstetrics and Gynecology*, **133**, 217–220

KAHN, A. and BLUM, D. (1982) Home monitoring of infants considered at risk for the sudden infant death syndrome. Four year's experience (1977–1981). *European Journal of Pediatrics*, **139**, 94–100

KAHN, A., BLUM, D., ENGELMAN, E. and WATERSCHOOT, P. (1982a) Effects of central apneas on transcutaneous PO_2 in control subjects, siblings of victims of sudden infant death syndrome, and near miss infants. *Pediatrics*, **69**, 413–418

KAHN, A., BLUM, D., WATERSCHOOT, P., ENGELMAN, E. and SMETS, P. (1982b) Effects of obstructive sleep apneas on transcutaneous oxygen pressure in control infants, siblings of suddent infant death syndrome victims, and near miss infants: comparison with the effects of central sleep apneas. *Pediatrics*, **70**, 852–857

KELLY, D. H. and SHANNON, D. C. (1979) Periodic breathing in infants with near-miss sudden infant death syndrome. *Pediatrics*, **63**, 355–359

KELLY, D. H., SHANNON, D. C. and O'CONNELL, K. (1978) Care of infants with near-miss sudden infant death syndrome. *Pediatrics*, **61**, 511–513

KELLY, D. H., WALKER, A. M., CAHEN, L. and SHANNON, D. C. (1980) Periodic breathing in siblings of sudden infant death syndrome victims. *Pediatrics*, **66**, 515–520

KRAUS, J. F. and BORHANI, N. O. (1972) Postneonatal sudden unexpected death in California; a cohort study. *American Journal of Epidemiology*, **95**, 497–510

KULKARNI, P., HALL, R. T., RHODES, P. G. and SHEEHAN, M. B. (1978) Postneonatal infant mortality in infants admitted to a neonatal intensive care unit. *Pediatrics*, **61**, 178–183

LEISTNER, H. L., HADDAD, G. G., EPSTEIN, R. A., LAI, T. L., EPSTEIN, M. A. F. and MELLINS, R. B. (1980) Heart rate and heart rate variability during sleep in aborted sudden infant death syndrome. *Journal of Pediatrics*, **97**, 51–55

LEWAK, N. (1975) Sudden infant death syndrome in a hospitalized infant on an apnea monitor. *Pediatrics*, **56**, 296–298

LIPSITT, L. P., STARNER, W. Q. and OH, W. (1979) Wolff–Parkinson–White and sudden infant death syndromes, letter. *New England Journal of Medicine*, **300**, 1111

McCULLOCH, K., BROUILLETTE, R. T., GUZZETTA, A. J. and HUNT, C. E. (1982) Arousal responses in near-miss sudden infant death syndrome and in normal infants. *Journal of Pediatrics*, **101**, 911–917

MONOD, N., CURZI-DASCALOVA, L., GUIDASCI, S. and VALENZUELA, S. (1976) Pauses respiratoires et sommeil chez le nouveau-né et le nourrisson. *Revue d'Electroencephalographie et de Neurophysiologie Clinique*, **6**, 105–110

NAEYE, R. L. (1977) Placental abnormalities in victims of the sudden infant death syndrome. *Biology of the Neonate*, **32**, 189–193

NAEYE, R. L., LADIS, B. and BRAGE, J. S. (1976) Sudden infant death syndrome. A prospective study. *American Journal of Diseases of Children*, **130**, 1207–1211

NAVELET, Y., BENOIT, O. and LACOMBE, J. (1979) Respiration et sommeil due nourrison. *Revue d'Electroencephalographie et de Neurophysiologie Clinique*, **9**, 258–265

NOGUES, B. and SAMSON-DOLLFUS, D. (1979) Etude comparative de la respiration pendant le sommeil chez des bébés temoins et des bébés a risque de mort subite (Enfants de 2 mois a 1 an). *Waking Sleeping*, **3**, 263–268

PETERSON, D. R., CHINN, N. M. and FISHER, L. D. (1980) The sudden infant death syndrome: repetitions in families. *Journal of Pediatrics,* **97,** 265–267

PETERSON, D. R., VAN BELLE, G. and CHINN, N. M. (1979) Epidemiological comparisons of the sudden infant death syndrome with other major components of infant mortality. *American Journal of Epidemiology,* **110,** 699–707

ROSEN, C. L., FROST, J. D. and HARRISON, G. M. (1983) Infant apnea: Polygraphic and follow-up monitoring. *Pediatrics,* **71,** 731–736

SALK, L., GRELLONG, B. A. and DIETRICH, J. (1974) Sudden infant death. Normal cardiac habituation and poor autonomic control. *New England Journal of Medicine,* **291,** 219–222

SCOTT, C. B., NICKERSON, B. G., SARGENT, C. W., DENNIES, P. C., PLATZKER, A. C. G. and KEENS, T. G. (1982) Diaphragm strength in near-miss sudden infant death syndrome. *Pediatrics,* **69,** 782–784

SHANNON, D. C., KELLY, D. H. and O'CONNELL, K. (1977) Abnormal regulation of ventilation in infants at risk for sudden-infant death syndrome. *New England Journal of Medicine,* **297,** 747–750

SOUTHALL, D. P. (1983) Home monitoring and its role in the sudden infant death syndrome. *Pediatrics,* **72,** 133–138

SOUTHALL, D. P., RICHARDS, J. M., RHODEN, K. J. *et al.* (1982) Prolonged apnea and cardiac arrhythmias in infants discharged from neonatal intensive care units: Failure to predict an increased risk for sudden infant death syndrome. *Pediatrics,* **70,** 844–851

STEIN, I. M., WHITE, A., KENNEDY, J. L., MERISALO, R. L., CHERNOFF, H. and GOULD, J. B. (1979) Apnea recordings of healthy infants at 40, 44, and 52 weeks postconception. *Pediatrics,* **63,** 724–730

STEINSCHNEIDER, A. (1972) Prolonged apnea and the sudden infant death syndrome: Clinical and laboratory observations. *Pediatrics,* **50,** 646–653

STEINSCHNEIDER, A. (1977) Prolonged sleep apnea and respiratory instability: A discriminative study. *Pediatrics,* **59,** 962–970

STEINSCHNEIDER, A. and WEINSTEIN, S. (1983) Sleep respiratory instability in term neonates under hyperthermic conditions: Age, sex, type of feeding, and rapid eye movements. *Pediatric Research,* **17,** 35–41

TEBERG, A. J., WU, P. Y. K., HODGMAN, J. E. *et al.* (1982) Infants with birth weight under 1500 g: physical, neurological, and developmental outcome. *Critical Care Medicine,* **10,** 10–14

THOMAN, E. B., FREESE, M. P., BECKER, P. T., ACEBO, C., MORIN, V. N. and TYNAN, W. D. (1978) Sex differences in the ontogeny of sleep apnea during the first year of life. *Physiology and Behavior,* **20,** 699–707

THOMAN, E. B., MIANO, V. N. and FREESE, M. P. (1977) The role of respiratory instability in the sudden infant death syndrome. *Developmental Medicine and Child Neurology,* **19,** 729–738

VAN SOMEREN, V. and STOTHERS, J. K. (1983) A critical dissection of obstructive apnea in the human infant. *Pediatrics,* **71,** 721–725

WARBURTON, D., STARK, A. R. and TAEUSCH, H. W. (1977) Apnea monitor failure in infants with airway obstruction. *Pediatrics,* **60,** 742–744

WERTHAMMER, J., KRASNER, J., DIBENEDETTO, J. and STARK, A. R. (1983) Apnea monitoring by acoustic detection of airflow. *Pediatrics,* **71,** 53–55

6
The flexible fiberoptic bronchoscope as a diagnostic and therapeutic tool in infants

Robert E. Wood

Pediatricians caring for infants with respiratory disease are often faced with challenging diagnostic or therapeutic dilemmas. The ability to examine the airway directly or to obtain specimens from the lower respiratory tract would be of great help, but is seriously hampered by technological considerations and by the small dimensions of the airway in infants. In most institutions, physicians have traditionally been reluctant to employ bronchoscopy in infants unless there are very clear indications for a procedure which is perceived as significantly invasive. Thus, in many cases questions go unanswered, or physicians must seek information in other indirect ways.

The development of the flexible fiberoptic bronchoscope in the late 1960s (first introduced into the United States in 1969) had a major impact on the practice of pulmonary medicine. This instrument allowed the performance of bronchoscopic examinations without the need for general anesthesia, and with a significant reduction in operative morbidity. However, the application of such technology to the pediatric population had to await the development of much smaller instruments than were initially available (Sackner, 1975; Wood and Fink, 1978; Wood and Sherman, 1980).

In order to perform bronchoscopy, some specific requirements must be met. The instrument must be sufficiently small that it can safely enter the trachea, which in a full-term newborn infant is approximately 5 mm in diameter. The instrument must have suitable optical characteristics, and must provide for illumination of the airways. Finally, the patient must be able to maintain arterial oxygenation during the procedure.

The rigid bronchoscope meets these criteria if it is sufficiently small. Bronchoscopes used in infants are usually '3 mm' or '3.5 mm' instruments, which have an external diameter of 4–5 mm (or slightly more). Ventilation is achieved through the bronchoscope, either with positive pressure inflation or with a venturi jet injection device. General anesthesia is usually used, although some operators prefer to proceed without anesthesia. If a glass rod telescope is used the lumen of the instrument is reduced, but the optics give a spectacular (and unexcelled) view of the airway (Benjamin, 1982).

The flexible bronchoscope differs from the rigid instruments in many ways. Most importantly, it is essentially solid, and thus the patient is required to breathe around, rather than through, the instrument. The overall diameter is smaller than the corresponding rigid bronchoscopes. The standard pediatric flexible broncho-scope in use today (BF3C4, Olympus Corporation) has an external diameter of 3.5 mm. Other instruments are now available which are smaller, but have more limited characteristics (*Table 6.1*). The tip of the flexible bronchoscope may be controlled remotely to flex in a single plane; movement from side to side is controlled by rotation of the shaft of the instrument.

Table 6.1 Flexible endoscopes suitable for use in the pediatric airway

Model	Diameter (mm)	Angulation	Suction channel (mm)	Comments
BF3C4	3.5	+160 −60	1.2	The pediatric standard
BF4B2	4.8	+180 −120	2.0	3–4 years and older
PF27	2.7	+180 −90	None	Special applications
PF22	2.3	None	None	Special applications
PF18	1.8	None	None	Special applications

Other instruments such as nasopharyngoscopes may be used for special applications.
Olympus Corp.

TECHNIQUES FOR FLEXIBLE BRONCHOSCOPY IN INFANTS

The following description of technique is based on my personal practice and experience; other bronchoscopists may use techniques which differ in some respects.

Procedures are performed under the most optimum conditions possible. Unless the patient cannot be moved from the intensive care unit, the procedures are done in an endoscopy laboratory, with all the necessary supplies and equipment readily at hand. In selected patients, such as infants in the neonatal intensive care unit, transporting the patient to the endoscopy facility would place the patient under undue stress and risk and so the procedures are done at the bedside.

Patients are fasted for at least 4 h prior to the procedure which is carried out with the patient in a prone position. A simple swaddling technique (Hughes and Buescher, 1980) is used which leaves the patient's chest free for observation and auscultation. An electronic monitor is used in selected patients. In addition, an assistant gently stabilizes the infant's head while observing the child throughout the procedure for signs of respiratory distress or other problems.

Infants who are very active or who are older than 1–2 months are sedated with intravenous meperidine $1–3 \text{ mg} \cdot \text{kg}^{-1}$. This usually produces a satisfactory level of sedation, from which the infants awaken within 30 min. Very small infants, those who are very ill or hypoxic, or who are already intubated with either an endotracheal tube or tracheostomy tube, are not sedated unless absolutely necessary. The addition of a very small dose $(1 \text{ mg} \cdot \text{kg}^{-1})$ of an ultrashort-acting barbiturate (e.g. methohexital) as an inducing agent can be very helpful in selected infants and in my experience has been associated with no complications.

It is essential to provide anesthesia of the upper airway. Topical 2% lidocaine is instilled into the nose before the bronchoscope is introduced, and then a second aliquot is deposited directly onto the larynx through the suction channel of the bronchoscope. If the 2.7-mm instrument is being used, the entire dose of lidocaine is placed in the nose; after several minutes the larynx is almost always sufficiently anesthetized to allow passage of the bronchoscope without difficulty. Additional small aliquots of lidocaine are sometimes required in the lower airway to control coughing.

The bronchoscope is passed transnasally in all patients unless there is a nasal anomaly which obliterates the nasal passage or the instrument is being inserted through an artificial airway such as a tracheostomy tube. The 3.5-mm bronchoscope will readily pass through the nose of infants as small as 700 g. The 2.7-mm instrument will pass easily through a 3.0-mm endotracheal tube or a no. 00 tracheostomy tube; the 3.5-mm bronchoscope will pass through a 4.5-mm endotracheal tube.

If collection of secretions or washings from the lower airway is contemplated, the patient is placed in a 15–20 degree head-down position prior to anesthetizing the upper airway. This minimizes the aspiration of oral secretions into the trachea. In addition, the bronchoscope is not used for suctioning until its tip reaches the carina. It is usually (although by no means always) possible to obtain specimens from the lower airway without significant contamination from the upper airway and mouth. This must be confirmed by microscopic examination of the specimen.

In almost all full-term infants the 3.5-mm bronchoscope allows adequate ventilation around the instrument (although it increases the airway resistance somewhat). As soon as the instrument is passed into the trachea, the infant is checked for adequacy of breath sounds and for retractions. Careful monitoring of the infant throughout the procedure is essential, as airway obstruction is a constant possibility. Supplemental oxygen may be given if desired, either through a face mask or by insufflating small volumes intermittently through the suction channel of the bronchoscope. This latter technique is capable of maintaining oxygenation relatively well even in very small infants, but carbon dioxide retention will result if the bronchoscope is kept below the glottis longer than 1–2 min. Therefore, it is probably better to perform the procedure with stopwatch timing than to rely on alternative methods of oxygen delivery. Infants smaller than about 3 kg cannot reliably ventilate around the bronchoscope. Therefore, the procedure must either be completed in a very short time or one of the smaller instruments must be used. In very small infants even the 2.7-mm instrument will obstruct the airway. Fortunately, in most cases a complete examination of the lower airway can be completed within 30–45 s after entering the trachea. If the patient cannot achieve adequate ventilation, the procedure is timed with a stopwatch and the bronchoscope is removed from the trachea within 45 s. Multiple insertions of the bronchoscope may be required in some patients for completion of the procedure. This is especially true if there are large quantities of mucus in the lower airway which require extensive suctioning. With careful monitoring and rapid completion of the procedure, however, bronchoscopy can be safely carried out under essentially apneic conditions without unduly stressing the patient.

EXPERIENCE WITH THE FLEXIBLE BRONCHOSCOPE IN INFANTS LESS THAN ONE YEAR OLD

Between November 1978 and February 1984, 613 infants less than one year of age underwent pulmonary endoscopy. The age distribution of these patients is shown in *Table 6.2*. The median age was 2.5 months, and the mean age was 3.6 months. The

Table 6.2 Age distribution of
patients undergoing pulmonary
endoscopic procedures

Age (months)	Number
0–1	118
1–2	71
2–3	85
3–4	63
4–5	57
5–6	65
6–7	38
7–8	32
8–9	27
9–10	26
10–11	16
11–12	15

smallest patient weighed 540 g, and was bronchoscoped with the 2.7-mm instrument. Sixteen patients weighed less than 1000 g, and 57 weighed between 1001 and 2000 g.

The indications for bronchoscopy and laryngoscopy in infants are considerably different from those usually listed for adults (Sackner, 1975). The primary indications for the procedures in this series are shown in *Table 6.3* and are discussed in the remainder of the text.

The flexible bronchoscope is ideally suited, with a few exceptions, for the evaluation of the infant with stridor. Because the instrument is passed through the nose, the entire upper airway is examined, and often significant abnormalities are found in the nose or posterior pharynx that would not be seen by rigid laryngoscopy or bronchoscopy. More importantly, the transnasal approach leaves the laryngeal structures in their natural state, without any distorting forces being applied. Thus, the dynamics of the larynx and pharynx are observed clearly. Furthermore, the fact that patients are examined with only mild sedation allows full evaluation of vocal

Table 6.3 Indications for pulmonary endoscopic procedures in 613 infants less than 12 months old

Indication	Number	Percentage
Stridor	204	33
Atelectasis	123	20
Tracheostomy evaluation	89	15
Wheezing	35	6
Endotracheal tube problems	25	4
Suspected airway compression	24	4
Miscellaneous lower airway	75	12
Miscellaneous upper airway	38	6

cord movement. Problems may arise, however, in patients in whom the upper airway and larynx collapse profoundly during inspiration. In some such patients, it is difficult to see the vocal cords without providing some mechanical support to the supralaryngeal structures. Occasionally it may also be difficult to evaluate the posterior commissure fully, due to the fact that the flexible bronchoscope approaches the larynx from a slightly posterior position (at least when it is passed transnasally).

When the glottis or subglottis are severely narrowed, the bronchoscope should not be passed through the glottis, so as to avoid producing edema and further obstruction. However, even when a cause for stridor is evident above the glottis, it is useful to continue the examination into the lower airway. In this series, 204 patients were evaluated for stridor and, in 81 of these, only laryngoscopy was performed. In the remaining 123 patients, the lower airway was also examined. The diagnostic findings are shown in *Table 6.4.* It is of note that 15% of the patients in

Table 6.4 Primary diagnostic findings in infants with stridor

Primary finding	Laryngoscopy only	Bronchoscopy
Upper airway		
Laryngomalacia	31	55
Laryngeal edema	8	10
Subglottic stenosis	13	10
Subglottic cyst	2	
Subglottic hemangioma	6	1
Vocal cord paralysis	6	16
Supraglottic hemangioma	4	
Supraglottic cyst	4	
Supraglottic sarcoma	1	
Pharyngeal collapse		4
Nasal obstruction	1	2
Normal larynx	5	
Lower airway		
Tracheomalacia		9
Tracheal compression		10
Tracheal stenosis		3
Inflammatory changes only		1
Central mucus plug		1
Esophageal foreign body		1
Normal examination		1

whom an upper airway cause of stridor was found also had significant findings in the lower airway (tracheomalacia, tracheal compression, compression of the left main bronchus, or granulation tissue). Twelve per cent of the patients had lower airway causes of stridor. In only 7 patients was no cause of the stridor found. In 5 of these, only laryngoscopy was done, and in all 7, the stridor was either intermittent or historical. In every patient who was stridorous at the time of the examination the cause of the stridor was demonstrated.

When should patients with stridor undergo a flexible fiberoptic examination? The answer is when someone is worried about the stridor. Even though the most common cause of stridor in infants is laryngomalacia, a self-limited disorder which only rarely requires treatment, continuing stridor often causes significant family stress and anxiety. A definitive diagnosis is often very reassuring, and can restore more normal family (if not airway) dynamics. Furthermore, in a number of patients who quite clearly had laryngomalacia on clinical grounds, flexible endoscopy revealed quite different diagnoses. These included subglottic stenosis, subglottic hemangiomas, subglottic and supraglottic cysts, and tracheal compression. On the other hand, it is not very useful to perform such examinations on such patients with typical croup. Only if the clinical presentation is unusual (very young age, unusual severity with rapid onset, prolonged symptoms), should such children undergo endoscopic examination. It is difficult to distinguish visually between subglottic edema and many forms of subglottic stenosis, and it is usually more productive (as well as safer) to postpone such an examination for several weeks after the acute episode has resolved, if the examination is necessary at all.

In principle it is very easy and efficient to use the flexible bronchoscope to perform transnasal intubation (Rucker, Silva and Worcester, 1979). In my experience the procedure usually requires about 30 s and yields an enormous amount of useful information in the process. It would appear attractive to use this technique in patients with suspected epiglottitis, and some endoscopists do so. However, I strongly recommend against this practice, since if the patient really needs intubation because of supraglottic edema it may very well not be possible to do so without physically displacing the epiglottis. A rigid laryngoscope and rigid bronchoscope are much more appropriate instruments in patients with suspected epiglottitis.

In the evaluation of the child with stridor, it may be useful to also examine the esophagus. This can be done easily with the flexible bronchoscope at the time of the laryngoscopy/bronchoscopy. In one patient in this series (and in several older subjects), the stridor was caused by foreign bodies in the esophagus compressing the trachea.

Atelectasis was the second most common indication for the use of the flexible bronchoscope in this series. In 7 patients, the examination was completely normal, and in 8 the lower airway was normal, but there were significant findings in the upper airway. Sixteen patients had lower airway findings which were probably unrelated to the atelectasis, while in 88 patients the cause of the atelectasis was demonstrated. The findings in these latter patients included central mucus plugs (67 patients), foreign bodies (2 patients), airway compression or stenosis (12 patients), and granulation tissue (7 patients). Secondary findings (mostly in infants with central mucus plugs) included tracheomalacia, bronchial compression, and inflammatory changes.

Bronchoscopy is indicated in patients with atelectasis for two reasons: diagnosis and therapy. Although foreign body is more common in patients over one year of age, 2 infants in this series had foreign bodies resulting in atelectasis. The patients with granulation tissue were all infants who had been intubated for ventilatory support with resultant mucosal trauma from suction catheters.

In patients with atelectasis, central mucus plugs (if present) were aspirated and the airways lavaged with 5- to 10-ml aliquots of sterile saline. In infants too small to ventilate around the bronchoscope (the majority of patients with central mucus plugs), the instrument was kept below the glottis for less than 45 s, including the time required for lavage and suctioning. Some of the mucus plugs were so tenacious that they could be removed intact, often with recognizable anatomical features (i.e. bronchial casts). Although these large plugs could not pass through the suction channel of the bronchoscope, a portion of the plug could be suctioned into the tip of the bronchoscope and then removed with the instrument. The largest of these plugs measured nearly 4 mm by 2 cm (*Figures 6.1* and *6.2*).

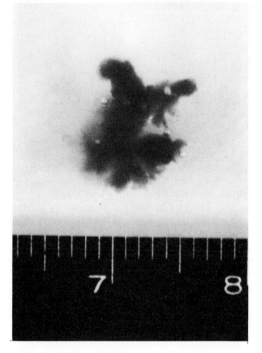

Figure 6.1 Bronchial cast of the right upper lobe removed from a 1-kg preterm infant via flexible bronchoscopy

The smaller the infant, the more likely that the atelectasis is massive, involving usually one entire lung, and due to central mucus plugs. The infants with central mucus plugs had a mean weight of 1700 g. Also, the more massive the atelectasis, the more likely it was to respond to bronchoscopic suctioning. Ninety four per cent of the patients with central mucus plugs had immediate resolution of the atelectasis. In all of these infants, previous therapy had included vigorous chest physiotherapy, and intubation and suctioning had been performed without success in many. The bronchoscope offers great advantages over intubation and suctioning with a catheter. Visual inspection of the airway, with the ability to direct the bronchoscope to the site of the mucus plug despite anatomical distortions caused by volume loss, and the fact that the bronchoscope has only a single end hole for suctioning, all contribute to the success of the technique. The results may be directly assessed, and other diagnoses established at the same time.

The results of bronchoscopy in the older infants with atelectasis were less rewarding than in the small infants with massive atelectasis and central mucus plugs. Overall, 61% of the procedures led to complete resolution. In another 15%,

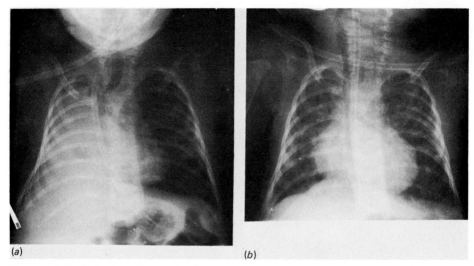

(a)   (b)

Figure 6.2 Radiological changes in the same infant with (*a*) massive atelectasis of the right lung and (*b*) re-expansion of the collapsed lung immediately following bronchoscopic removal of the cast depicted in *Figure 6.1*. (Reproduced from Fanaroff, A. and Martin, R. J., 1983, *Behrman's Neonatal–Perinatal Medicine*, St. Louis: CV Mosby, by courtesy of the Authors and Publishers)

an etiological anatomical diagnosis was established, and unrelated diagnoses were made in 11%. In 5% of the patients, a microbiological or cytological diagnosis was made, and in the remainder of the patients no diagnosis was made. Infants with single lobe atelectasis (especially the right upper lobe) were much less likely to achieve resolution of the atelectasis.

Infants with tracheostomies present very special problems to the pediatrician. It is often difficult to determine whether the tube is of the correct length, and radiographs can be misleading at times. The use of one of the ultrathin bronchoscopes *through the tracheostomy tube* yields immediate verification not only of the location of the tip of the tube, but also its relationship to the tracheal wall. In many infants with tracheostomies, persistent wheezing is a problem. Inspection through the tube has often revealed that the tube was partially obstructed by the tracheal wall, either by hypertrophic mucosa, granulation tissue, or simply by tracheomalacia. In other children, the flexible bronchoscope can be used to determine the suitability of the patient for attempted decannulation. The larynx and upper trachea are examined from above and, if they appear satisfactory, the lower airway is then examined. Often, granulation tissue or collapse of the upper trachea is found, which requires surgical intervention prior to successful decannulation. I believe that all children should undergo bronchoscopy prior to attempted decannulation. This may be done with either the rigid bronchoscope (Filston, Johnson and Crumrine, 1978) or the flexible bronchoscope. The flexible instrument seems more amenable to outpatient procedures. If the airway appears suitable for decannulation, the dynamics of the larynx and trachea are observed after the tracheostomy tube has been withdrawn. If the patient remains stable for at least 30 min in the bronchoscopy laboratory, he/she is then admitted to the hospital for observation at least overnight prior to discharge. The study of infants with the flexible bronchoscope at intervals of 2–4 months can lead to earlier decannulation and the avoidance of some serious complications. Patients in whom the upper trachea is obstructed with granulation tissue are referred for degranulation, as it is felt that this situation places the patient at greater risk in the event of accidental decannulation.

In the evaluation of the infant with a tracheostomy, it may be useful to pass the bronchoscope through the glottis (if there is sufficient room) and then alongside the tracheostomy tube. Occasionally, it will be necessary to temporarily replace the tracheostomy tube with a smaller tube (e.g. a 2.5-mm endotracheal tube) passed through the stoma, but I have never encountered a problem using this technique. Because the patient breathes through the tracheostomy tube, the bronchoscope may be left in the lower airway without obstructing ventilation. Thus the lower airway can be examined at leisure, and the dynamics observed undisturbed by increased airway resistance.

As would be expected in patients with tracheostomies, a high frequency of anatomical problems was found. More than a third of the patients had granulation tissue in the lower airway, and another third had significant tracheomalacia. Subglottic stenosis was the most common upper airway lesion, occurring in more than 40% of the patients.

Persistent or recurrent wheezing is often a cause for concern on the part of families and pediatricians. When wheezing occurs in the first year of life, anatomical abnormalities are usually suspected. In 20 of the 35 patients examined for this indication, anatomical abnormalities were found in the major airways. Tracheomalacia or bronchomalacia (7 patients) were the most common findings, followed by tracheal compression (5 patients), or bronchial compression (6 patients). The larynx was the site of the anatomical problem in 5 patients, while in 7 patients (20%) the examination was completely normal.

The use of the flexible bronchoscope in these 613 patients aged less than one year was associated with a relatively small number of complications. One infant with congenital cystadenomatoid malformation developed a lung abscess following a bronchogram performed in preparation for lobectomy. Two infants developed pneumothoraces. One occurred in a 960-g infant with massive atelectasis whose pneumothorax was minor and asymptomatic. The other pneumothorax occurred in a 3 month old with a stenotic mainstem bronchus in whom I (unwisely) attempted to dilate the stenosis with the bronchoscope. This infant required a chest tube. One infant developed transient laryngospasm when the lidocaine was deposited onto the larynx; this resolved very quickly without treatment and the procedure was continued. Three infants had mild epistaxis. The most frequent complication was transient bradycardia (12 patients). This occurred in very small infants or very sick infants with major anatomical abnormalities. In no case was active resuscitation required.

In summary, the flexible fiberoptic bronchoscope provides an extremely useful tool for the evaluation and, to some extent, treatment of infants with pulmonary problems. Although bronchoscopy is clearly an invasive procedure, the benefits in almost all cases clearly outweigh the risks, and as we have gained more experience with the procedure the indications for bronchoscopy in infants and children have been considerably liberalized. In infants, the all-too-common major uncertainties regarding the possibility of foreign body, congenital abnormalities or other problems can be resolved quickly and efficiently by the application of this diagnostic technique.

References

BENJAMIN, B. (1982) An Atlas of Pediatric Endoscopy. Oxford: Oxford University Press

FILSTON, H. C., JOHNSON, D. G. and CRUMRINE, R. S. (1978) Infant tracheostomy. A new look with a solution to the difficult decannulation problem. *American Journal of Disease in Childhood*, **132,** 1172–1176

HUGHES, W. T. and BUESCHER, E. S. (1980) *Pediatric Procedures*. Philadelphia: W. B. Saunders Co.

RUCKER, R. W., SILVA, W. J. and WORCESTER, C. C. (1979) Fiberoptic bronchoscopic nasotracheal intubation in children. *Chest, 76,* 56

SACKNER, M. A. (1975) State of the art: bronchofiberscopy. *American Review of Respiratory Disease,* **111,** 62

WOOD, R. E. and FINK, R. J. (1978) Applications of flexible fiberoptic bronchoscopes in infants and children. *Chest, 73,* 737

WOOD, R. E. and SHERMAN, J. M. (1980) Pediatric flexible bronchoscopy. *Annals of Otology, Rhinology, and Laryngology, 89,* 414

7
Diagnosis and management of upper airway obstruction

Anthony Olinsky and Peter D. Phelan

Upper airway obstruction, both acute and chronic (persistent), are common and at times life-threatening problems in infancy and childhood. Several factors contribute to this situation: the presence of congenital abnormalities, the anatomy of the upper airway and the increased incidence of acute infection, particularly viral, in this age group. Congenital abnormalities of the nasopharynx, oropharynx, larynx and trachea can all cause obstruction to airflow. It is not our intention to discuss all these lesions but to highlight some of the more common problems.

There are anatomical differences in the upper airway between children and adults and the size of the larynx in infants is an important determinant in the predisposition to airway obstruction with inflammatory lesions of the upper airway. In young children, the narrowest part of the larynx is at the level of the vocal cords with the triangular opening of the glottis measuring about 7×4 mm. The subglottic region is even smaller, by approximately 1–2 mm (Pelton and Whalen, 1972). Beneath the mucosa of the larynx and immediate subglottic region is a layer of loose areolar tissue which swells with trauma or inflammation and quickly decreases the airway size. The cricoid area of the larynx is surrounded by a complete ring of cartilage which limits the extension of any mucosal or submucosal swelling thereby further narrowing the lumen.

The classic clinical sign of extrathoracic upper airway obstruction is inspiratory stridor. Airflow through an unobstructed upper airway is generally quiet, but when obstruction to airflow occurs stridor develops. Stridor is usually a harsh low-pitched whistling sound occurring predominantly during inspiration. It can vary in intensity and at times it may be higher pitched and musical. It results from the increased velocity and turbulence of airflow that develops from laryngeal or tracheal obstruction. The two main factors producing stridor are: (1) narrowing or obstruction of the laryngeal opening or subglottic region and vibration of the aryepiglottic folds or vocal cords; (2) narrowing of the extrathoracic trachea from dynamic compression during inspiration which results from the negative intratracheal pressure immediately below the obstruction. Stridor indicates substantial narrowing or obstruction of either the larynx or trachea. In minor degrees of narrowing, breathing may be quiet at rest, but with increased activity and consequent increased velocity of airflow, stridor may develop. In lesions causing narrowing at the level of the vocal cords or above, the stridor is predominantly inspiratory, but in some infants with subglottic lesions, particularly if there is involvement of the upper trachea as well, prolonged expiratory stridor is marked. A harsh (croupy) cough is common in children with lesions involving the vocal cords and with some tracheal lesions.

Upper airway obstruction usually presents in one of two ways. First, a fairly sudden onset of stridor in a previously well child (acute 'acquired' obstruction) and, secondly, in a more subacute or chronic presentation with a history of symptoms evolving over a period of time (chronic or persistent (*see Table 7.1*).

When presented with a previously well child who has signs of upper airway obstruction, it should be possible to make the appropriate clinical diagnosis and institute the correct management in the majority of cases without resorting to detailed special investigations. Acute obstruction should be regarded as a potential medical emergency and approached accordingly. By far the most common cause of acute upper airway obstruction is acute laryngotracheobronchitis.

ACUTE LARYNGOTRACHEOBRONCHITIS (CROUP)

Acute laryngotracheobronchitis (croup) is the major cause of acute laryngeal obstruction in childhood in temperate climates and is due to viral infection of the larynx, trachea, bronchi and rarely bronchioles. The parainfluenza viruses are the principal agents responsible for acute laryngotracheobronchitis and account for over 50% of the cases. The remainder are caused by respiratory syncytial virus, rhinovirus, influenza A and B, measles and adenovirus. The peak age incidence is in the second year of life and 70% are male. It occurs throughout the year with peaks in autumn and early winter and in early spring.

Clinical features and management

The child usually has 1 or 2 days of coryzal symptoms before developing the harsh barking (croupy) cough and a hoarse voice indicating laryngeal involvement, as well as stridor due to the inflammatory narrowing of the subglottic region. When severe airway obstruction is present, indrawing of the chest wall occurs and the stridor is both inspiratory and expiratory. Tachycardia, tachypnoea, restlessness and eventually cyanosis may occur as a result of hypoxia. Some children may become physically exhausted due to the increased respiratory work.

The majority of children have a relatively mild illness and signs of obstruction disappear after 1–2 days, but the cough may persist for 1–2 weeks. In a recent survey over a 12-month period in 1982, 489 children were admitted with a diagnosis of acute laryngotracheobronchitis, to our unit, which serves a population of about 3 million. Seventy per cent were male and the median age was 20 months. The majority (58%) were mild (stridor at rest without chest wall retraction), 32% were classified as moderate (stridor at rest plus chest wall retraction) and 10% were severe (severe respiratory distress with stridor and retraction) and required admission to the intensive care unit. Children with very mild croup (stridor on exertion but not at rest) were not included as they were routinely managed as outpatients.

Most children with acute laryngotracheobronchitis require no specific treatment and simply need close observation. Investigations are rarely necessary. Humidification of the environment is widely used as the cornerstone of management and may help relieve the symptoms, although much of the evidence supporting this is anecdotal. It is felt by some that warm moist air is more beneficial than cool moist air, but this is without sound scientific basis. There are no data to indicate that particulate water vapour (mist or steam) is especially helpful. Minimal disturbance and careful observation of pulse rate, respiratory rate, colour, degree of agitation and degree of chest wall and soft tissue retractions are essential if the early signs of hypoxia are to be detected. While there are some theoretical objections to the use of oxygen because it will delay the appearance of the signs of hypoxia in a child with severe obstruction, there is an additional reason for not recommending its routine use. It is very difficult to provide a high ambient concentration of oxygen for a child in the toddler age group in a way that will not upset him. He will rarely tolerate a face mask and any form of enclosing oxygen tent must be kept closed for long periods if concentrations of oxygen much above 25% are to be achieved. Blood gas analysis has almost no role in the management of children with acute laryngeal obstruction. The decision that relief of obstruction is indicated is made on clinical evidence.

About 2–5% of admitted patients require mechanical relief of obstruction. This may be achieved either by endotracheal tube, which we prefer, or tracheostomy. Of the 489 recent admissions, 7% were intubated. When patients intubated at other hospitals and transferred to the Royal Children's Hospital were excluded, only 4.5% of the admissions required an artificial airway. None of the children who were classified as mild on admission required intubation. In our experience the average duration of intubation is about 3 days but varies over 1–10 days.

No drugs favourably alter the course of the illness. Antibiotics are not necessary because the disease is viral in aetiology. Corticosteroids have been claimed to be of benefit. However, as yet there have been no satisfactory trials to substantiate their value and their use cannot be recommended (Cherry, 1979; Tunnessen and Feinstein, 1980). Nebulized racemic adrenaline (a mixture of the L- and R-isomers of adrenaline) will often give temporary relief of acute laryngeal obstruction (Taussig, Castro and Beaudry, 1975; Fogel *et al.*, 1982). This drug should rarely be used as definitive management and it should never be used in ambulatory patients who are sent home soon after an inhalation. Its major place is probably in giving temporary relief of obstruction in children who require transfer from one hospital to another, in children in whom temporary relief is required while facilities are organized to provide some form of artificial airway, in children in whom sudden unexpected deterioration occurs and in whom secretion retention is thought to be a major factor, and in children with other laryngeal anomalies, such as subglottic stenosis, in whom it is thought desirable to avoid any form of artificial airway. It also has a place in the management of postintubation stridor. Inhalations may be repeated every few hours, but deterioration following frequent inhalations would warrant an artificial airway.

PSEUDOMEMBRANOUS CROUP

Another uncommon type of acute infectious croup is an entity that has been labelled pseudomembranous croup (Henry, Mellis and Benjamin, 1983). The condition is more often seen in slightly older children, usually more than 5 years of age. The child presents with symptoms extending over several days. A croupy cough, high fever and marked toxicity with severe upper airway obstruction are typical features. Pathologically the supraglottic structures are normal but the mucosa of the glottis, subglottis and trachea is inflamed, oedematous and ulcerated, while the lumen is filled with thick mucopurulent material giving the appearance of a membrane. The mucopus can sometimes be seen as radio-opaque material in the airway on a lateral radiograph of the neck. In most cases, *Staphylococcus aureus* has been cultured from the secretions but there is some controversy as to whether it is a primary bacterial infection or secondary infection following acute viral laryngotracheobronchitis.

Most of the children have severe upper airway obstruction and will require mechanical relief of the obstruction in addition to appropriate anti-staphylococcal antibiotics. Endoscopy and tracheal aspiration often result in a marked improvement but this is usually short-lived. Following the placement of an endotracheal tube, meticulous endotracheal toilet is required. However, despite frequent suctioning and humidification, the tube may become obstructed and need replacement. In a few children, tracheostomy may be needed particularly if there is a problem maintaining an adequate airway with an endotracheal tube. The artificial airway is frequently required for several days or even longer. Healing usually occurs without scarring and the long-term outlook is good.

The differential diagnosis should include acute epiglottitis, diphtheria, infectious mononucleosis and an inhaled foreign body. The high fever and toxicity and upper airway obstruction may be confused with acute epiglottitis, but the relatively longer history and the presence of a croupy cough are features against the diagnosis of acute epiglottitis as well as the obvious normal supraglottic structures on endoscopy. A history of adequate immunization makes the diagnosis of diphtheria unlikely, as well as the fact that the membrane in pseudomembranous croup strips easily and without bleeding, unlike that of diphtheria. Although infectious mononucleosis may at times present with signs of upper obstruction, there are usually sufficient other systemic clinical signs present to make the diagnosis of infectious mononucleosis. The presence of radio-opaque material in the upper airway may be mistaken for an inhaled foreign body; however, the high fever and toxicity are signs that favour an acute infection.

RECURRENT CROUP

There is a group of children who develop recurrent episodes of acute laryngeal obstruction. The term 'spasmodic croup' has been applied to the typical episodes that occur in a child with recurrent croup. These episodes often occur without any obvious respiratory infection. Typically the child, having gone to bed perfectly well, wakes during the night with a harsh cough, hoarse voice and inspiratory stridor. Signs of laryngeal obstruction may last for several hours but have usually cleared by morning. The episodes may recur over the next 1–2 nights. Occasionally, an episode may become sufficiently severe to require mechanical relief but most will settle quickly with reassurance and warm, moist atmosphere. At direct laryngoscopy, the only abnormality detected is pale watery oedema of the subglottic tissue.

We studied a large number of children with a history of recurrent croup and compared them to children who had had only 1 or 2 episodes (Zach, Erben and Olinsky, 1981). We found that in the children with recurrent croup there was: (1) a greater proportion of males (6 : 1 compared to 1.6 : 1), (2) a tendency to experience the first attack earlier in life, (3) a greater association with allergy as documented by a positive history of atopic disease and positive skin test to environmental allergens, (4) a tendency towards subsequent development of asthma, (5) slightly lower flow rates in baseline pulmonary function tests, (6) a greater association with airways hyper-reactivity as assessed by histamine inhalation challenge and (7) a familial predisposition towards the development of recurrent croup. In another study we evaluated 17 children with recurrent croup who had had their last episode within the previous 12 months (Zach, Schnall and Landau, 1980). Fourteen of the 17 had a positive histamine inhalation challenge. In addition to the characteristic decrease in expiratory flow rates on the flow–volume loops with the positive histamine challenge, they also showed, unlike the asthmatic subjects, a 'cut-off' or plateau formation of the inspiratory curve. A plateau formation of the maximal inspiratory flow–volume curve is considered evidence of extrathoracic upper airway obstruction. The histamine-induced reaction in these children with recurrent croup suggests a widespread narrowing involving both upper (extrathoracic) and lower (intrathoracic) airways (*Figure 7.1*).

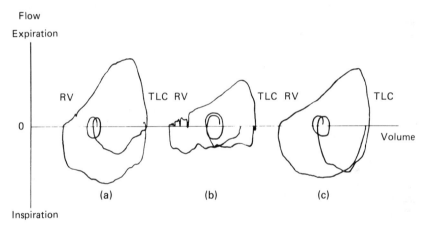

Figure 7.1 Histamine response in a child with recurrent croup. (*a*) Flow–volume loop before histamine inhalation challenge. (*b*) Flow–volume loop following a positive histamine response showing a significant fall in maximum inspiratory flow rate with plateau formation of the inspiratory curve. There is also some fall in maximum expiratory flow rate. (*c*) Partial recovery 12 min after histamine inhalation. The inspiratory curve is almost back to normal while the expiratory flow has increased but not yet returned to baseline values. RV = residual volume; TLC = total lung capacity. (Reproduced from Zach, Schnall and Landau, 1980, by courtesy of the Publishers, *American Review of Respiratory Disease*)

Thus there appears to be a fair amount of evidence suggesting that recurrent or spasmodic croup has many features in common with asthma. These include a male predominance, a genetic predisposition, the frequent coexistence of allergy, a tendency for the episodes to occur at night and the presence of bronchial hyper-reactivity. It seems likely therefore that recurrent croup and asthma share, at least in part, the same pathophysiological basis.

The approach to the management of recurrent croup is as for acute laryngotracheobronchitis. There is no evidence that antihistamines, sympatho-mimetic drugs or corticosteroids are of any benefit.

ACUTE EPIGLOTTITIS

Acute epiglottitis is a severe, life-threatening illness in children caused almost exclusively by infection with *Haemophilus influenzae* type B. Acute inflammatory hyperaemia and gross oedema of the epiglottitis and aryepiglottitic folds, which does not extend below the vocal cords, is responsible for the airway obstruction. In addition to the local infection, septicaemia almost always occurs and is responsible for most of the constitutional features of the condition. The median age of our patients is 30 months and 60% are boys.

The onset is usually rapid over several hours although some children may have a mild preceding upper respiratory tract infection. The child appears unwell, is feverish and lethargic. He refuses to eat or drink and may complain of a sore throat. Signs of upper airway obstruction soon develop with a soft inspiratory stridor and a characteristic sonorous expiratory noise. There is a tachycardia and the child prefers to sit upright and breathes through an open mouth and drooling of saliva is often seen. Typically, there is no harsh cough such as in acute laryngotracheobronchitis, and the voice and cry are muffled rather than hoarse.

The diagnosis of acute epiglottitis should be made on history, general appearance of the child and the quality of the stridor. It can be confirmed by direct visualization of the epiglottitis which is oedematous and cherry red. This procedure may precipitate an acute obstructive episode and should only be done if there is doubt about the diagnosis and there are facilities at hand to immediately relieve the acute obstruction, should it occur. A lateral radiograph of the neck is fairly diagnostic, but again this is not to be recommended as a routine, as the manipulation necessary to obtain adequate films may be very disturbing and could precipitate acute obstruction and should only be done in an intensive care situation.

From January 1975 to December 1979, an average of 14 cases per year were treated at the Royal Children's Hospital, Melbourne. In 1980, 1981 and 1982 the incidence increased to 47, 51 and 54, respectively. An analysis of the cases up to 1979 and those in the more recent years failed to reveal any differences apart from the absolute increase in the number. We could find no evidence to suggest altered referral practices, a changing disease pattern, nor evidence for a changing host resistance or antibiotic usage within the community. Over the same period a similar but less marked increase occurred with *Haemophilus influenzae* type B meningitis, bacteraemia and untyped *Haemophilus influenzae* respiratory tract cultures.

The child with acute epiglottitis is at grave risk of laryngeal obstruction and immediate transfer to a hospital with facilities appropriate to the management of acute laryngeal obstruction in children should be arranged. Until decisions on definitive management are made, the child should be propped up with pillows. Lying flat on the back may cause complete obstruction.

An antibiotic to which *Haemophilus influenzae* type B is sensitive should be given as soon as the diagnosis is suspected. For many years chloramphenicol in an initial dosage of 40–50 mg · kg^{-1} intravenously or intramuscularly and repeated in a dose of 20–25 mg · kg^{-1} 6-hourly for 3–4 days has been used with very satisfactory results and there have been no complications. Ampicillin has been suggested as an alternative, but the increasing incidence of *Haemophilus influenzae* type B resistant to ampicillin has affected the popularity of this therapy.

In most centres, introduction of an artificial airway as soon as the diagnosis is established is the appropriate management. The risk of severe obstruction is very high. Our intubation rate is 70% and the duration of intubation about 6–18 hours.

Provided the diagnosis is made promptly and an artificial airway introduced, the outcome should be satisfactory. However, a small number of children with epiglottitis die, most commonly before they reach a hospital with appropriate facilities. Prompt recognition is the best method of reducing mortality. A few patients develop acute pulmonary oedema, probably as a complication of the severe hypoxia. Such children usually need prolonged endotracheal intubation, mechanical ventilation with high oxygen concentrations and positive end-expiratory pressures.

OTHER CAUSES OF ACUTE UPPER AIRWAY OBSTRUCTION

Apart from the conditions already discussed, the differential diagnosis in a child presenting with acute obstruction should include other infections such as diphtheria, infectious mononucleosis and retropharyngeal abscess as well as inhaled foreign bodies. Differentiating these conditions from acute laryngo-tracheobronchitis, recurrent croup and epiglottitis is usually not difficult, but unless borne in mind one is likely to miss the diagnosis in the occasional child.

Diphtheria

Diphtheria, although uncommon nowadays in developed countries, still occurs and one should be alerted to the unimmunized child presenting with stridor, a serosanguineous nasal discharge, a pseudomembrane on the posterior pharyngeal wall and significant cervical lymphadenopathy. Although faucial diphtheria is more common, in about one-quarter of the cases there is involvement of the larynx and trachea with significant airway obstruction.

Infectious mononucleosis

Infectious mononucleosis occurs fairly frequently in childhood and at times the presentation may be confused with diphtheria. Malaise, fever, fatigue and sore throat with cervical lymphadenopathy and splenomegaly and a skin rash are typical manifestations. About 50% of children will have some otolaryngological involvement and, in a small number of these, there will be signs of upper airway obstruction (Snyderman, 1981). Airway obstruction is caused by hypertrophy of Waldeyer's ring of lymphoid tissue that encircles the naso- and oropharynx. There may be massive tonsillar enlargement and a membrane may be present. Significant cervical lymphadenopathy is often present as well. Most children will settle without any specific treatment although a few may require an artificial airway for a short period of time. Steroids have been advocated by some but this is controversial. Emergency tonsillectomy has also been proposed but the potential risks and complications do not support this form of therapy.

Retropharyngeal abscess

This is a suppurative lesion in one or more of the retropharyngeal lymph nodes and is usually secondary to a nasopharyngeal infection or, rarely, trauma. It occurs most commonly in early infancy usually in children less than 2 years of age. The clinical presentation is often abrupt with dysphagia, head retraction, open mouth, stridor and high fever. A bulge may be visible and/or palpable on the posterior pharyngeal wall. Palpation is an important part of the clinical examination. A lateral radiograph of the neck will show widening of the retropharyngeal space with anterior displacement of the airway. Treatment should include antibiotics. Surgical drainage of the abscess and an artificial airway may be required.

Foreign bodies

An inhaled foreign body presenting a clinical picture of pure upper airway obstruction is uncommon. A foreign body lodged in the larynx can produce stridor and a distressing cough. The patient is often aphonic. Symptoms usually begin suddenly while the child is playing or eating. More commonly, however, the foreign body is inhaled into the trachea, or main stem bronchi and other signs, such as cough and wheeze, are more prominent than stridor. It is important to remember that a foreign body lodged in the upper oesophagus may compress the trachea and present with either acute but more commonly persistent (chronic) stridor.

PERSISTENT (CHRONIC) UPPER AIRWAY OBSTRUCTION

Chronic upper airway obstruction in childhood may be caused by a variety of conditions. The majority are congenital in origin and are listed on *Table 7.1*. This is not a comprehensive list of all the possible causes. Most of the conditions present in early infancy usually within the first couple of months of life. By far the most common is a condition called infantile larynx.

Infantile larynx

Infantile larynx or laryngomalacia as the condition is commonly named in North America is the commonest cause of persistent stridor in early infancy. The onset of stridor occurs frequently within the first 4 weeks of life, often very soon after birth. The stridor is fairly characteristic being described as a jerky or cogwheel inspiratory crowing noise. It varies in intensity from breath to breath, is loudest when the infant is crying or in the supine position and may disappear when the infant is quiet and in the prone position. The stridor usually becomes less after 12 months of age and the majority of infants have lost the noise by 24 months of age. In a few children it persists into the second or third year of life. It is very rare for babies with an infantile larynx to develop respiratory obstruction of a sufficient degree to require an artificial airway. The stridor is more often annoying than worrying. If severe obstruction occurs in a baby in whom a clinical diagnosis of infantile larynx has been made, then further investigation to determine the cause is essential.

In most infants a fairly reliable presumptive diagnosis can be made clinically. The definitive diagnosis is made on direct laryngoscopy. The larynx is small and anteriorly placed. The epiglottitis is long and omega-shaped (*Figure 7.2*). During inspiration, the epiglottis and especially the arytenoids and aryepiglottitic folds collapse into and cover the glottic orifice. These floppy tissues intermittently

Table 7.1 Causes of upper airway obstruction

Acute	
Acute laryngotracheobronchitis	Very common
Pseudomembranous croup	Uncommon
Recurrent or spasmodic croup	Common
Acute epiglottitis	Common
Infectious mononucleosis	Uncommon
Retropharyngeal abscess	Rare
Diphtheria	Uncommon
Foreign body	Uncommon
Chronic (persistent)	
(1) Supraglottic	
Adenotonsillar hypertrophy	Common
Cysts: glossal, aryepiglottic	Rare
(2) Laryngeal	
Infantile larynx	Very common
Vocal cord palsy	Uncommon
Laryngeal webs	Rare
Laryngocele	Rare
Laryngeal cleft	Rare
Laryngeal papillomata	Rare
(3) Subglottic	
Subglottic stenosis	Common
Subglottic haemangioma	Common
Subglottic cysts	Uncommon
(4) Tracheal	
Vascular ring	Uncommon
Tracheal stenosis	Uncommon

obstruct the entrance of air and vibrate, thus causing the stridor. On expiration, the positive pressure of air from below blows them apart. No significant treatment is required but parental reassurance is important.

Congenital subglottic stenosis

This is of two types. The commonest type consists of thickening of the soft tissues in the subglottic area and sometimes the true cords themselves. The point of greatest obstruction is generally 2–3 mm below the level of the true cords. Except in mild obstruction inspiratory and expiratory stridor are persistent. If obstruction is marked, severe respiratory distress occurs. Recurrent episodes of 'croup' may be the only indication of mild obstruction. In these mild cases, a careful history often discloses that the parents have noticed a mild stridor when the child hyperventilates, as after running, but have accepted this as normal. Most subglottic stenoses improve with growth of the larynx and active surgical measures should be avoided if at all possible.

The other type of rare subglottic stenosis is congenital malformation of the cricoid cartilage. It usually consists of a shelf-like plate of cartilage with a very small posterior airway. Infants with this anomaly are usually in severe respiratory distress at birth and require tracheostomy. There have been reports that there is a progressive increase in the size of the airway with growth of the child. Various surgical procedures have been tried but none are completely satisfactory.

Subglottic stenosis can be acquired by prolonged intubation, and a high incidence (1%) has been found in survivors of mechanical ventilation with birth weights less than 1.5 kg. This may be due to the extremely small size of the trachea in the very-low-birth-weight infant. Although some mucosal damage can occur during the act of intubation, the greatest damage is probably caused by repetitive up-and-down movements of the endotracheal tube related to mechanical ventilation and nursing manipulations. Damage is also likely to occur if the tube is excessively large or cuffed and may be aggravated by airway infections or hypoperfusion (Ratner and Whitfield, 1983).

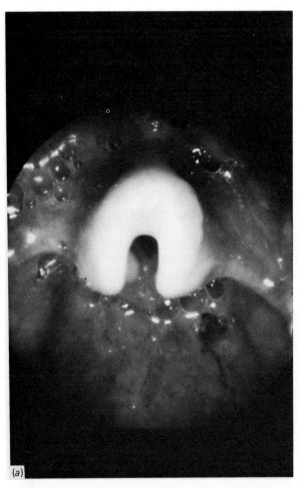

(a)

Figure 7.2 Infantile larynx. (*a,b*) Note the long curved epiglottitis and the deep interarytenoid cleft; (*c*) note the beginning of prolapse of the arytenoids into the glottic orifice

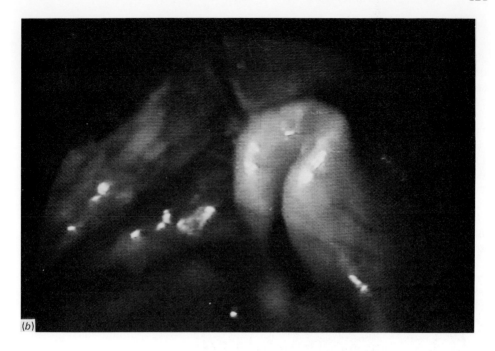

(b)

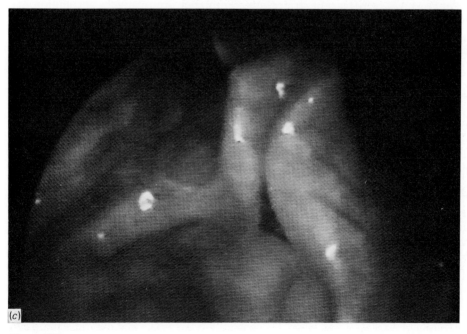

(c)

Figure 7.2

Haemangioma of the larynx

Although subglottic haemangioma is said to be an uncommon cause of laryngeal obstruction in infancy, in our experience it ranks after infantile larynx and subglottic stenosis as being the third most common cause of persistent stridor in early infancy.

The symptoms are usually not present at birth but appear at about 2–3 months of life. A variable inspiratory and expiratory stridor develops and there is a progressive increase in severity during the ensuing few weeks or months. Depending on the size of the haemangioma, severe respiratory obstruction may develop particularly with intercurrent infections. The diagnosis is made on endoscopy. The appearance of the subglottic region can be quite variable. The haemangiomas vary in size and may totally obstruct the airway. The cords may occasionally be involved. The overlying mucosa is pale rather than deep red and the haemangioma is soft and compressible either with an endotracheal tube or bronchoscope.

The haemangiomas tend to regress spontaneously over 1–2 years. Various forms of therapy including surgery, radiotherapy, corticosteroids, injection of sclerosing material and laser surgery have been advocated. Because of the potential risk of the various interventions our approach has essentially been a conservative one. In those infants with relatively large haemangiomas obstructing the airway we would do a tracheostomy and leave it *in situ* for 1–2 years allowing spontaneous regression of the haemangioma to occur. This approach has proved highly satisfactory and without residual complications. If after 18 months the haemangioma is still of sufficient size for a tracheostomy to be needed, we would then consider surgical treatment with laser therapy.

Other causes of persistent stridor in early infancy are relatively uncommon and will not be discussed but details can be found in the referred text (Phelan, Landau and Olinsky, 1982). The conditions include vocal cord palsy, congenital laryngeal webs, cysts and laryngoceles, laryngeal cleft and laryngeal papillomatosis.

Vascular ring

Tracheal compression from vascular anomalies can be divided into 3 main types. These are (1) some form of double aortic arch, (2) rings in which the aorta and a combination of other vessels and rudimentary structures such as the ligament arteriosum cause the obstruction, and (3) a major artery of anomalous origin.

The clinical significance of compression by an artery of anomalous origin is always difficult to prove. There are documented cases in which removal of an anomalous right subclavian artery has been claimed to cure clinical symptoms suggestive of tracheal compression, but usually the anomalous vessel indenting the oesophagus and trachea causes no significant obstruction. An anomalous left pulmonary artery passing between trachea and oesophagus may cause symptoms of significant tracheal compression. However, these usually settle as the child grows and surgical intervention is generally not indicated. There is frequently an associated tracheal stenosis which is responsible for much of the symptomatology.

The main symptom of vascular rings is soft inspiratory stridor which is often like a prolonged inspiratory wheeze. There is usually an associated expiratory wheeze. Both sounds probably arise at the site of the obstruction though there may be associated downstream compression of the intrathoracic trachea during expiration. There is frequently a brassy cough and there may be difficulty in swallowing because of the associated oesophageal compression. These symptoms usually begin within the first few weeks of life. The diagnosis can be established by barium swallow examination followed by aortography.

The treatment is surgical division of the ring. Cough, wheeze and rattling breathing may persist for a number of years after surgery as there is poor development of the tracheal cartilages in the region of the ring. Tracheomalacia is responsible for the inspiratory stridor and expiratory wheeze and cough. Excess secretions may be associated with superimposed respiratory infections.

INVESTIGATION OF CHILD WITH PERSISTENT OR RECURRENT STRIDOR

Provided appropriate facilities and experienced personnel are available, infants with persistent stridor should be investigated to establish a precise diagnosis, so that appropriate treatment can be planned and an accurate prognosis can be given to the parents. The only exception is the child with the typical features of infantile larynx in whom symptoms are mild. If there are any unusual features investigation is essential.

The two important investigations are radiological examination of the airway, especially with barium swallow, and endoscopy. A barium swallow examination should be considered in every infant with persistent stridor, particularly if there is an expiratory component, as the diagnosis of a vascular ring can then be established. Radiographs of the neck and chest should usually be taken as cystic lesions compressing the respiratory passages may very rarely have stridor as the only symptom.

Laryngoscopy is indicated in most other infants with persistent stridor. In a small weak baby or in one with respiratory distress this procedure is difficult and should only be undertaken by highly skilled staff. Ideally, the first examination should be without anaesthesia to demonstrate vocal cord movement. At times an infantile larynx can also be more easily identified in the unanaesthetized infant. If a diagnosis cannot be made during this examination, direct laryngoscopy should be carried out under general anaesthesia. If the cause of the stridor cannot be identified in the supraglottic and glottic regions, bronchoscopy is indicated. Before introducing the bronchoscope, it is wise to determine the size of the subglottic region with a soft rubber endotracheal tube.

At times it is difficult to decide whether to investigate an infant in whom stridor develops some weeks or months after birth. Such a child usually presents with a history of respiratory infection preceding the development of stridor. Stridor due to viral laryngotracheobronchitis can last for up to 2 weeks in an infant under the age of 12 months and further investigation is rarely indicated unless stridor persists longer than this period in such an infant.

A more difficult decision is when to investigate a child with recurrent croup. The reason for investigating such children is to determine whether a minor degree of subglottic stenosis is an important factor in leading to the development of stridor with minor respiratory infections. If the child has had episodes of severe or prolonged stridor and especially if there has been a history of mild stridor in infancy, endoscopy should be carried out. Parental anxiety is also an important factor in determining whether to examine a child with recurrent stridor, especially if the possibility has been suggested by the family doctor. In the child with recurrent episodes of croup of short duration it is rare, at laryngoscopy and bronchoscopy, to find an aetiological factor and the approach to investigate in such a child should be conservative unless parents are very anxious about the diagnosis.

OBSTRUCTIVE SLEEP APNOEA

In the context of upper airway obstruction in children, we should also consider the entity of airway obstruction occurring during sleep. Chronic upper airway obstruction occurring in sleep and associated with hypertrophy of the nasopharyngeal lymphoid tissue (tonsils and adenoids) is not an uncommon problem in early childhood. The true incidence is unknown and may be masked by the fact that when the child is examined during the day and in the awake state he may appear normal. Physical abnormalities are late manifestations. Because of these features, failure to recognize the syndrome is common and overt parental anxiety often results from this delay in the diagnosis.

The age of onset is variable and may be as early as 6 months. The child may present with a wide range of symptoms. The most common complaint is usually one of noisy breathing occurring during sleep. The parents will often state that the child snores a great deal and that there are periods when the noise ceases, but the child continues to make breathing movements which are often exaggerated. This is then followed by a gasp and partial arousal with resumption of the snoring. Other less specific presenting complaints may be: failure to thrive, lethargy, daytime somnolence, behaviour disturbance and chest wall deformity. In a review of 20 cases seen over a recent 4-year period at the Royal Children's Hospital, noisy breathing was the presenting complaint in 12, 3 presented with acute life-threatening obstructive episodes and cyanosis, 2 with failure to thrive, 2 with features of congestive cardiac failure and in 1 a chest wall deformity was the presenting complaint.

Symptoms elicited on systematic enquiry showed that, in all 20, snoring was present. Sixteen reported irregular breathing at night, 12 were restless with disturbed sleep and in 11 periods of apnoea occurred. Heaving of the chest was noted in 11. Failure to thrive in 11 and 9 had morning irritability, while 8 had lethargy and tired quickly and in 6 daytime somnolence occurred.

Studies during sleep in children with obstructive sleep apnoea have shown that the soft palate falls backwards against the posterior pharynx, the tongue moves posteriorly and the lateral walls of the hypopharynx approximate medially during inspiration. The majority of children have moderately enlarged tonsils and adenoids but not all of them do. The fact that not all children with large tonsils and adenoids have obstructive sleep apnoea suggests that other factors, and in particular central nervous system control of respiration and muscle tone, may play a significant role in this entity.

Physical findings in the awake child may be deceiving and some will be normal. Mouth breathing may be present and there may be moderate enlargement of the tonsillar tissue. Growth failure may be evident and there may be signs of pulmonary hypertension and rarely cor pulmonale and congestive cardiac failure. In our series of 20 cases, 12 had moderate enlargement of the tonsils, 6 were grossly enlarged while 2 were normal. Features of cor pulmonale were present in 4 children.

The most important part of the assessment is observation of the child while asleep. Monitoring of the breathing pattern during sleep, cardiac rate and continuous oxygen saturation measurements are useful parameters if the facilities are available but not essential. Simple observation of the child while asleep will provide sufficient information to confirm the diagnosis of obstructive sleep apnoea. A lateral radiograph of the neck provides useful information with respect to tonsil and adenoid size.

Although the tonsillar and adenoidal lymphoid tissue itself is not the sole cause of the obstruction, and the neuromuscular control of upper airway patency is probably an important factor, removal of the tonsils and adenoids will nevertheless relieve the obstruction in the majority of infants. Adenoidectomy alone may relieve the obstruction in many children. However, most will subsequently require tonsillectomy due to continuing or recurring obstruction and it is probably best to remove both tonsils and adenoids initially. There is a small group of children in whom the underlying neuromuscular aberration is the major component and removal of adenoids and tonsils will not relieve the obstruction. In most instances these children will need a tracheostomy.

References

CHERRY, J. W. (1979) The treatment of croup: continued controversy due to failure of recognition of historic, ecologic and clinical perspective. *Journal of Pediatrics*, **94**, 352–354

FOGEL, J. M., BERG, I. J., GERBER, M. A. and SHERTER, C. B. (1982) Racemic epinephrine in the treatment of croup: nebulization alone versus nebulization with intermittent positive pressure breathing. *Journal of Pediatrics*, **101**, 1028–1031

HENRY, R. L., MELLIS, C. M. and BENJAMIN, B. (1983) Pseudomembranous croup. *Archives of Disease in Childhood*, **58**, 180–183

PELTON, D. A. and WHALEN, J. S. (1972) Airway obstruction in infants and children. *International Anesthesiology Clinics*, **10**, 123–150

PHELAN, P. D., LANDAU, L. I. and OLINSKY, A. (1982) Respiratory noises. In *Respiratory Illness in Children*, 2nd ed. pp. 104–131. London: Blackwell Scientific Publications

RATNER, I. and WHITFIELD, J. (1983) Acquired subglottic stenosis in the very low birth weight infant. *American Journal of Diseases of Children*, **137**, 40–43

SNYDERMAN, N. L. (1981) Otorhinolaryngologic presentations of infectious mononucleosis. *Pediatric Clinics of North America*, **28**, 1011–1016

TAUSSIG, L. M., CASTRO, O. and BEAUDRY, P. H. (1975) Treatment of laryngotracheobronchitis (croup). Use of intermittent positive pressure breathing and racemic epinephrine. *American Journal of Diseases of Children*, **129**, 790–793

TUNNESSEN, W. W. and FEINSTEIN, A. R. (1980) The steroid–croup controversy: an analytic review of methadologic problems. *Journal of Pediatrics*, **96**, 751–756

ZACH, M., ERBEN, A. and OLINSKY, A. (1981) Croup, recurrent croup, allergy and airways hyper-reactivity. *Archives of Disease in Childhood*, **56**, 336–341

ZACH, M., SCHNALL, R. P. and LANDAU, L. I. (1980) Upper and lower airway hyper-reactivity in recurrent croup. *American Review of Respiratory Disease*, **121**, 979–983

8
The lung in immunological disease

Don M. Roberton

The respiratory tract is subjected to challenge by particulate matter, chemical agents and microbial organisms from a very early stage in human development. Efficient pulmonary defence and repair mechanisms are required to maintain normal lung function in the face of these challenges. The lung as a site of primary antigenic exposure also has a role in the development of a normal local and systemic immune response.

Damage to the lung may occur as a consequence of an overwhelming insult by micro-organisms or other agents, as a result of a primary or secondary deficiency of pulmonary defence mechanisms, or because of a poorly controlled immunological response. The purpose of this chapter is to review pulmonary abnormalities that arise as a result of alteration of host defence mechanisms.

PULMONARY DEFENCE MECHANISMS

Anatomy

The respiratory tract provides a continuous epithelial cell barrier to the entry of particulate matter and micro-organisms. The basic structure of the lining of the trachea and bronchi is a pseudostratified columnar epithelium containing ciliated cells and goblet cells with smaller numbers of several other types of specialized cells. The alveoli are lined by squamous type I pneumocytes interspersed with cuboidal type II pneumocytes (Breeze and Wheeldon, 1977).

The anatomical configuration of the upper and lower respiratory tracts determines velocity and turbulence of airflow (Newhouse, Sanchis and Bienenstock, 1976a). Lymphoid tissue aggregates within the respiratory tract tend to be situated where particle deposition occurs at sites of increased turbulence.

Secretions

Airway mucus is a complex mixture of water, glycoproteins, immunoglobulins, lipids and salts (Gail and Lenfant, 1983). The major source of mucus is the submucosal glands in the walls of larger airways; there is also secretion from

126

epithelial goblet cells and serous cells. The mucous blanket consists of two layers. The periciliary fluid adjacent to the luminal side of the epithelial cells and surrounding the cilia has the physical characteristics of a sol. A gel layer of lower shear characteristics and with greater visco-elasticity is situated superficial to this (Newhouse, Sanchis and Bienenstock, 1976a). Serous cells may contribute to the periciliary fluid and are also thought to secrete lysozyme and neutral glycoprotein (Gail and Lenfant, 1983).

The mucous coat forms a barrier for particles and microbial organisms and prevents the attachment of organisms to epithelial cell surfaces. Other specific secretions such as lysozyme, lactoferrin and α_1-anti-trypsin have a role in pulmonary defence. Alpha-1 antitrypsin is probably of particular importance in inactivation of the proteases produced by phagocytic cells. Very little is known about the control of production of secretions.

Flow

Very large particles are filtered in the nasal airway; those that escape this mechanism impact at the site of large airway divisions in the lower respiratory tract. Over 90% of particles more than 2–3 µm in diameter are deposited in the mucus overlying the ciliated epithelium (Kaltreider, 1976). Ciliated cells are present from the level of the trachea to the sixteenth generation of bronchioles (terminal bronchioles) (Pavia, Bateman and Clarke, 1980). These cells are the most abundant of all airway epithelial cells. Each cell has approximately 200 cilia, the cilia decreasing progressively in length more peripherally in the airways. Each cilium contains 2 tubules forming a central core, with a peripheral arrangement of 9 further pairs of tubules or doublets. These outer tubules connect to a basal body which anchors each cilium to the cell cytoplasm (Gail and Lenfant, 1983). Dynein arms which are ATPase containing extend from the A tubule of each doublet and are thought to be important in the production of ciliary movement (*Figure 8.1*).

Ciliated cells are responsible to a large extent for mucus transport towards the central airway. Cilia on contiguous cells beat in a coordinated fashion producing metachronal waves. Most ciliary movement occurs in the periciliary layer; only the

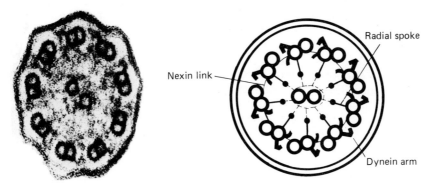

Radial spoke

Nexin link

Dynein arm

Figure 8.1 Ciliary ultrastructure. Normal ciliary ultrastructure is represented diagrammatically on the right. In the electron micrograph of a cilium contained in a nasal biopsy from a child with Kartagener's triad on the left, the inner and most of the outer dynein arms are absent

tips of the cilia move in the thicker, more viscous gel layer. Ciliary beat frequency is probably more rapid in the central airway (Rutland, Griffin and Cole, 1982).

Mucociliary transport can be assessed by measuring the rate of transport of a deposited bolus of a labelled substance such as technetium-labelled microspheres in large airways, or by measuring total lung clearance of labelled inhaled particles (Yeates *et al.*, 1975; Pavia, Bateman and Clarke, 1980). Ciliary activity can be observed *in vitro* following biopsy of nasal epithelium (Rutland and Cole, 1980) or biopsy of bronchial epithelium (Rutland, Griffin and Cole, 1982). Other factors contributing to mucus transport are coughing and airway movement during the phases of respiration.

Particles with a diameter of 0.5–3 µm tend to be deposited on the non-ciliated epithelial surfaces distal to the terminal bronchioles (Kaltreider, 1976). Here airflow rates fall dramatically and particle deposition is by sedimentation (Newhouse, Sanchis and Bienenstock, 1976a). Alveolar macrophages are important in the removal of inhaled substances from these distal airways.

Cells involved in immune responses

Lymphoid tissues are found throughout the respiratory tract, extending from the nasopharynx to the respiratory bronchioles and alveolar ducts. Antibody of all immunoglobulin classes is found within the secretions of the respiratory tract, although IgM concentrations are usually extremely low. The upper respiratory tract secretions contain high concentrations of secretory IgA and there are many IgA-producing plasma cells within lymphoid tissue. More peripherally IgG may become the predominant immunoglobulin class within secretions. Production of specific antibody within the secretions of the respiratory tract may result either from stimulation of local lymphoid aggregates by inhaled antigen or may follow the homing of committed IgA secreting B-lymphocytes from other mucosally associated lymphoid tissues.

Local cell-mediated responses also occur within the respiratory tract (Newhouse, Sanchis and Bienenstock, 1976b), and phagocytic cells (neutrophils and macrophages) are important in ingestion of particulate matter and killing of organisms.

ABNORMALITIES OF PULMONARY DEFENCES

Non-specific abnormalities of the pulmonary defence mechanisms include anatomical defects, abnormalities of secretions or flow of secretions and some abnormalities of specialized cells within the respiratory tract. Recently recognized defects which are included in this category are the abnormalities of mucociliary clearance due to defective ciliary motility. These will be considered before discussing immunodeficiency disorders and specific pulmonary disease arising from immunological disorders.

Abnormal ciliary motility

The first description of a structural ciliary defect causing abnormal motility was by Afzelius in 1976. Investigation of the ultrastructure of immotile sperm tails in infertile men demonstrated an absence of dynein arms. Three of the four subjects had defective mucociliary transport in association with recurrent respiratory tract infections and situs inversus totalis. Eliasson *et al.* (1977) confirmed the association of defective mucociliary clearance and the absence of dynein arms from respiratory tract cilia.

Several groups of investigators have since described a variety of defects of cilia as determined by electron microscopy (Katz *et al.,* 1977; Rooklin *et al.,* 1980; Sturgess, Chao and Turner, 1980; Turner *et al.,* 1981). A proposed classification of the ultrastructural abnormalities is: defective dynein arms, defective radial spokes, and microtubular transposition (Sturgess, Chao and Turner, 1980).

Defects of the dynein arms themselves show marked heterogeneity (Chao, Turner and Sturgess, 1982). In some patients there is a complete dynein defect in which cilia lack all inner and outer dynein arms. In others there is a partial dynein defect in which 60–70% of the inner and outer arms are absent, whereas some patients have absent inner arms only or absent outer arms only. Within the group of patients with dynein-deficient cilia, the lack of both inner and outer arms and the lack of outer arms alone are the most prevalent specific defects (Chao, Turner and Sturgess, 1982). Total aplasia of respiratory tract cilia has been described recently (Gotz and Stockinger, 1983).

Patients presenting with respiratory disease associated with abnormal cilia have frequently had recurrent sinusitis, bronchiectasis and situs inversus (Kartagener's triad). Recurrent otitis media may be seen in this condition and abnormal middle ear cilia have been described (Fischer *et al.,* 1978). Some patients have presented with neonatal respiratory distress (Whitelaw, Evans and Corrin, 1981). Cilia with major ultrastructural defects are usually immotile when examined under appropriate conditions immediately after biopsy, although in some motility is abnormal rather than absent (Rossman, Forrest and Newhouse, 1980). The defective ciliary movement is thought to relate to abnormal tubular linkage in the peripheral tubules (Veerman *et al.,* 1980) and is perhaps also due to an inability to utilize ATP because of the absence of ATPase activity consequent upon the loss of dynein arms.

Secondary structural changes may be seen within some cilia in children with recurrent pulmonary infection; these later return to normal (Corbee *et al.,* 1981). For accurate diagnosis, therefore, it is recommended that the same abnormality must be present in over 50% of cilia before it can be considered to be significant (Sturgess, Chao and Turner, 1980). Children with Kartagener's syndrome have also been described who have normal ciliary ultrastructure (Schidlow and Katz, 1983).

Structural ciliary abnormalities have a close but not absolute relationship with mucociliary clearance. Eliasson *et al.* (1977) found decreased lung clearance of radiolabelled particles in adults with an immotile-cilia syndrome over a 2-h period when coughing was suppressed. In contrast, Pullan *et al.* (1983) demonstrated an increased total pulmonary clearance over 24 h in children with Kartagener's syndrome which may be accounted for by effective coughing. Pulmonary clearance and mucosal transport rates may also be affected by extrinsic agents in the presence of normal ciliary structure. Influenza A virus and *Mycoplasma pneumoniae* cause reversible damage to ciliated cells. Sulphur dioxide and some hair sprays lead to a decrease in clearance (Pavia, Bateman and Clarke, 1980). Aspirin causes a small but significant decrease in both tracheal mucociliary transport rate and lung clearance of urates (Gerrity *et al.,* 1983). Smoking appears to have an inconstant effect, while steroids may improve clearance (Pavia, Bateman and Clarke, 1980).

IMMUNODEFICIENCY DISORDERS

The immunodeficiency disorders include abnormalities of lymphocyte-dependent antigen-specific mechanisms (adaptive immunity), defects of the complement system and deficiencies of phagocytic cell function. Disorders of adaptive immunity range from isolated antibody deficiencies to the total immunological failure of some forms of severe combined immunodeficiency disease.

Each component of the immune response is closely dependent upon normal function of others. Antibody production to many antigens is T-cell dependent in that macrophages present antigen to both T and B cells, with a subpopulation of T cells being responsible for subsequent antigen-specific amplification of B-cell responses. Later suppression of antibody production is again mediated by T-lymphocyte-dependent mechanisms. Antigen–antibody complexes lead to complement activation; complement products recruit phagocytic cells and amplify the inflammatory response.

The result of a deficiency of any of these components of the immune system is recurrent infection, often caused by organisms which are normally of low pathogenicity. Because of the close and complex inter-relationships of each of the above areas of the immune and inflammatory responses, specific types of infection are often not characteristic of particular immunodeficiencies. The lung, as an important site of primary antigen exposure, is the organ involved most commonly in infection resulting from immunodeficiency disorders followed closely by involvement of the skin and gastrointestinal tract. The specific features of the primary and secondary immunodeficiency disorders are described below, followed by a description of the pulmonary disorders common to immunodeficiency disease.

Primary immunodeficiency disorders

Specific disorders are grouped according to the classification presented in a report prepared for the WHO by a scientific group on immunodeficiency (Rosen *et al.*, 1983). The characteristics of infections seen in these and other immunodeficiency states are described later in this chapter.

Predominantly cell-mediated immunity defects

SEVERE COMBINED IMMUNODEFICIENCY SYNDROMES
This heterogeneous group of disorders is characterized by a profound defect of cell-mediated immune responses in association with a usually severe deficiency of immunoglobulin and antibody production. It is likely that there is a wide variety of aetiologies, but in the majority a specific defect has yet to be found. In some there is probably a failure of development of lymphoid stem cells, but in others, particularly those with some immunoglobulin production, the primary defect may be of T-cell function.

Almost all children present within the first 6 months of life, the clinical features being failure to thrive, diarrhoea and lower respiratory tract infection. Common infecting agents are *Pneumocystis carinii*, cytomegalovirus, measles, varicella, and parainfluenza viruses. Systemic bacterial infections such as meningitis or septicaemia occur frequently. The aetiology of the diarrhoea is often difficult to determine but probably relates to infection. Recalcitrant oral candidiasis is very common. Some may present with the features of graft versus host disease if blood transfusions or fresh plasma have been given. Skin infections may be associated with a generalized seborrheic dermatitis.

The usual laboratory features in the severe combined immunodeficiency (SCID) syndromes are lymphopaenia, low T-cell numbers as defined by sheep red-cell rosette formation or anti-T-cell monoclonal antibodies, failure of lymphocyte responses to mitogens or allogeneic cell stimulation, and panhypogammaglobulin-aemia with absent antibody formation. Variants of these findings include normal lymphocyte numbers, panhypogammaglobulinaemia with elevated IgE levels, and normal immunoglobulins with either partial or complete failure of antibody production. These variations emphasize that this collection of disorders represents a syndrome rather than a specific disease.

The severe combined immunodeficiency syndromes may be inherited as sex-linked disorders, as an autosomal recessive disorder particularly if associated with specific enzyme abnormalities as in adenosine deaminase (ADA) deficiency or purine nucleoside phosphorylase (PNP) deficiency, or they may occur as a spontaneous event. Analysis of fetal cord blood lymphocyte surface membrane antigens, lymphocyte proliferative activity and red cell or amniotic fluid fibroblast ADA or PNP activity allows for antenatal diagnosis in subsequent pregnancies.

Details of some of the better characterized severe combined immunodeficiency syndromes are described below.

Reticular dysgenesis
This rare condition may occur because of a severe lymphomyeloid maturation defect. It appears to have an autosomal recessive inheritance. There is a profound neutropaenia and a reduction or absence of myeloid precursors in the bone marrow. Early death has prevented extensive investigation but T- and B-cell numbers and function are markedly deficient. One patient has been transplanted successfully with allogeneic bone marrow (Levinsky and Tiedeman, 1983).

Adenosine deaminase deficiency
Deficiency of this purine salvage pathway enzyme was shown to be associated with severe combined immunodeficiency by Giblett *et al.* in 1972. This disorder has an autosomal recessive mode of inheritance and may account for 15–20% of cases of SCID. It appears likely that impairment of T-cell function arises from accumulation of adenosine or deoxyadenosine (Simmonds, Panayi and Corrigall, 1978) or other metabolites (Herschfield *et al.*, 1979) within lymphocytes. The clinical features are similar to other forms of SCID; treatment with frozen irradiated red cells as a source of exogenous ADA (Dyminski *et al.*, 1979; Yulish, Stern and Polmar, 1980) has allowed improvement in clinical and laboratory parameters in a few affected children but in general has been disappointing. Bone marrow transplantation remains the treatment of choice.

Purine nucleoside phosphorylase deficiency
Deficiency of this enzyme leads to a predominantly T-cell defect due to intracellular accumulation of metabolites (Giblett *et al.*, 1975). Immunoglobulin levels are normal or raised. There may be a progressive defect in lymphocyte function and a progressive lymphopaenia; clinical presentation may therefore be later than in other combined immunodeficiency disorders.

Bare lymphocyte syndrome

Some infants with combined immunodeficiency fail to express HLA-A and -B antigens on lymphocytes (Schuurman *et al.*, 1979). These antigens are important in the cell–cell interactions of specific immune responses. T-lymphocyte numbers are decreased and there is a variable hypogammaglobulinaemia.

Treatment of SCID depends upon successful bone marrow transplantation. Because of the problems of graft versus host disease (GVHD), the marrow donor must be matched at the HLA-A and -B loci and the mixed leucocyte reaction must be non-reactive for successful transplantation. *In vitro* removal of alloreactive T lymphocytes from donor marrow may allow a wider choice of donors in the future (Reinherz *et al.*, 1982); however, at present the only practical donors are tissue-matched siblings. Because only one in four siblings will have satisfactory tissue matches, the majority of children with SCID have no potential donor. Rarely some such children have been treated successfully with fetal liver transplants (Kenny and Hitzig, 1979).

Many children have now been reconstituted successfully by matched bone marrow transplantation (Kenny and Hitzig, 1979). Graft-versus-host disease still causes morbidity and death, probably because of non-identity of other 'minor' tissue antigens. Supportive therapy involves the use of intravenous gammaglobulin infusions (Winston *et al.*, 1982). Blood and plasma must be irradiated before use to destroy residual lymphocytes capable of causing GVHD. Cotrimoxazole is useful prophylaxis for *Pneumocystis carinii* pneumonia and should be commenced at the time of diagnosis and continued until at least 3 months after successful engraftment.

Predominantly antibody defects

X-LINKED AGAMMAGLOBULINAEMIA

This disorder was known initially as Bruton's disease. Affected boys become susceptible to bacterial infections as maternally derived antibody concentrations diminish in the first few months of life. Upper and lower respiratory tract infections are particularly common, and the most usual reasons for seeking medical attention are recurrent otitis media and a persistent productive cough. Many children have undergone repeated surgical procedures with respect to their ear infections. The repeated infections lead to poor growth. A family history of infection-related early male death on the maternal side of the family may be an important clue to diagnosis.

Nasal obstruction due to a chronic purulent rhinitis is frequent and a persistent low grade conjunctivitis is common. Other complicating infections may be septic arthritis, osteomyelitis and meningitis. Some affected boys seem to be uniquely susceptible to a slowly progressive and ultimately fatal echovirus encephalitis which is associated with a dermatomyositis-like illness. Another unusual infectious agent is *Ureaplasma* which may cause multifocal septic arthritis. Vaccine-associated poliomyelitis has been reported with a higher frequency in these patients (Wright *et al.*, 1977).

Tonsils and lymph nodes are small or absent. Adenoidal tissue is absent from lateral X-rays of the oropharynx. The laboratory features of this disorder are very low IgG concentrations, absent IgA, IgM and IgE and absent antibody formation. T-lymphocyte and phagocytic cell function are normal. B cells as defined by cells bearing surface membrane immunoglobulin or by B-cell specific monoclonal antibodies are absent or present in only low numbers in peripheral blood. Plasma cells and B cells are also absent from lymphoid tissue, including that associated with the gut and the respiratory tract. However, pre-B cells, i.e. cells containing intracytoplasmic immunoglobulin or reacting with B-lineage precursor antibodies, are found in the bone marrow. The differentiative defect responsible for this disorder has yet to be defined.

Pulmonary disease is the major cause of morbidity in this condition. Untreated patients or patients receiving inadequate replacement therapy have recurrent episodes of pneumonia, often due to *Pneumococcus* or *Haemophilus influenzae*. Affected boys remain susceptible to infections with organisms such as *Bordetella pertussis* because they fail to produce antibody in response to infection or immunization. Pulmonary infections with *Mycoplasma* may run a prolonged course.

Immunoglobulin replacement therapy prevents many of the infections in early life, but some degree of bronchiectasis is still common in the second and third decades even in those treated from birth. The extent and rate of progression of pulmonary disease in later life remains uncertain; intravenous gamma-globulin preparations may allow a further reduction in hospital admissions and morbidity from infection (Roberton and Hosking, 1983a) and frequent subcutaneous gamma-globulin infusions may prevent the wide fluctuations of IgG levels seen with present therapy (Roord *et al.*, 1982).

IMMUNOGLOBULIN DEFICIENCY WITH INCREASED IgM

Patients with this disorder, often inherited in X-linked fashion, have infections similar to those experienced by boys with X-linked agammaglobulinaemia with the important addition of an increased susceptibility to *Pneumocystis carinii* pneumonia (Rao and Gelfand, 1983). Recurrent mouth ulcers and neutropaenia occur. Tonsillar tissue is usually present. IgG and IgA are absent but there are normal or even elevated levels of IgM; some of this IgM is monomeric. Lymphocytes bearing surface membrane IgM are present in the peripheral blood.

IgA DEFICIENCY

Studies of adult members of the population or of blood donors suggest a prevalence of IgA deficiency of 1 : 500 to 1 : 800 individuals (Holt, Tandy and Anstee, 1977). IgA production is slow to mature in early childhood with the result that adult serum concentrations of IgA are not attained normally until approximately 9 years of age. Some younger children have very low concentrations of IgA in their serum for some years, although adult levels are attained eventually (Ostergaard, 1980). The clinical associations of this partial and transient IgA deficiency have yet to be documented adequately.

A higher incidence of some diseases has been associated with selective IgA deficiency in some individuals. The ascertainment of the true risk of association is difficult because of selection bias in many of these studies. IgA deficiency may be associated only weakly with respiratory tract infections if at all (Koistinen, 1975). A low serum IgA has been found with greater frequency among children undergoing tonsillectomy (Ostergaard, 1976). Recurrent infections may also be more common in asthmatic children with IgA deficiency than in children with asthma who have normal IgA levels (Ostergaard, 1977). In interpreting such studies it is important to remember that most have measured the association of symptomatic infection with serum IgA concentrations. These may not necessarily bear a direct relationship to IgA concentrations in secretions.

Recent studies have shown an increased frequency of infections in individuals with IgA deficiency if there is also an associated IgG_2 deficiency (Oxelius *et al.*, 1981).

TRANSIENT HYPOGAMMAGLOBULINAEMIA OF INFANCY

In some children there is delay in the initial production of all immunoglobulins. The hypogammaglobulinaemia persists beyond the age of 6 months, but eventually there is spontaneous recovery, often before the age of 2 years. During the period of hypogammaglobulinaemia these children are susceptible to infections of the respiratory tract and other organ systems. Such infections may be life threatening. Lymphoid tissue is present as are circulating B cells. The primary defect may be a delay in the maturation of T-cell help for immunoglobulin production (Siegel *et al.*, 1981).

ANTIBODY DEFICIENCY SYNDROMES

Rarely children are seen who have normal immunoglobulin concentrations but who are either unable to form antigen-specific antibody or who manufacture only a very restricted range of specific antibodies. The basis of this defect is unknown; diagnosis depends on the demonstration of a failure of specific antibody responses after known antigenic exposure.

Treatment of all the defects mentioned above, with the exception of isolated IgA deficiency, depends upon administration of adequate volumes of replacement immunoglobulin. The most conveniently used preparation currently is intravenous gamma-globulin (Ammann *et al.*, 1982a; Roberton and Hosking, 1983a). Minor reactions are common during infusions but newer preparations have a lower incidence of side effects (Ochs *et al.*, 1980). We commence treatment with a loading dose of $10–15 \, ml \cdot kg^{-1}$ of a 6% solution followed by maintenance therapy of 4-weekly infusions of $7.5 \, ml \cdot kg^{-1}$ commencing 10 days after the loading dose. Supplementary infusions are given during any major infections or at the time of surgery. This therapy is designed to maintain pre-infusion IgG concentrations above $35 \, IU \cdot ml^{-1}$ (Roberton and Hosking, 1983a). Weekly subcutaneous infusions of 16% gamma-globulin solutions can achieve high IgG levels and may be the treatment of choice in the future (Roord *et al.*, 1982).

Common variable immunodeficiency

This disorder is also known as late onset hypogammaglobulinaemia or varied immunodeficiency. The major features are onset usually after the first 2 years of life, hypogammaglobulinaemia and variable defects of cell-mediated immunity. Nomenclature remains unsatisfactory because of the often indeterminate age of onset and heterogeneity of the laboratory findings.

Respiratory tract infections predominate. Lymph nodes and tonsils are present. Several associated conditions may occur including splenomegaly, neutropenia, lymphomas, malabsorption, giardiasis and nodular lymphoid hyperplasia.

Serum concentrations of more than one immunoglobulin class are low. Although some residual antibody production may remain the response to immunization is poor. In many patients lymphocyte responses to mitogens are deficient; in some, T-lymphocyte numbers are also low. There are probably several different aetiologies. Maturation and differentiation of B cells is probably deficient in some patients, while in others lymphocyte coculture techniques have demonstrated a lymphocyte-induced suppression of immunoglobulin production or inefficient T-cell help.

Pulmonary disease in this form of immunodeficiency is again predominantly due to bacterial infection. There is a higher incidence of malignancy in this group of patients in comparison with other forms of immunoglobulin deficiency. Lymphomas are common and are often gut associated, but may present as a mediastinal mass.

Treatment is by replacement of IgG as for other forms of hypogammaglobulinaemia described above.

Immunodeficiency associated with other major defects

THIRD AND FOURTH ARCH SYNDROME (DIGEORGE ANOMALAD)

Primary thymic aplasia in association with hypoparathyroidism and congenital cardiac defects is known as the DiGeorge anomalad. Abnormal development of the third and fourth pharyngeal pouches in early fetal life explains the inter-relationship of these disorders. In many instances, the cardiac malformation leads to death in the neonatal period. Hypocalcaemia secondary to the absence of the parathyroid glands may cause convulsions or tetany which respond to calcium supplementation. The thymic shadow may be absent from the chest X-ray, but this is not of use in diagnosis as thymic involution occurs rapidly in many ill infants. Of more diagnostic usefulness is the absence of thymic tissue noted at the time of cardiac surgery.

Lymphocyte maturation is deficient because of the absence of the epithelial component of the thymus. T-cell numbers are usually low and lymphocyte proliferative responses are deficient. B cells are present and immunoglobulin levels are normal but specific antibody formation may be defective.

Pulmonary disease plays a less prominent part in this immunodeficiency disorder than in many others, probably because many die early of the congenital heart disease before pulmonary infection becomes fully established. Pneumocystis pneumonia and viral infections may occur. Cardiac failure also has a part to play in pulmonary dysfunction. In some affected infants, spontaneous resolution of the immunological defect has been noted (Asherson and Wester, 1980); this may be due to function of small remnants of thymic tissue. Pabst *et al.* (1976) described two children with substantial cell-mediated immunity. The occurrence of spontaneous resolution makes it difficult to judge the effects of therapy such as thymosin or cultured fetal thymic epithelial cell transplantation (Thong *et al.*, 1978).

ATAXIA TELANGIECTASIA

This autosomal recessive disorder consists of ataxia of cerebellar origin, telangiectases of bulbar conjunctivae and skin especially over the pinnae and nose, and progressive immunological dysfunction. Neurological features are often present in the first 5 years; telangiectases become progressively more noticeable in the second 5 years of life. Lymphopenia develops and lymphocyte responses to mitogens deteriorate. IgE levels are usually low or IgE is completely absent; IgA deficiency is frequent. When peripheral blood chromosome preparations are studied an increased frequency of chromatid breaks is noted. The number of breaks can be increased markedly *in vitro* by exposure of the cells to a radiation source. This can be a useful ancillary diagnostic test and may be of help in carrier detection. Abnormalities of DNA repair may be responsible for the high incidence of tumours in these children. Serum α-fetoprotein levels are usually elevated.

Most patients have problems with recurrent respiratory tract infections with later development of bronchiectasis. Malignancy such as lymphoma or lymphosarcoma may involve the mediastinum and respiratory tract.

WISKOTT–ALDRICH SYNDROME

The cardinal features of this sex-linked disorder are eczema, symptomatic thrombocytopaenia and recurrent infections due to an associated progressive immunodeficiency disorder. The primary defect remains unknown. Severe bleeding often leads to presentation in infancy. Platelet granules are deficient and platelet aggregation is defective.

Pneumonia is common and the most common cause of death is infection (Perry *et al.*, 1980). The inability to form antibody to polysaccharide antigens means that pathogens such as pneumococci have a greater potential to cause disease. IgM levels are low and isohaemagglutinin titres which form as a result of cross-reactivity with enteric flora tend to be low or absent. IgE concentrations are elevated. Cellular immunity becomes progressively impaired. The only successful treatment has been bone marrow transplantation following marrow ablation. Supportive therapy involves gamma-globulin, prophylactic antibiotics and possibly splenectomy.

Defects of phagocytic cells and complement

Quantitative or qualitative defects of neutrophils or complement components affect amplification of the inflammatory response and lead to infection.

CHRONIC GRANULOMATOUS DISEASE

This disorder is caused by an inability of polymorphonuclear phagocytes to initiate microbial killing by oxidative mechanisms (Holmes *et al.*, 1966). It is inherited as a sex-linked recessive disorder although autosomal recessive inheritance may account for the few cases seen in girls. The primary defect appears to be an abnormality of cytochrome b_{245} (Segal *et al.*, 1983). In males with chronic granulomatous disease (CGD) cytochrome b_{245} is undetectable; obligatory heterozygote females have reduced concentrations of the cytochrome. In patients who have a probable autosomal recessive mode of inheritance, the cytochrome is present but non-functional (Segal *et al.*, 1983).

Affected children experience persisting or recurring infections with specific bacteria (staphylococci, *Klebsiella* sp., *Serratia* sp.) of skin, lymph nodes, bones, liver and lungs in the early years of life. In a series of 168 patients reviewed by Johnston and Newman (1977), pneumonitis occurred in 80%. *Aspergillus* and other fungal infections of lung or bones are becoming recognized with increasing frequency. Among 245 cases of chronic granulomatous disease, fungal infection occurred in 20.4% (Cohen *et al.*, 1981). Organisms encountered included *Aspergillus, Torulopsis* and *Candida* and most had fungal pneumonia or widely disseminated disease. Recently clinically milder forms of CGD presenting at a somewhat later age have been recognized (Frayha and Bigger, 1983).

Assays of phagocytic cell oxidative metabolism give abnormally low results. Bacterial killing assays show very poor microbicidal activity. Carrier females have intermediate levels.

OTHER PHAGOCYTIC CELL DEFECTS

In the Chediak–Higashi syndrome, neutrophil movement is impaired and there is defective lysosomal degranulation. Respiratory tract infections are common. Leucocyte function in this condition can be corrected *in vitro* and *in vivo* by ascorbic acid (Boxer *et al.*, 1976). The defect of neutrophil mobility associated with recurrent infections, delayed umbilical cord separation and a neutrophil membrane glycoprotein abnormality (GP 180 deficiency) (Hayward *et al.*, 1979) can also be corrected by ascorbate.

COMPLEMENT DEFECTS

The complement sequence generates a large number of biological activities which are important in the inflammatory response (Rosen *et al.*, 1983). Defects may be associated with recurrent infections or with systemic lupus erythematosus (SLE)-like syndromes. Genetic defects, usually inherited in an autosomal recessive manner, have been described for almost all the complement components. C1q deficiency may also been seen in hypogammaglobulinaemia and severe combined immunodeficiency and appears to be due to an increased catabolic rate of C1q. Deficiency of C3 leads to recurrent pyogenic infections as does deficiency of C3b inactivator (factor I). Recurrent infections including meningitis and pneumonia have been described in association with C3 nephritic factor and hypocomplementaemia (Edwards *et al.*, 1983).

Acquired immune deficiency syndrome (AIDS)

This recently recognized form of progressive immunological attrition has an increased frequency of expression in homosexuals and recipients of blood products. Opportunistic bacterial, fungal and parasitic infections occur (Editorial, 1983a). AIDS has been described in children, either following exchange transfusions (Ammann *et al.*, 1982b), platelet transfusions, in infants of Haitian mothers (Joncas *et al.*, 1983) and in infants of mothers with AIDS or at risk for AIDS (Editorial, 1983a).

Immunodeficiency secondary to other disease

In contrast to the primary immunodeficiency disorders, immunodeficiency secondary to other disease is relatively common. Treatment of the underlying disorder will usually allow resolution of the immunodeficiency, as for example in malnutrition or in the nephrotic syndrome, but acquired immunodeficiency disorders may also arise as a consequence of the treatment procedures themselves, as in the treatment of many forms of malignancy.

Malnutrition

The increased incidence and severity of infective illness in children with severe protein–calorie malnutrition has been recognized for many years.

In malnourished children the thymus is small and there is a depletion of lymphoid cells in the thymus and in the thymus-dependent areas of spleen and lymph nodes. Cell-mediated immune responses are abnormal and there are also alterations in neutrophil bactericidal function, complement activity and secretory IgA responses (Chandra, 1983). Cells bearing an antigen recognized by the OKT 4 antibody are decreased in number. Mortality from measles is high in malnutrition, particularly before the age of one year (Editorial, 1983b). *Pneumocystis carinii* infection is more common in protein–calorie malnutrition (Hughes *et al.*, 1974). Deficiencies of specific substances may also lead to immunodeficiency: zinc deficiency is associated with effector T-cell dysfunction (Good, 1981) and a zinc-responsive defect of neutrophil and monocyte chemotaxis may be seen in acrodermatitis enteropathica (Weston *et al.*, 1977).

Loss of immunological mediators

Loss of protein in burned patients, children with the nephrotic syndrome and children with protein-losing enteropathies is associated with an increased susceptibility to infection. This relates not only to loss of immunoglobulin, but probably also to loss of other acute phase reactant proteins whose function is understood poorly. Lymphocyte and protein losses in gastrointestinal lymphangiectasia may also be associated with an increased susceptibility to infection.

Splenectomy results in removal of a large amount of lymphoid tissue and is associated with an increased risk of bacterial infections. There is a high risk of overwhelming pneumococcal infection in the subsequent few years particularly in children (Editorial, 1978). Severe cytomegalovirus (CMV) infection with pneumonitis has been reported recently in patients undergoing splenectomy and receiving multiple transfusions for trauma (Baumgartner *et al.*, 1982).

Preceding infection

Some infections, particularly viral infections, lead to an alteration of the integrity of the immune response with a subsequent, usually transient, increased susceptibility to other infections. Measles virus may lead to a transient and sometimes severe immunodeficiency of several weeks duration due to direct infection of lymphocytes (Coovadia, Wesley and Brain, 1978). Experimental evidence suggests interference with helper T-cell function and thus an effect on the inductive phase of the immune response (Pelton, Hylton and Denman, 1982). Serum factors inhibiting lymphocyte responses to mitogens and to specific antigens have been demonstrated in patients with pulmonary tuberculosis and paracoccidioidomycosis (Barclay *et al.*, 1979).

Malignancy

Widespread invasion of immunological tissues by malignant cells of extrinsic origin leads directly to immunosuppression. Consequently infection is a common cause of death in disseminated malignancy. Malignancy may also arise from cells of the immune system directly with subsequent abnormalities of the immune response as seen in lymphomas (Kumar and Penny, 1982). Immunodeficiency occurs as a result of the treatment of malignant disease particularly with use of high dose chemotherapy, total body irradiation and bone marrow transplantation. Cytotoxic drugs and radiation therapy both have major effects on normal bone marrow function. In bone marrow transplantation for the treatment of malignancy, recipient marrow and lymphoid function has to be ablated entirely prior to successful transplantation. The subsequent reconstitution of full immunological function takes many months and complications, such as GVHD, lead to further immunological dysfunction and susceptibility to infection.

PULMONARY ABNORMALITIES AND IMMUNODEFICIENCY DISORDERS

Specific infections

The most important consequence of immunodeficiency, irrespective of cause, is an increased susceptibility to infection. The respiratory tract is the most common site of involvement. In primary immunodeficiencies, especially, the patient may experience several infections before an immunodeficiency disorder is suspected. Although some infections are more prevalent in particular disorders, most can occur in a wide range of immunodeficiency states. The features of specific immunodeficiency disorders have been delineated above: the pulmonary diseases attributable to particular infective agents in these disorders are now described.

Pneumocystis carinii infection

This protozoan organism is of very low virulence in the immunologically normal host but may cause severe disease in the immunodeficient individual. Serological studies suggest that antibody titres to the organism appear at an early age, presumably as a consequence of very mild or subclinical infection in early childhood. Acquisition of serum antibody to *P. carinii* occurs progressively with age; by 4 years, two-thirds of normal children in cross-sectional and longitudinal studies had antibody in titres of $1:16$ or greater (Pifer *et al.*, 1978). Clinical infection with *P. carinii* may also be more common than previously recognized in normal children in the first 3 months of life. Stagno *et al.* (1981) studied 104 infants between 1 and 3 months of age hospitalized with pneumonitis. Infection with one or more potential respiratory pathogens was recognized in 63%; *P. carinii* infection was demonstrated in 19 of the 104 infants (18%). Clinical, radiological and laboratory characteristics of the pneumonitis syndrome associated with *Chlamydia trachomatis*, CMV and *P. carinii* were indistinguishable.

Culture of the organism is difficult. However, corticosteroid-treated Sprague–Dawley rats become infected readily. This has allowed isolation and continued propagation *in vitro* in embryonic chick epithelial lung-cell cultures (Pifer, Hughes and Murphy, 1977). The infection in rats provides a model for the determination of antibiotic efficacy.

Pneumocystis carinii pneumonia is a common infection in severe combined immune deficiency disease, in patients with haematological or other malignancies receiving bone marrow transplants, and in hypogammaglobulinaemia with normal or elevated IgM levels (Rao and Gelfand, 1983). The condition is also seen in malnourished children as described above and was common in Europe in the 1930s. In patients with secondary immunodeficiences it is probable that lung disease results from activation and replication of latent organisms (Hughes, 1977).

The onset of pneumonia is usually relatively slow in comparison with viral and bacterial pulmonary infections. Over a period of 2–4 weeks there is progressive dyspnoea, tachypnoea and a non-productive cough. Cyanosis develops, pneumothoraces are common and untreated patients die of respiratory failure. Radiologically there may be early hyperinflation with generalized perihilar opacification. These changes are not specific but with progression of the infection there is more widespread pulmonary opacification, often with a granular appearance (*Figure 8.2*).

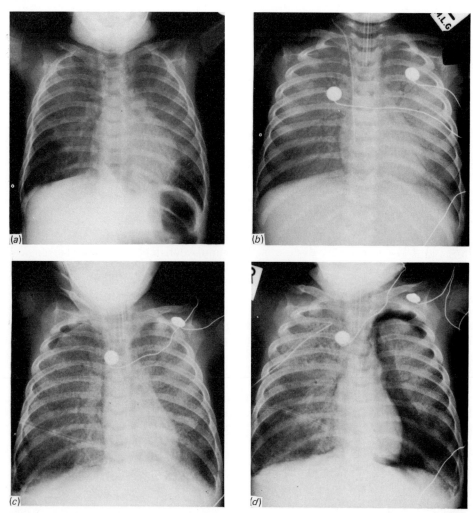

Figure 8.2 Unresponsive *Pneumocystis carinii* pneumonia in a 7-month-old child with SCID. (*a*) At presentation; (*b*) day 11; (*c*) day 23; (*d*) day 23

Diagnosis can be confirmed only by demonstration of the cysts, often containing merozoites, in pulmonary secretions or tissue. Sputum only rarely contains the organism in known *P. carinii* pneumonia. Open lung biopsy is the most effective means of obtaining tissue and has the greatest likelihood of providing a specific aetiological diagnosis in immunocompromised patients with radiological evidence of pulmonary infiltrates. In a study of 53 biopsies in such patients, open biopsy confirmed a specific aetiology in 81% (Jaffe and Maki, 1981). Transbronchial and trephine lung biopsies had lower rates of identification (32 and 20%, respectively); tracheal aspirates also have a relatively low success rate although they may be useful in following the response to therapy (Trigg *et al.*, 1983).

Haematoxylin–eosin preparations characteristically show intra-alveolar foam, but in patients who are markedly immunosuppressed this typical exudate may not be seen on lung biopsy (Weber, Askin and Dehner, 1977). With appropriate staining (Gomori silver methenamine and Giemsa), two major forms of the organism are recognized (Nash, 1982). The largest and most easily identified is the encysted form, 6–8 μm in diameter and containing up to 8 merozoites, often arranged in a circle. Trophozoites are smaller (2–5 μm) and are seen as free-living groups in the intra-alveolar foam, although they have also been seen in the septa (Weber, Askin and Dehner, 1977). The trophozoites appear to attach selectively to type I pneumocytes and later evolve to form cysts. After the cysts detach, they rupture leaving empty crescentic forms and releasing further trophozoites (*Figure 8.3*).

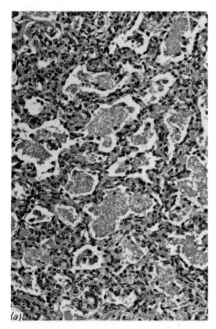 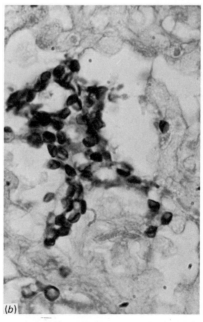

Figure 8.3 Pneumocystis carinii pneumonia: pulmonary histology of a lung biopsy from a 7-month-old male with immunoglobulin deficiency with increased IgM. (*a*) Haematoxylin–eosin stain showing foamy intra-alveolar infiltrate (×50); (*b*) silver methenamine stain showing cystic forms of the organism (×128)

Pentamidine has been used for some years for treatment of *P. carinii* pneumonia. At an intramuscular dose of $4\,mg\cdot kg^{-1}\cdot d^{-1}$ in two divided doses, 60–75% of patients respond. However, there is some morbidity associated with the use of pentamidine. The injections are painful and hypoglycaemia, hypotension, vomiting, and hallucinations may occur (Hughes, 1977). Within recent years the combination of trimethoprim and sulphamethoxazole has been shown to be effective in 70–80% of patients with *P. carinii* pneumonia (Hughes, 1977; Winston *et al.*, 1980). The recommended intravenous or oral dose is $20\,mg\cdot kg^{-1}\cdot d^{-1}$ of trimethoprim and $100\,mg\cdot kg^{-1}\cdot d^{-1}$ of sulphamethoxazole in 4 equally divided doses. Some immunocompromised children with *P. carinii* infection have not responded to either drug even when used in combination. Rifampicin $15\,mg\cdot kg^{-1}$ $\cdot d^{-1}$ has been suggested as a possible alternative following apparent improvement with treatment of 4 children with infection in the first 6 months of life (Szychowska, Prandota-Schoepp and Chabudzinska, 1983), but the aetiology of the infection in these children, although suggestive according to serological responses, had not been proven by biopsy. Rifampicin has not been shown to be protective in the corticosteroid-treated rat model (Hughes, 1983).

Because of the high risk of *P. carinii* in immunosuppressed patients undergoing bone marrow transplantation, cotrimoxazole in two divided doses (Hughes, 1977) has a place as prophylaxis given at the commencement of the conditioning regime and continued for 3 months following transplantation. Similar prophylaxis is useful following the diagnosis of severe combined immunodeficiency, commencing at the time of diagnosis and continuing until at least three months after transplantation. Lung parenchymal recovery is usually complete following successful treatment of *P. carinii* pneumonia.

Viral infections

Viral infections are usually associated with diffuse alveolar damage. Clinical and radiological signs in the immunocompromised host are often non-specific; concurrent infections with other viral agents, bacteria or fungi may be present (Williams, Krick and Remington, 1976a).

CYTOMEGALOVIRUS INFECTION

In the normal host CMV infection is usually mild or asymptomatic. However, in the compromised host, and particularly in patients undergoing renal, cardiac or marrow transplantation, CMV infection is an important cause of morbidity and mortality. Infections may be associated with pneumonia, choreoretinitis and hepatitis (Hirsch *et al.*, 1983). Cytomegalovirus infection also further increases the likelihood of bacterial, protozoan and fungal superinfection (Baar, 1955; Hirsch *et al.*, 1983). In bone marrow transplantation for acute myelogenous leukaemia, interstitial pneumonitis occurred in 31 (23%) of a series of 133 patients reported by Gale *et al.* (1982). Cytomegalovirus was the causal agent in 13.

Infection may occur due to reactivation of latent virus during the period of immunosuppression (Neiman *et al.*, 1977). Transmission of virus by blood transfusion is possibly also an important source of infection.

Infection is characterized by fever, tachypnoea and respiratory distress, but there are few abnormalities on auscultation of the chest. Lung biopsy affords the most accurate method of diagnosis; diffuse alveolar damage is seen and the typical large cells up to 40 µm in diameter with basophilic or eosinophilic nuclear inclusions up to 17 µm are diagnostic (Nash, 1982). A clear halo is seen which separates the inclusion from the nuclear membrane; this imparts the owl's eye appearance. Other diagnostic techniques are immunofluorescence of biopsy tissue, electron microscopy, culture of tissue, secretions or buffy coat of blood on human fibroblasts, or measurement of IgM antibodies in serum. A method for rapid detection and quantitation of human cytomegalovirus in urine from cardiac-transplant recipients employing DNA hybridization has been described (Chou and Merigan, 1983). Application of this form of highly antigen-specific rapid microbiological diagnosis to other body tissues has major implications for the future.

Treatment of CMV infection remains difficult. Screening of blood donors and blood products may prevent infection, as may protective isolation particularly from other patients that are known to be excreting virus. Hyperimmune immunoglobulin pooled from donors with known high titres of anti-CMV antibody has been shown to be useful in active disease in transplant recipients when given by intravenous and subcutaneous infusion (Nicholls *et al.*, 1983). Conventional antiviral agents seem to offer little benefit in CMV infection in the immunocompromised host, and acyclovir is either not useful (Wade *et al.*, 1982) or has only limited benefit (Balfour *et al.*, 1982). *In vitro* tests of arildone however appear promising. This new antiviral agent is reported to have broad spectrum activity against several RNA and DNA viral pathogens. It may prevent viral replication by preventing virion uncoating. It has been able to block infection of embryonic lung fibroblast cells by a laboratory-adapted isolate of CMV at low concentrations (Jeffries and Tyms, 1983). Interferon alpha has been effective at reducing the frequency of CMV syndromes in recipients with pre-renal transplantation CMV-antibody titres of >1 : 8; opportunistic superinfections were also reduced (Hirsch *et al.*, 1983). An effective form of therapy is needed urgently; infection, particularly with CMV, remains a primary cause of treatment failure in transplantation (Gale *et al.*, 1982).

MEASLES

Patients with antibody deficiency syndromes usually cope with measles virus infection well. In those who are receiving immunoglobulin replacement therapy measles infection is uncommon, because of passive acquisition of protective titres of anti-measles antibody from the donor population. However, measles infection causing giant cell pneumonia in patients with severe abnormalities of cell-mediated immunity can be catastrophic. This virus, therefore, is a significant cause of mortality in patients on immunosuppressive therapy.

Pulmonary infection, causing a high fever, cough and a rise in respiratory rate, occurs 3–4 weeks after exposure to measles. Often there is no pre-existing rash. Crepitations are audible and there are generalized coarse opacities on chest X-ray (*Figure 8.4*). Measles virus can be demonstrated by immunofluorescence studies of pharyngeal secretions or can be cultured. The pneumonitis is almost always progressive with eventual death.

Measles infection without giant cell pneumonia may still cause respiratory disease because of further immunosuppression secondary to the viral infection (Coovadia, Wesley and Brain, 1978; Pelton, Hylton and Denman, 1982). Bacterial bronchopneumonia in association with primary measles infection is common (Gremillion and Crawford, 1981). There is no available effective antimicrobial treatment for measles pneumonitis. Prevention depends upon avoidance of contact with other children excreting virus, or early administration of normal human

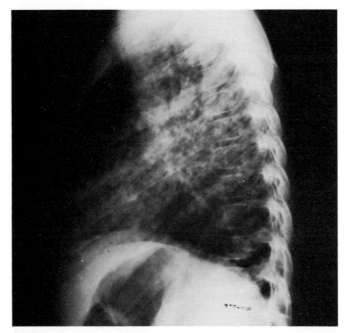

Figure 8.4 Measles pneumonia in a 5-year-old girl with acute lymphoblastic leukaemia

immunoglobulin if contact does occur. Immunoglobulin is probably not useful if given once clinical signs of infection are present. Antibiotics should be used to treat secondary bacterial pulmonary infection; common organisms are *Staphylococcus aureus, Haemophilus influenzae* and *Streptococcus pyogenes* (Gremillion and Crawford, 1981).

HERPES SIMPLEX VIRUS

Herpes simplex virus (HSV) can produce significant disease in the compromised host. Most cases of pulmonary disease are thought to be due to type 1 HSV because of the presumed oropharyngeal origin of the infection. It may cause disease at a variety of sites following bone marrow transplantation; mucocutaneous herpes simplex infection may occur in as many as 40–50% of patients receiving transplants as treatment for malignancy (Hann *et al.*, 1983). Of 525 transplant recipients reported from Seattle, 12 died of HSV pneumonia (Buchner *et al.*, 1982). Infection is thought to be due to reactivation of latent virus; evidence for this is the observation that there is a lower incidence of HSV infection in those with low titres of HSV antibodies prior to transplantation (Hann *et al.*, 1983).

Herpes simplex involves the lung as either a localized or disseminated infection (Nash, 1982). The localized form is more common; this causes a necrotizing laryngotracheobronchitis and may be associated with bronchopneumonia. This pattern of infection is probably initiated by aspiration of the organism from the oropharynx with subsequent extension via the airways to the pulmonary parenchyma (Williams, Krick and Remington, 1976b). Disseminated pulmonary parenchymal infection may result from haematogenous spread. Ulceration and necrosis of airway mucosa occurs; there may also be necrosis of alveolar walls.

Eosinophilic intranuclear inclusions (Cowdrey type A) are seen in epithelial cells at the ulcer edges and in seromucous glands in the base of ulcers (Nash, 1982). However, similar inclusions may be seen in other infections, as in varicella zoster, and ultimately diagnosis depends on viral isolation of material not contaminated by oropharyngeal herpetic infection. Radiological findings are not specific.

Until recently, adenine arabinoside $15 \, \text{mg} \cdot \text{kg}^{-1} \cdot \text{d}^{-1}$ (given as two 12-hourly doses) (Williams, Krick and Remington, 1976b) has been the treatment of choice. Acycloguanosine (acyclovir) has now been shown to be particularly effective in HSV infection and varicella-zoster infection. This drug becomes activated by a virus-induced thymidine kinase and subsequently inhibits viral DNA polymerase 10–30 times more effectively than host-cell DNA polymerase (Editorial, 1980a). Oral prophylaxis with acyclovir during bone marrow transplantation in a double-blind study of 39 consecutive patients given 200 mg 6-hourly demonstrated complete protection against HSV in the treated group, including those patients with high anti-HSV antibody titres prior to transplantation (Gluckman *et al.*, 1983). In contrast, HSV infection developed in 68% of the placebo-treated group. A further double-blind randomized trial used intravenous acyclovir in a dose of $5 \, \text{mg} \cdot \text{kg}^{-1}$ twice daily throughout the period of neutropaenia in 39 patients receiving remission induction therapy for malignancy and in 20 patients receiving allogeneic bone marrow transplants (Hann *et al.*, 1983). Among transplant recipients, acyclovir prevented HSV infection completely in the treated group in comparison with a 50% incidence of infection in those receiving placebo. There was also a significantly lower incidence of HSV in the acyclovir-treated non-transplantation group.

Resistant isolates of HSV from patients treated with acyclovir have been described in several reports (Burns *et al.*, 1982; Crumpacker *et al.*, 1982; Field and Wildy, 1982). Resistance is thought to be due to mutations of the virally induced enzymes.

VARICELLA-ZOSTER

Initial infection in the form of varicella or reinfection in the form of herpes-zoster may be seen in primary immunodeficiency states as in SCID or in secondary immunodeficiency disorders as in the treatment of nephrotic syndrome with immunosuppressive agents or in malignancy. The incidence of varicella-zoster pneumonia in immunocompromised patients is much less than that for CMV or HSV. Of 1132 children treated for neoplasia at St Judes Children's Research Hospital, 101 (9%) developed herpes-zoster. The incidence of infection was highest in patients with Hodgkin's disease (22%) and lowest in patients with acute myelogenous leukaemia (Feldman, Hughes and Kim, 1973). Only 3 of these 101 children developed zoster pneumonitis, but all died.

A further study in children with cancer from the same institution demonstrated a high incidence of disseminated viral disease with primary varicella infection whereas herpes-zoster tended to remain localized. Nineteen of 60 patients with varicella receiving active anti-tumour therapy had visceral dissemination with 15 of these 19 having lung involvement (Feldman, Hughes and Daniel, 1975). Four children died (7%); deaths occurred only in patients with acute leukaemia or lymphosarcoma and only in children with pneumonitis.

The rash usually precedes the respiratory tract symptoms of a dry cough, dyspnoea and chest pain. Visceral dissemination is more likely to occur in patients with low lymphocyte counts (Feldman, Hughes and Daniel, 1975; Prober, Kirk and

Keeney, 1982). Radiology demonstrates a bilateral peribronchiolar nodular infiltrate (Williams, Krick and Remington, 1976b) (*Figure 8.5*). The diagnosis can be confirmed by examination of vesicle fluid from the rash by immunofluorescence, electron microscopy or culture.

Zoster-immune globulin is effective in prevention if given within 72 h of exposure, but is not effective in established disease. Adenine arabinoside has been useful; intravenous idoxuridine 40–80 mg · kg^{-1} · d^{-1} in 4 doses for 5 days appeared to prevent new lesions appearing in 9 patients with pneumonitis but a further 2 patients died (Feldman, Hughes and Daniel, 1975). Acyclovir is protective in

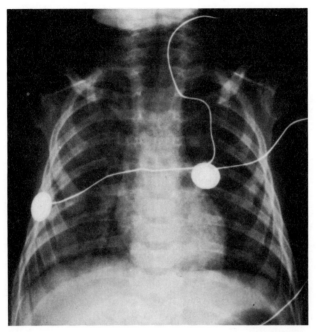

Figure 8.5 Varicella pneumonia in a 5-month-old child with SCID

that none of 8 acyclovir-treated patients with varicella-zoster, but 5 of 11 placebo-treated patients, developed pneumonitis (Prober, Kirk and Keeney, 1982). However, the numbers in this study were small and further studies are needed. Live varicella vaccine has been given to children with lymphoreticular malignancies who had been in remission for at least 1 year and half of whom were still receiving therapy. Seroconversion occurred in all (Brumell *et al.*, 1982). This may afford some protection from infection in the later stages of therapy.

OTHER VIRAL DISEASES

Adenovirus pneumonia may be seen in immunosuppressed patients (Williams, Krick and Remington, 1976a; Nash, 1982). There may be diffuse alveolar damage, bronchitis or bronchopneumonia. Fatal parainfluenza pneumonia has been reported in severe combined immune deficiency (Jarvis, Middleton and Gelfand, 1979) as has RSV pneumonitis (Gelfand *et al.*, 1983). Aerosolized ribavirin has been used in both of these latter infections (Gelfand *et al.*, 1983).

Bacterial infection

Many types of bacterial infection are seen in immunodeficiency states, tending to be more frequent in the hypogammaglobulinaemic disorders. Untreated hypogammaglobulinaemic children present with recurrent or persistent pulmonary infection leading to bronchiectasis. Because of the frequent use of antibiotics, colonization of upper and lower airways with ampicillin-resistant *Haemophilus influenzae* has been common.

Staphylococcal lung disease is seen in chronic granulomatous disease; *Klebsiella pneumoniae* is also a common pulmonary pathogen in this condition. These catalase-producing organisms survive within neutrophils because of the neutrophil metabolic defect and hence extensive local infection as well as disseminated infection can occur. Treatment of established infection requires prolonged courses of antibiotics and often surgical drainage is necessary. Antibiotics which penetrate cells such as rifampicin may be useful, as may granulocyte transfusions in otherwise unresponsive infections. Long-term prophylaxis with sulphonamides may be helpful in reducing bacterial infections in CGD (Frayha and Bigger, 1983). Johnston *et al.* (1975) demonstrated improved bactericidal activity of CGD neutrophils towards sulphisoxazole-resistant *Escherichia coli* and *Staph. aureus* in the presence of sulphisoxazole. However the mechanism of this improvement remains unexplained as none of the metabolic parameters of neutrophil function (iodination, ^{14}C glucose oxidation, superoxide generation or chemiluminescence) were altered.

Gram-negative bacterial pneumonias are common in patients with malignancy and following transplantation (Matthay and Greene, 1980). Mycobacterial infections are common in patients with malignancy (Kaplan, Armstrong and Rosen, 1974). Reactivation of latent disease is an important factor in some, particularly in adults (Williams, Krick and Remington, 1976b). Atypical mycobacteria may also give rise to caseous pulmonary nodules, miliary lesions or pleural effusions in patients with malignancy (Feld, Bodey and Groschel, 1976).

The relative immunodeficiency of the young infant allows infection with organisms not seen commonly in later life. Neutropenia is associated with bacterial lower respiratory tract infections. *Nocardia*, a Gram-positive acid-fast bacillus, may be seen in patients with malignancy particularly those with lymphomas (Matthay and Greene, 1980), but also occurs in primary immunodeficiency states such as CGD or hypogammaglobulinaemia (Williams, Krick and Remington, 1976a).

Fungal infections

Fungal infections of the lung are common in patients with leukaemia and lymphoma and following transplantation. *Candida* and *Aspergillus* are the predominant organisms.

CANDIDA ALBICANS

This organism is found in the gastrointestinal tract of most normal individuals and numbers of organisms increase in immunosuppression and with alteration of other flora during the administration of antibiotics. Pulmonary infection with *Candida* may occur either as a result of aspiration from the oropharynx with endobronchial infection, or as a result of haematogenous spread.

Polymorphonuclear leucocytes have been thought to be important in defence against systemic candidiasis but some clinical disease states suggest other mechanisms are also involved. Neutrophils from patients with CGD have defective candidacidal activity in comparison with neutrophils from normal individuals but systemic candida infection is relatively uncommon in this condition. Neutrophil metabolic activity towards *Candida albicans* has been shown to be normal in patients with chronic mucocutaneous candidiasis (Roberton and Hosking, 1983b); such patients often have specific lymphocyte defects with respect to *Candida* and therefore cell-mediated responses are responsible in part for control of candida infection. However, 20 of 25 immunosuppressed patients dying of pulmonary candidiasis in one series were granulocytopaenic in the week before death (Dubois, Myerowitz and Allen, 1977).

If pulmonary infection has occurred as a result of haematogenous spread, macroscopic nodular lesions are found throughout both lungs, as well as dissemination to other organs such as liver, spleen and kidneys. Endobronchial pulmonary candidiasis is characterized by mucosal infection of the larynx or trachea and proliferation of *Candida* within the bronchial lumen. In this form of infection lower lobe involvement is predominant. No specific radiographic patterns are seen because of the small size of the lesions and the high frequency of other infections as well as oedema and haemorrhage (Dubois, Myerowitz and Allen, 1977). Endobronchial candidiasis in immunosuppressed patients is often secondary to intubation.

The presence of *Candida* in sputum or other respiratory secretions is an unreliable guide to pulmonary infection because of the frequent carriage of *Candida* in the oropharynx of normal individuals. Lung biopsy specimens may be useful if pseudohyphae of *Candida* can be seen in the bronchial lumen or the lung parenchyma. Excretion of *Candida* in urine may lead to suspicion of disseminated candidiasis (Williams, Krick and Remington, 1976a).

Treatment of systemic infection due to *Candida* requires consideration of the site of dissemination; removal of central venous catheters, urinary catheters or peripheral intravenous lines may be required. Amphotericin B, with or without 5 fluorocytosine, has been the standard form of chemotherapy until recently (Medoff and Kobayashi, 1980). Ketoconazole, an imidazole derivative, is now the drug of choice for systemic infection (Medoff and Kobayashi, 1980; Hay, 1982), although a higher dose ($400–500\,mg \cdot d^{-1}$ in adults) than that originally recommended may be required for some fungal diseases (Graybill *et al.*, 1982).

ASPERGILLUS

The species causing clinical disease most commonly is *Aspergillus fumigatus*. Pulmonary infection is usually caused by inhalation of spores. Aspergillosis may occur during the secondary immunosuppression of treatment for leukaemia and is less common in Hodgkin's disease or lymphoma. Of the primary immunodeficiency disorders, infections with *Aspergillus* are most common in chronic granulomatous disease, suggesting that phagocytic cells may be an important defence mechanism against this organism, although this has not been supported experimentally (Lehrer and Jan, 1970).

Patients with pulmonary infection due to *Aspergillus* present with an unremitting fever, tachypnoea and a non-productive cough. Bronchopneumonic changes are common radiologically (*Figure 8.6*); cavitation and interstitial pneumonitis may occur. In one series of 93 patients with neoplastic disease, aspergillosis was common following *Pseudomonas aeruginosa* infection (Meyer *et al.*, 1973). It was also noted in this study that Aspergillus precipitins correlated well with invasive disease but that pulmonary infection could still be present in the absence of precipitins.

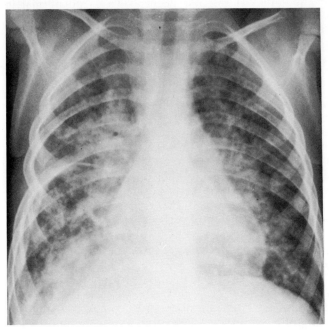

Figure 8.6 Aspergillus pneumonia in a 3-year-old boy with CGD. He had presented with a staphylococcal pneumonia 7 months previously

Diagnosis is dependent upon the histological demonstration of fungus in viable lung tissue as well as identification on culture (Williams, Krick and Remington, 1976a). Positive culture alone may reflect laboratory contamination of samples or colonization of the respiratory tract rather than true infection.

Amphotericin B has been used for many years for treatment, but results have been disappointing. Meyer *et al.* (1973) noted that survival in 14 patients treated with amphotericin alone was not related to the total dosage of amphotericin B administered, but rather to the outcome of the primary disease process.

OTHER FUNGAL INFECTIONS

Pulmonary disease due to other fungal agents in immunodeficient patients is in general much less common, although there are geographical variations. Histoplasmosis, blastomycosis, coccidioidomycosis and cryptococcosis may all occur. Ketoconazole is useful in coccidioidomycosis, histoplasmosis, chromomycosis and paracoccidioidomycosis (DeFelice *et al.*, 1982; Graybill *et al.*, 1982). Prophylactic therapy with ketoconazole afforded significantly better protection against all fungal infections in 72 severely immunocompromised patients in comparison with nystatin used in conjunction with amphotericin B in a study reported recently by Hann *et al.* (1982).

Other pulmonary abnormalities and immunodeficiency disease

Several types of pulmonary abnormality are seen in association with disorders related to acquired immunodeficiency states or disorders arising during the treatment of immunodeficiency. These may be confused with infective processes or may lead subsequently to infection. Each of the following conditions causes pulmonary damage and each leads to local and systemic alteration of the immune response.

Drug toxicity

Several drugs used as immunosuppressants have direct and indirect effects on the lung. It is over 20 years since busulphan was noted to be associated with interstitial pulmonary fibrosis (Oliner *et al.*, 1961). Several other drugs are now known to cause direct pulmonary toxicity; these include methotrexate, cyclophosphamide, 6-mercaptopurine, bleomycin and azathioprine. The characteristic lesion is a chronic interstitial pneumonia although the exact pathogenesis remains unknown (Nash, 1982). The one exception is bleomycin toxicity in which large atypical cells with hyperchromatic nuclei and prominent nucleoli are seen. Bleomycin toxicity is potentiated by oxygen therapy in experimental animals (Tryka *et al.*, 1982). Corticosteroids, used in the treatment of connective tissue disorders, nephrotic syndrome, the therapy of malignancy and in transplantation are potent immunosuppressants and thus are responsible for many infections. Anti-thymocyte globulin, used to promote graft acceptance, also predisposes to pulmonary infection (Salaman, 1983). Cyclosporin A, a drug with a selective effect on cytotoxic T cells, appears to be useful in renal, hepatic and marrow transplantation for potentiation of graft survival. This drug also leads to accentuation of immunosuppression and therefore may predispose to further infection (Editorial, 1983c).

Some antibiotics have been implicated as being immunosuppressive agents, not only by altering normal flora, but by direct effects on cells modulating the immune response (Miller and North, 1981; Hauser and Remington, 1982).

Irradiation

Radiation pneumonitis has been recognized for many years (Nash, 1982). High risk patients are those receiving field radiation to the chest. Alveolar damage with subsequent interstitial changes relates not only to the total dose received but to the time interval over which radiotherapy is administered. In bone marrow transplantation, the maximum dose of total body irradiation is limited principally by the risk of pulmonary toxicity that starts within days or weeks of irradiation. However, interstitial pneumonitis is rare below a total dose of 8 Gy (Editorial, 1983d), although others have suggested a lower dose should be given at least in marrow transplantation for acute leukaemia (Bortin *et al.*, 1982). Some drugs such as cyclophosphamide and methotrexate may lead to enhancement of the radiation injury (Phillips, Wharam and Margolis, 1975; Bortin *et al.*, 1982).

Tumour invasion

Lymphoproliferative disease may give rise to an interstitial infiltrate of lymphoid cells in the lung. Abnormal cells tend to surround blood vessels and invade the walls of bronchi, extending as far as the pleura (Nash, 1982). The lungs may also be involved diffusely in histiocytosis X; interstitial pulmonary disease may be the presenting feature of this condition (Stempel *et al.*, 1982).

Bone marrow transplantation

Interstitial pneumonitis occurred in 20% of 176 patients with acute leukaemia receiving bone marrow transplants between 1977 and 1980 who were documented by the International Bone Marrow Transplant Registry (Bortin *et al.*, 1982). The disease was fatal in 58% of those affected. Apart from the effect of radiation as described above, the risk of interstitial pneumonitis was lower when cyclosporin A rather than methotrexate was employed for post-transplantation immunosuppression, and when female cells were given to female recipients. In another study from the same group, 55% of 31 patients with interstitial pneumonitis after transplantation for acute leukaemia had no identifiable aetiological agent (Gale *et al.*, 1982). A further study of 80 patients receiving allogeneic bone marrow grafts for the treatment of acute leukaemia and aplastic anaemia demonstrated that GVHD significantly increases the incidence and lethality of interstitial pneumonia (Neiman *et al.*, 1977).

Interstitial pneumonitis and GVHD remain a major cause of treatment failure in bone marrow transplantation (Gale *et al.*, 1983). Graft-versus-host disease causes further immunosuppression directly and also allows a greater susceptibility to infection by causing damage to mucosal surfaces in the lung and in the gastrointestinal tract (Editorial, 1980b; Storb *et al.*, 1983a). In a study of 130 patients with aplastic anaemia receiving bone marrow transplants from HLA identical siblings, 11% had transient grade I acute GVHD and 34% had more severe GVHD. There was no association of GVHD with HLA-A antigens, but those with B8 antigen had an incidence of acute GVHD that was three times that of recipients who did not have the B8 antigen (Storb *et al.*, 1983b). The incidence of GVHD was reduced in those patients who had undergone bacterial decontamination and who had been treated in laminar airflow rooms.

Other lung disorders in immunosuppressed patients

Pulmonary haemorrhage may occur as a result of clotting disorders caused by therapy of the underlying condition (Nash, 1982). Fat embolization has been recorded after marrow transplantation (Paradinas *et al.*, 1983). Twelve of 35 patients receiving mismatched bone marrow from family donors for leukaemic conditions died of pulmonary oedema which was thought to be related to pulmonary vascular lesions occurring after transplantation (Powles *et al.*, 1983).

IMMUNOLOGICALLY MEDIATED LUNG DISEASE

A number of disorders of unknown aetiology may affect the lung parenchyma, the airway and the pleura. In these disorders the pulmonary disease is presumed to have an immunological basis, through the action of specific cells or their soluble products, antibodies directed against pulmonary tissues or in the form of immune complexes, or through complement activation. There is a close inter-relationship and interdependence of antibody, complement and phagocytic cells in the production of these inflammatory lesions.

Several of these disorders have been shown to be associated with a higher prevalence of particular loci within the major histocompatibility locus, suggesting that they may arise as a result of suboptimal or abnormal immunoregulation.

Disorders with specific immunological involvement

Goodpasture's syndrome

In this condition pulmonary and glomerular disease is caused by antibodies directed against basement membrane at these sites. Tissue damage is mediated by complement activation and antibody-dependent cellular cytotoxicity (Dreisin, 1981). Immunofluorescence of pulmonary tissue shows a linear deposition of IgG and complement along the basement membrane of the alveolar septae and this appearance is virtually diagnostic. IgG from serum from affected patients will attach to the basement membrane of normal lung tissue. There is a strong association between the HLA antigen DR2 and Goodpasture's syndrome (Rees *et al.*, 1978).

Systemic lupus erythematosus

Pulmonary disease, particularly pleuritis and pleural effusions, are common in systemic lupus erythematosus (SLE). In a review of the clinical and autopsy records of 120 patients aged between 8 and 79 years seen at the Johns Hopkins Hospital, pleuritis was present in 36 and was directly attributable to SLE in 22 (61%) (Haupt, Moore and Hutchins, 1981). Twenty-two patients in this series had moderate or severe pulmonary parenchymal disease, mainly interstitial pneumonitis and interstitial fibrosis. They noted that there are no pathognomic pulmonary findings in SLE. Secondary infection is common and is due to the immunosuppression related to treatment, although advanced disease also causes immunosuppression associated with uraemia.

Acute lupus pneumonitis is associated with fever, cough and hypoxia; infiltrates are seen on X-ray. IgG, IgM and complement components may be seen in the alveolar septae (Pertschuk *et al.*, 1977). However, it is difficult to be certain whether the immunoglobulin deposition is primary or occurs following pulmonary parenchymal damage due to other causes. Deposits containing DNA in association with antibody suggest a pathogenetic role for immune complexes (Eagan *et al.*, 1979). Patients with SLE without clinical pulmonary disease do not have such deposits. Changes may also be seen within pulmonary vessels as part of a widespread vasculitis. Pleural effusion fluid has low C3 and C4 levels: in studies of adult patients a pleural fluid to serum ratio of C3 and C4 of less than 0.15 was suggestive of a diagnosis of either SLE or rheumatoid arthritis (Hunger, McDuffie and Hepper, 1972).

Rheumatoid arthritis

Primary lung disease is rare in juvenile chronic arthritis although it may be seen in seropositive polyarticular disease. Immune complexes and rheumatoid factor are present in pleural effusions in adults while complement levels are low (Dreisin, 1981). Interstitial pneumonitis and fibrosis occur; airflow obstruction has been shown to be due to mononuclear cell infiltration of peribronchiolar tissue with subsequent obliteration of the small airways by fibrosis (Begin *et al.*, 1982).

Idiopathic interstitial pneumonitis and fibrosis

The morphological features of chronic interstitial pneumonia may be the final result of many differing pulmonary lesions in immunosuppressed patients (Nash, 1982). The pathological features are usually non-specific, with diffuse alveolar damage resulting in an exudative inflammatory response and a subsequent proliferative phase. The histological features have given rise to a number of different subclassifications. In bone marrow transplantation 40–55% of episodes of pneumonitis are idiopathic in nature (Neiman *et al.*, 1977; Gale *et al.*, 1982).

Several studies suggest an immunological basis for idiopathic pulmonary fibrosis (Snider, 1983). The frequency of the HLA antigen DR2 was 65% in 20 patients studied by Libby *et al.* (1983) in comparison with a frequency of this antigen of 26% in 200 healthy blood donors used as controls. Circulating T lymphocytes from some patients with idiopathic pulmonary fibrosis have been shown to be sensitized to type I collagen (Kraves *et al.*, 1976). Immune complexes found in bronchoalveolar lavage fluid from patients are able to stimulate alveolar macrophages to secrete neutrophil chemotactic factor. Neutrophils recruited to the site of inflammation may be an important cause of further pulmonary damage; oxygen-derived free radicals produced by neutrophils may be cytotoxic (Fantone and Ward, 1981) and proteases and myeloperoxidase released from neutrophils may cause further damage (Cohen, Chenoweth and Hugli, 1982; Snider, 1983). One of the major functions of α_1-anti-trypsin may be to protect the lung interstitium from neutrophil enzymes (Cohen, Chenoweth and Hugli, 1982).

Eosinophilia and pulmonary infiltrative disease

Peripheral blood eosinophilia may be seen in association with pulmonary disease due to infection (e.g. allergic bronchopulmonary aspergillosis), drug reactions (e.g. nitrofurantoin, sulphonamides), parasitic infestation, neoplasia, connective tissue diseases or unknown causes. In most of these entities a pulmonary eosinophilia also occurs but the role of the eosinophil in pathogenesis is uncertain (Schatz, Wasserman and Patterson, 1981).

Sarcoidosis

Sarcoidosis is much less common in childhood than in adults. The characteristic immunological abnormality is a generalized hyperimmunoglobulinaemia associated with deficiency of cell-mediated responses manifested by cutaneous anergy. Helper T-cell activity appears to be accentuated at sites of disease activity in the lungs (James and Williams, 1982), resulting in markedly increased local immunoglobulin production (Rankin *et al.*, 1983). Macrophages are also activated; circulating immune complexes are demonstrable but their presence is not closely correlated with pulmonary disease (Saint-Remy, Mitchell and Cole, 1983).

Hypersensitivity pneumonitis

Hypersensitivity pneumonitis or extrinsic allergic alveolitis arises in some individuals following the inhalation of organic dusts. Bird fancier's disease is the most common form seen in children. Precipitating antibodies directed against the causative antigen are present in the serum, but are not necessarily diagnostic as they may be found in normal children. Immune complex injury and cell-mediated immune responses are involved in the pathogenesis of the pulmonary disease (Davies, 1983).

References

AFZELIUS, B. A. (1976) A human syndrome caused by immotile cilia. *Science*, **193**, 317–319

AMMANN, A. J., ASHMAN, R. F., BUCKLEY, R. H. *et al.* (1982a) Use of intravenous γ-globulin in antibody immunodeficiency: results of a multicenter controlled trial. *Clinical Immunology and Immunopathology*, **22**, 60–67

AMMANN, A. J., COWAN, M. J., WARA, D. *et al.* (1982b) Acquired immunodeficiency in an infant: possible transmission by means of blood products. *Lancet*, **1**, 956–958

ASHERSON, G. L. and WEBSTER, A. D. B. (1980) *Diagnosis and treatment of Immunodeficiency Diseases: DiGeorge Syndrome.* pp. 175–179. London: Blackwell Scientific Publications

BAAR, H. S. (1955) Interstitial plasmacellular pneumonia due to *Pneumocystis carinii. Journal of Clinical Pathology*, **8**, 19–24

BALFOUR, H. H., BEAN, B., MITCHELL, C. D., SACHS, G. W., BOEN, J. R. and EDELMAN, C. K. (1982) Acyclovir in immunocompromised patients with cytomegalovirus disease. *American Journal of Medicine*, **73**, (no 1A), 241–248

BARCLAY, G. R., KELLER, A. J., VAN SOMEREN, V. and URBANIAK, S. J. (1979) Serum inhibition of lymphocyte transformation in a case of pulmonary tuberculosis. *Clinical Immunology and Immunopathology*, **14**, 449–455

BAUMGARTNER, J. D., GLAUSER, M. P., LURGO-BLACK, A. L., BLACK, R. D., PYNDIAH, N. and CHIDERO, R. (1982) Severe cytomegalovirus infection in multiply transfused, splenectomised, trauma patients. *Lancet*, **2**, 63–66

BEGIN, R., MASSE, S., CONTIN, M., MENARD, H. A. and BUREAU, M. A. (1982) Airway disease in a subset of nonsmoking rheumatoid patients. Characterization of the disease and evidence for an autoimmune pathogenesis. *American Journal of Medicine*, **72**, 743–750

BORTIN, M. M., KAY, H. E. M., GALE, R. P. and RIMM, A. A. (1982) Factors associated with interstitial pneumonitis after bone-marrow transplantation for acute leukaemia. *Lancet*, **1**, 437–439

BOXER, L. A., WATANABE, A. M., RISTER, M., BESCH, H. R., ALLEN, J. and BAEHNER, R. L. (1976) Correction of leucocyte function in Chediak–Higashi syndrome by ascorbate. *New England Journal of Medicine*, **295**, 1041–1045

BREEZE, R. G. and WHEELDON, E. B. (1977) The cells of the pulmonary airways. *American Review of Respiratory Disease*, **116**, 705–777

BRUMELL, P. A., SHEHAB, Z., GEISER, C. and WAUGH, J. E. (1982) Administration of live varicella vaccine to children with leukaemia. *Lancet*, **2**, 1069–1072

BUCHNER, C. D., CLIFT, R. A., FEFER, A. *et al.* (1982) Bone marrow transplantation. In *Recent Advances in Haematology*. Ed. A. V. Huffbrand. pp. 143–159. Edinburgh: Churchill Livingstone

BURNS, W. H., SARAL, R., SANTOS, G. W. *et al.* (1982) Isolation and characterisation of resistant herpes simplex virus after acyclovir therapy. *Lancet*, **1**, 421–423

CHANDRA, R. K. (1983) Nutrition, immunity and infection: present knowledge and future directions. *Lancet*, **1**, 688–691

CHAO, J., TURNER, J. A. P. and STURGESS, J. M. (1982) Genetic heterogeneity of dynein-deficiency in cilia from patients with respiratory disease. *American Review of Respiratory Disease*, **126**, 302–305

CHOU, S. and MERIGAN, T. C. (1983) Rapid detection and quantitation of human cytomegalovirus in urine through DNA hybridization. *New England Journal of Medicine*, **306**, 921–925

COHEN, A. B., CHENOWETH, D. E. and HUGLI, T. E. (1982) The release of elastase, myeloperoxidase and lysozyme from human alveolar macrophages. *American Review of Respiratory Disease*, **126**, 241–247

COHEN, M. S., ISTURIZ, R. E., MALECH, H. E. *et al.* (1981) Fungal infection in chronic granulomatous disease. The importance of the phagocyte in defense against fungi. *American Journal of Medicine*, **71**, 59–66

COOVADIA, H. M., WESLEY, A. and BRAIN, P. (1978) Immunological events in acute measles influencing outcome. *Archives of Disease in Childhood*, **53**, 861–867

CORBEEL, L., CORNILLIE, F., LAUWERYNS, J., BOEL, M. and VAN DEN BERGHE, G. (1981) Ultrastructural abnormalities of bronchial cilia in children with recurrent airways infections and bronchiectasis. *Archives of Disease in Childhood*, **56**, 929–933

CRUMPACKER, C. S., SCHNIPPER, L. E., MARLOWE, S. I., KOWALSKY, P. N., HERSHEY, B. J. and LEVIN, M. J. (1982) Resistance to antiviral drugs of herpes simplex isolated from a patient treated with acyclovir. *New England Journal of Medicine*, **306**, 343–346

DAVIES, D. (1983) Bird fancier's disease. *British Medical Journal*, **287**, 1239–1240

DEFELICE, R., GALGIANI, J. N., CAMPBELL, S. C. *et al.* (1982) Ketoconazole treatment of nonprimary coccidioidomycosis. Evaluation of 60 patients during three years of study. *American Journal of Medicine*, **72**, 681–687

DREISIN, R. B. (1981) Lung diseases associated with immune complexes. *American Review of Respiratory Disease*, **124**, 748–752

DUBOIS, P. J., MYEROWITZ, R. L. and ALLEN, C. M. (1977) Pathoradiologic correlation of pulmonary candidiasis in immunosuppressed patients. *Cancer*, **40**, 1026–1036

DYMINSKI, J. W., DAOUD, A., LAMPKIN, B. C. *et al.* (1979) Immunological and biochemical profiles in response to transfusion therapy in an adenosine deaminase deficient patient with severe combined immunodeficiency disease. *Clinical Immunology and Immunopathology*, **14**, 307–326

EAGAN, J. W., ROBERTS, J. L., SCHWARTZ, M. M. and LEWIS, E. J. (1979) The composition of pulmonary immune deposits in systemic lupus erythematosus. *Clinical Immunology and Immunopathology*, **12**, 204–219

EDITORIAL (1978) After splenectomy. *British Medical Journal*, **2**, 1042–1043

EDITORIAL (1980a) Antiviral treatment of varicella zoster and herpes simplex. *Lancet*, **1**, 1337–1339

EDITORIAL (1980b) Preventing graft-versus-host disease. *Lancet*, **2**, 1343–1344

EDITORIAL (1983a) Acquired immunodeficiency syndrome. *Lancet*, **1**, 162–164

EDITORIAL (1983b) Measles morbidity and malnutrition. *Lancet*, **2**, 661

EDITORIAL (1983c) Cyclosporin and neoplasia. *Lancet*, **1**, 1083

EDITORIAL (1983d) Total body irradiation preceding bone marrow transplantation. *Lancet*, **1**, 803–804

EDWARDS, K. M., ALFORD, R., GEWURZ, H. and MOLD, C. (1983) Recurrent bacterial infections associated with C3 nephritic factor and hypocomplementemia. *New England Journal of Medicine*, **308**, 1138–1141

ELIASSON, R., MOSSBERG, M., CAMNER, P. and AFZELIUS, B. A. (1977) The immotile-cilia syndrome: a congenital ciliary abnormality as an etiologic factor in chronic airway infections and male sterility. *New England Journal of Medicine*, **297**, 1–6

FANTONE, J. C. and WARD, P. A. (1981) Experimental studies of immune complex injury to the lung. *American Review of Respiratory Disease*, **124**, 743–748

FELD, R., BODEY, G. P. and GROSCHEL, D. (1976) Mycobacteriosis in patients with malignant disease. *Archives of Internal Medicine*, **136**, 67–70

FELDMAN, S., HUGHES, W. T. and DANIEL, C. B. (1975) Varicella in children with cancer: seventy-seven cases. *Pediatrics*, **56**, 388–397

FELDMAN, S., HUGHES, W. T. and KIM, H. Y. (1973) Herpes zoster in children with cancer. *American Journal of Diseases of Children*, **126**, 178–184

FIELD, H. J. and WILDY, P. (1982) Clinical resistance of herpes simplex virus to acyclovir. *Lancet*, **1**, 1125

FISCHER, T. J., MCADAMS, J. A., ENTIS, G. N., COTTON, R., GHORY, J. E. and AUSDENMOORE, R. W. (1978) Middle ear ciliary defect in Kartagener's syndrome. *Pediatrics,* **62,** 443–445

FRAYHA, H. H. and BIGGER, W. D. (1983) Chronic granulomatous disease of childhood: a changing pattern? *Journal of Clinical Immunology,* **3,** 287–291

GAIL, D. B. and LENFANT, C. J. M. (1983) Cells of the lung: biology and clinical implications. *American Review of Respiratory Disease,* **127,** 366–387

GALE, R. P., KAY, H. E. M., RIMM, A. A. and BORTIN, M. M. (1982) Bone-marrow transplantation for acute leukaemia in first remission. *Lancet,* **2,** 1006–1008

GALE, R. P., KERSEY, J. H., BORTIN, M. M. *et al.* (1983) Bone-marrow transplantation for acute lymphoblastic leukaemia. *Lancet,* **2,** 663–666

GELFAND, E. W., MCCURDY, D., RAO, C. P. and MIDDLETON, P. J. (1983) Ribavirin treatment of viral pneumonitis in severe combined immunodeficiency disease. *Lancet,* **2,** 732–733

GERRITTY, T. R., COTROMANES, E., GARRARD, C. S., YEATES, D. B. and LOURENCO, R. V. (1983) The effect of aspirin on lung mucociliary clearance. *New England Journal of Medicine,* **308,** 139–141

GIBLETT, E. R., AMMAN, A. J., WARA, D. W., SANDMAN, R. and DIAMOND, L. K. (1975) Nucleoside-phosphorylase deficiency in a child with severely defective T-cell immunity and normal B-cell immunity. *Lancet,* **1,** 1010–1013

GIBLETT, E. R., ANDERSON, J. E., COHEN, F., POLLARA, B. and MEUWISSEN, H. J. (1972) Adenosine-deaminase deficiency in two patients with severely impaired cellular immunity. *Lancet,* **2,** 1067–1069

GLUCKMAN, E., LOTSBERG, J., DEVERGIE, A. *et al.* (1983) Prophylaxis of herpes infections after bone-marrow transplantion by oral acyclovir. *Lancet,* **2,** 706–708

GOOD, R. A. (1981) Nutrition and immunity. *Journal of Clinical Immunology,* **1,** 3–11

GOTZ, M. and STOCKINGER, L. (1983) Aplasia of respiratory tract cilia. *Lancet,* **1,** 1283

GRAYBILL, D. R., CRAVEN, P. C., DONOVAN, W. and MATTHEW, E. B. (1982) Ketoconazole therapy for systemic fungal infections: inadequacy of standard dosage regimes. *American Review of Respiratory Disease,* **126,** 171–174

GREMILLION, D. H. and CRAWFORD, G. E. (1981) Measles pneumonia in young adults: an analysis of 106 cases. *American Journal of Medicine,* **71,** 539–542

HANN, I. M., PRENTICE, H. G., BLACKLOCK, H. A. *et al.* (1983) Acyclovir prophylaxis against herpes virus infections in severely immunocompromised patients: randomised double blind trial. *British Medical Journal,* **287,** 384–388

HANN, I. M., PRENTICE, H. G., CORRINGHAM, R. *et al.* (1982) Ketoconazole versus nystatin plus amphotericin B for fungal prophylaxis in severely immunocompromised patients. *Lancet,* **1,** 826–829

HAUPT, H. M., MOORE, G. W. and HUTCHINS, G. M. (1981) The lung in systemic lupus erythematosus. Analysis of the pathologic changes in 120 patients. *American Journal of Medicine,* **71,** 791–798

HAUSER, W. E. and REMINGTON, J. S. (1982) Effect of antibiotics on the immune response. *American Journal of Medicine,* **72,** 711–716

HAY, R. (1982) Ketoconazole. *British Medical Journal,* **285,** 584–585

HAYWARD, A. R., HARVEY, B. A. M., LEONARD, J., GREENWOOD, M. C., WOOD, C. B. S. and SOOTHILL, J. F. (1979) Delayed separation of the umbilical cord, widespread infections and defective neutrophil mobility. *Lancet,* **1,** 1099–1101

HERSCHFIELD, M. S., KREDICH, N. M., OWNBY, D., OWNBY, H. and BUCKLEY, R. (1979) *In vitro* inactivation of erythrocyte *S*-adenosylhomocysteine hydrolase by 2′-deoxyadenosine in adenosine deaminase-deficient patients. *Journal of Clinical Investigation,* **63,** 807–811

HIRSCH, M. S., SCHOOLEY, R. T., COSIMI, A. B. *et al.* (1983) Effects of interferon-alpha on cytomegalovirus reactivation syndrome in renal transplant recipients. *New England Journal of Medicine,* **308,** 1489–1493

HOLMES, B., QUIE, P. G., WINDHORST, D. B. and GOOD, R. A. (1966) Fatal granulomatous disease of childhood. An inborn abnormality of phagocytic function. *Lancet,* **1,** 1225–1228

HOLT, P. D. J., TANDY, N. P. and ANSTEE, D. J. (1977) Screening of blood donors for IgA deficiency: a study of the donor population of south-west England. *Journal of Clinical Pathology,* **30,** 1007–1010

HUGHES, W. T. (1977) *Pneumocystis carinii* pneumonia. *New England Journal of Medicine,* **297,** 1381–1383

HUGHES, W. T. (1983) Rifampicin for *Pneumocystis carinii* pneumonia. *Lancet,* **2,** 162

HUGHES, W. T., PRICE, R. A., SISKO, F. *et al.* (1974) Protein–calorie malnutrition: a host determinant for *Pneumocystis carinii* infection. *American Journal of Diseases of Children,* **128,** 44–52

HUNDER, G. G., MCDUFFIE, F. C. and HEPPER, N. G. G. (1972) Pleural fluid complement in system lupus erythematosus and rheumatoid arthritis. *Annals of Internal Medicine,* **76,** 357–363

JAFFE, J. P. and MAKI, D. G. (1981) Lung biopsy in immunocompromised patients: one institution's experience and an approach to management of pulmonary disease in the compromised host. *Cancer,* **48,** 1144–1153

JAMES, D. G. and WILLIAMS, W. J. (1982) Immunology of sarcoidosis. *American Journal of Medicine*, **72**, 5–8

JARVIS, W. R., MIDDLETON, P. J. and GELFAND, E. W. (1979) Parainfluenza pneumonia in severe combined immunodeficiency disease. *Journal of Pediatrics*, **94**, 423–425

JEFFRIES, D. J. and TYMS, A. S. (1983) Arildone, a potent inhibitor of cytomegalovirus infection. *Lancet*, **1**, 1214–1215

JOHNSTON, R. B., WILFERT, C. M., BUCKLEY, R. H., WEBB, L. S., DECHATELET, L. R. and MCCALL, C. E. (1975) Enhanced bactericidal activity of phagocytes from patients with chronic granulomatous disease in the presence of sulphisoxozole. *Lancet*, **1**, 824–827

JOHNSTON, R. B. and NEWMAN, S. L. (1977) Chronic granulomatous disease. *Pediatric Clinics of North America*, **24**, 365–376

JONCAS, J. H., DELAGE, G., CHAD, Z. and LAPOINTE, N. (1983) Acquired (or congenital) immunodeficiency syndrome in infants born of Haitian mothers. *New England Journal of Medicine*, **308**, 842

KALTREIDER, H. B. (1976) Expression of immune mechanisms in the lung. *American Review of Respiratory Disease*, **113**, 347–379

KAPLAN, M. H., ARMSTRONG, D. and ROSEN, P. (1974) Tuberculosis complicating neoplastic disease: a review of 201 cases. *Cancer*, **33**, 850–858

KATZ, S. M., DAMJANOV, I., CARVER, J. et al. (1977) Kartagener's syndrome and abnormal cilia. *New England Journal of Medicine*, **297**, 1011–1012

KENNY, A. B. and HITZIG, W. A. (1979) Bone marrow transplantation for severe combined immunodeficiency disease. *European Journal of Pediatrics*, **131**, 155–177

KOISTINEN, J. (1975) Selective IgA deficiency in blood donors. *Vox Sanguinis*, **29**, 192–202

KRAVES, T. C., AHMED, A., BROWN, T. E., FULMER, J. D. and CRYSTAL, R. G. (1976) Pathogenic mechanisms in pulmonary fibrosis. *Journal of Clinical Investigation*, **58**, 1223–1232

KUMAR, R. K. and PENNY, R. (1982) Cell-mediated immune deficiency in Hodgkin's disease. *Immunology Today*, **3**, 269–273

LEHRER, R. I. and JAN, R. G. (1970) Interaction of *Aspergillus fumigatus* spores with human leucocytes and serum. *Infection and Immunity*, **1**, 345–350

LEVINSKY, R. J. and TIEDEMAN, K. (1983) Successful bone marrow transplantation for reticular dysgenesis. *Lancet*, **2**, 671–673

LIBBY, D. M., GIBOFSKY, A., FOTINO, M., WATERS, S. J. and SMITH, J. P. (1983) Immunogenetic and clinical findings in idiopathic pulmonary fibrosis: association with the B-cell alloantigen HLA-DR2. *American Review of Respiratory Disease*, **127**, 618–622

MATTHAY, R. A. and GREENE, W. H. (1980) Pulmonary infections in the immunocompromised patient. *Medical Clinics of North America*, **64**, 529–551

MEDOFF, G. and KOBAYASHI, G. S. (1980) Strategies in the treatment of systemic fungal infections. *New England Journal of Medicine*, **302**, 145–155

MEYER, R. D., YOUNG, L. S., ARMSTRONG, D. and YU, B. (1973) *Aspergillus* complicating neoplastic disease. *American Journal of Medicine*, **54**, 6–15

MILLER, T. E. and NORTH, D. K. (1981) Clinical infections, antibiotics and immunosuppression: a puzzling relationship. *American Journal of Medicine*, **71**, 334–336

NASH, G. (1982) Pathologic features of the lung in the immunocompromised host. *Human Pathology*, **13**, 841–858

NEIMAN, P. E., REEVES, W., RAY, G. et al. (1977) Prospective analysis of interstitial pneumonitis and opportunistic viral infections among recipients of allogeneic bone marrow grafts. *Journal of Infectious Diseases*, **136**, 754–767

NEWHOUSE, M., SANCHIS, J. and BIENENSTOCK, J. (1976a) Lung defense mechanisms. *New England Journal of Medicine*, **295**, 990–998

NEWHOUSE, M., SANCHIS, J. and BIENENSTOCK, J. (1976b) Lung defense mechanisms. *New England Journal of Medicine*, **295**, 1045–1052

NICHOLLS, A. J., BROWN, C. B., EDWARD, N., CUTHBERTSON, B., YAP, P. L. and MCCLELLAND, D. B. L. (1983) Hyperimmune immunoglobulin for cytomegalovirus infections. *Lancet*, **1**, 532–533

OCHS, H. D., BUCKLEY, R. H., PIROFSKY, B. et al. (1980) Safety and patient acceptability of intravenous immune globulin in 10% maltose. *Lancet*, **2**, 1158–1159

OLINER, H., SCHWARTZ, R., RUBIO, F. and DAMESHEK, W. (1961) Interstitial pulmonary fibrosis following busulfan therapy. *American Journal of Medicine*, **31**, 134–139

OSTERGAARD, P. A. (1976) IgA levels and carrier rate of *Haemophilus influenzae* and beta-haemolytic streptococci in children undergoing tonsillectomy. *Acta Pathologica et Microbiologica Scandinavica (C)*, **84**, 290–298

OSTERGAARD, P. A. (1977) IgA levels, bacterial carrier rate and the development of bronchial asthma in children. *Acta Pathologica et Microbiologica Scandinavica (C)*, **85**, 187–195

OSTERGAARD, P. A. (1980) Clinical and immunological features of transient IgA deficiency in children. *Clinical and Experimental Immunology*, **40**, 561–565

OXELIUS, V. A., LAURELL, A. B., LINDQUIST, B. *et al.* (1981) IgG subclasses in selective IgA deficiency. *New England Journal of Medicine*, **304**, 1476–1477

PABST, H., WRIGHT, W. C., LERICHE, J. and STIEHM, E. R. (1976) Partial di-George syndrome with substantial cell mediated immunity. *American Journal of Diseases of Children*, **130**, 316–319

PARADINAS, F. J., SLOANE, J. P., DEPLEDGE, M. H. *et al.* (1983) Pulmonary fat embolisation after bone marrow transplantation. *Lancet*, **1**, 715–716

PAVIA, D., BATEMAN, J. R. and CLARKE, S. W. (1980) Deposition and clearance of inhaled particles. *Bulletin Europeen de Physiopathologie Respiratoire*, **16**, 335–366

PELTON, B. K., HYLTON, W. and DENMAN, A. M. (1982) Selective immunosuppressive effects of measles virus infection. *Clinical and Experimental Immunology*, **47**, 19–26

PERRY, G. S., SPECTOR, B. D., SCHUMAN, L. M. *et al.* (1980) The Wiskott–Aldrich syndrome in the United States and Canada. *Journal of Pediatrics*, **97**, 72–78

PERTSCHUK, L. P., MOCCIA, L. F., ROSEN, Y. *et al.* (1977) Acute pulmonary complications in systemic lupus erythematosus, immunofluorescence and light microscopic study. *American Journal of Clinical Pathology*, **68**, 553–557

PHILLIPS, T. L., WHARAM, M. D. and MARGOLIS, L. W. (1975) Modification of radiation injury to normal tissues by chemotherapeutic agents. *Cancer*, **35**, 1678–1684

PIFER, L. L., HUGHES, W. T. and MURPHY, M. J. (1977) Propagation of *Pneumocystis carinii in vitro. Pediatric Research*, **11**, 305–316

PIFER, L. L., HUGHES, W. T., STAGNO, S. and WOODS, D. (1978) *Pneumocystis carinii* infection: evidence for high prevalence in normal and immunosuppressed children. *Pediatrics*, **61**, 35–41

POWLES, R. L., MORGENSTERN, G. R., KAY, H. E. M. *et al.* (1983) Mismatched family donors for bone-marrow transplantation as treatment for acute leukaemia. *Lancet*, **1**, 612–615

PROBER, C. G., KIRK, L. E. and KEENEY, R. E. (1982) Acyclovir therapy of chickenpox in immunosuppressed children – a collaborative study. *Journal of Paediatrics*, **101**, 622–625

PULLAN, C. R., ROBERTON, D. M., MILNER, A. D., ROBINSON, G., PERKINS, A. and CAMPBELL, A. C. (1983) Investigation of children with abnormal cilia. *European Journal of Respiratory Disease*, **64** (Suppl. 128), 466–469

RANKIN, J. A., NAEGEL, G. P., SCHRADER, C. E., MATTHAY, R. A. and REYNOLDS, H. Y. (1983) Air-space immunoglobulin production and levels in bronchoalveolar lavage fluid of normal subjects and patients with sarcoidosis. *American Review of Respiratory Disease*, **127**, 442–448

RAO, C. P. and GELFAND, E. W. (1983) *Pneumocystis carinii* pneumonitis in patients with hypogammaglobulinaemia and intact T-cell immunity. *Journal of Paediatrics*, **103**, 410–412

REES, A. J., PETERS, D. K., COMPSTON, D. A. S. and BATCHELOR, J. P. (1978) Strong association between HLA-DRW2 and antibody mediated Goodpasture's syndrome. *Lancet*, **1**, 966–969

REINHERZ, E. L., GEHA, R., RAPPEPORT, J. M. *et al.* (1982) Reconstitution after transplantation with T-lymphocyte-depleted HLA hapolotype-mismatched bone marrow for severe combined immunodeficiency. *Proceedings of the National Academy of Science USA*, **79**, 6047–6051

ROBERTON, D. M. and HOSKING, C. S. (1983a) Epidemiology and treatment of hypogammaglobulinaemia, Victoria, Australia. *Primary Immunodeficiency Diseases, Birth Defects Original Articles Series*, **19**, 223–227

ROBERTON, D. M. and HOSKING, C. S. (1983b) Ketoconazole treatment of nail infection in chronic mucocutaneous candidiasis. *Australian Pediatric Journal*, **19**, 178–181

ROOKLIN, A. R., MCGEADY, S. J., MIKAELIAN, D. O., SORIANO, R. Z. and MANSMANN, H. C. (1980) The immotile cilia syndrome: a cause of recurrent pulmonary disease in children. *Pediatrics*, **66**, 526–531

ROORD, J. J., VAN DER MEER, J. W. M., KUIS, W. *et al.* (1982) Home treatment in patients with antibody deficiency by slow subcutaneous infusion of gammaglobulin. *Lancet*, **1**, 689–690

ROSEN, F. S., WEDGWOOD, R. J., AIUTI, F. *et al.* (1983) Primary immunodeficiency diseases: report prepared for the WHO by a Scientific Group on Immunodeficiency. *Clinical Immunology and Immunopathology*, **28**, 450–475

ROSSMAN, C., FORREST, J. and NEWHOUSE, M. (1980) Motile cilia in 'immotile cilia' syndrome. *Lancet*, **1**, 1360

RUTLAND, J. and COLE, P. J. (1980) Non-invasive sampling of nasal cilia for measurement of beat frequency and study of ultrastructure. *Lancet*, **2**, 564–565

RUTLAND, J., GRIFFIN, W. M. and COLE, P. J. (1982) Human ciliary beat frequency in epithelium from intrathoracic and extrathoracic airways. *American Review of Respiratory Disease*, **125**, 100–105

SAINT-REMY, J. M., MITCHELL, D. N. and COLE, P. J. (1983) Variation in immunoglobulin levels and circulating immune complexes in sarcoidosis: correlation with extent of disease and duration of symptoms. *American Review of Respiratory Disease*, **127**, 23–27

SALAMAN, J. R. (1983) Steroids and modern immunosuppression. *British Medical Journal,* **286,** 1373–1375

SCHATZ, M., WASSERMAN, S. and PATTERSON, R. (1981) Eosinophils and immunologic lung disease. *Medical Clinics of North America,* **65,** 1055–1071

SCHIDLOW, D. V. and KATZ, S. M. (1983) Immotile cilia syndrome. *New England Journal of Medicine,* **308,** 595

SCHUURMAN, R. K. B., VAN ROOD, J. J., VOSSEN, J. M. *et al.* (1979) Failure of lymphocyte-membrane HLA-A and -B expression in two siblings with combined immunodeficiency. *Clinical Immunology and Immunopathology,* **14,** 418–434

SEGAL, A. W., CROSS, A. R., GARCIA, R. C. *et al.* (1983) Absence of cytochrome b_{245} in chronic granulomatous disease: a multicenter European evaluation of its incidence and relevance. *New England Journal of Medicine,* **308,** 245–251

SIEGEL, R. L., ISSEKUTZ, T., SCHWABER, J., ROSEN, F. S. and GEHA, R. S. (1981) Deficiency of T-helper cells in transient hypogammaglobulinemia of infancy. *New England Journal of Medicine,* **305,** 1307–1313

SIMMONDS, H. A., PANAYI, G. S. and CORRIGALL, V. (1978) A role for purine metabolism in the immune response: adenosine deaminase activity and deoxyadenosine catabolism. *Lancet,* **1,** 60–63

SNIDER, G. L. (1983) Interstitial pulmonary fibrosis – which cell is the culprit? *American Review of Respiratory Disease,* **127,** 535–539

STAGNO, S., BRASFIELD, D. M., BROWN, M. B., CASSELL, G. H., PIFER, L. L. and WHITLEY, R. J. (1981) Infant pneumonitis associated with CMV, *Chlamydia, Pneumocystis* and *Ureaplasma*: a prospective study. *Pediatrics,* **68,** 322–329

STEMPEL, D. M., VOLBERG, F. M., PORTER, B. R. and LEWISHAM, N. J. (1982) Malignant histiocytosis presenting as interstitial pulmonary disease. *American Review of Respiratory Disease,* **126,** 726–728

STORB, R., PRENTICE, R. L., BUCKNER, C. D. *et al.* (1983a) Graft-versus-host disease and survival in patients with aplastic anemia treated by marrow grafts from HLA-identical siblings. *New England Journal of Medicine,* **308,** 302–307

STORB, R., PRENTICE, R. L., HANSEN, J. A. and THOMAS, E. D. (1983b) Association between HLA-B antigens and acute graft versus host disease. *Lancet,* **2,** 816–819

STURGESS, J. M., CHAO, J. and TURNER, J. A. P. (1980) Transposition of ciliary microtubules – another cause of impaired ciliary motility. *New England Journal of Medicine,* **303,** 318–322

SZYCHOWSKA, Z., PRANDOTA-SCHOEPP, A. and CHABUDZINSKA, S. (1983) Rifampicin for *Pneumocystis carinii* pneumonia. *Lancet,* **1,** 935

THONG, Y. H., ROBERTSON, E. F., RISCHBIETH, H. G. *et al.* (1978) Successful restoration of immunity in DiGeorge syndrome with fetal thymic epithelial transplant. *Archives of Diseases in Childhood,* **53,** 580–584

TRIGG, M. E., KOHN, D. B., SONDEL, P. M. and CHESNEY, P. J. (1983) Tracheal aspirate examination for *Pneumocystis carinii* cysts as a guide to therapy in pneumocystis pneumonia. *Journal of Paediatrics,* **102,** 881–883

TRYKA, A. F., SKORNIK, W. A., GODLESKI, J. J. and BRAIN, J. D. (1982) Potentiation of bleomycin-induced lung injury by exposure to 70% oxygen. *American Review of Respiratory Disease,* **126,** 1074–1079

TURNER, J. A. P., CORKEY, C. W. B., LEE, J. Y. C., LEVISON, H. and STURGESS, J. (1981) Clinical expressions of immotile cilia syndrome. *Pediatrics,* **67,** 805–810

VEERMAN, A. J. P., VAN DELDEN, L., FEENSTRA, L. and LEENE, W. (1980) The immotile cilia syndrome: phase contrast light microscopy, scanning and transmission electron microscopy. *Pediatrics,* **65,** 698–702

WADE, J. C., HINTZ, M., MCGUFFIN, R. W., SPRINGMEYER, S. C., CONNOR, J. D. and MEYERS, J. D. (1982) Treatment of cytomegalovirus pneumonia with high dose acyclovir. *American Journal of Medicine,* **73,** 249–256

WEBER, W. R., ASKIN, F. B. and DEHNER, L. P. (1977) Lung biopsy in *Pneumocystis carinii* pneumonia: a histopathologic study of typical and atypical features. *American Journal of Clinical Pathology,* **67,** 11–19

WESTON, W. L., HUFF, J. C., HUMBERT, J. R., HAMBRIDGE, M., NELDNER, K. H. and WALRAVENS, P. A. (1977) Zinc correction of defective chemotaxis in acrodermatitis enteropathica. *Archives of Dermatology,* **113,** 422–425

WHITELAW, A., EVANS, A. and CORRIN, B. (1981) Immotile cilia syndrome: a new cause of neonatal respiratory distress. *Archives of Disease in Childhood,* **56,** 432–435

WILLIAMS, D. M., KRICK, J. A. and REMINGTON, J. S. (1976a) Pulmonary infection in the compromised host. *American Review of Respiratory Disease,* **114,** 359–394

WILLIAMS, D. M., KRICK, J. A. and REMINGTON, J. S. (1976b) Pulmonary infection in the immunocompromised host. *American Review of Respiratory Disease,* **114,** 593–627

WINSTON, D. J., HO, W. G., RASMUSSEN, L. E. *et al.* (1982) Use of intravenous immune globulin in patients receiving bone marrow transplants. *Journal of Clinical Immunology*, **2**, 42S–47S

WINSTON, D. J., LAU, W. K., GALE, R. P. and YOUNG, L. S. (1980) Trimethoprim-sulfamethoxazole for the treatment of *Pneumocystis carinii* pneumonia. *Annals of Internal Medicine*, **92**, 762–769

WRIGHT, P. F., HATCH, M. H., KASSELBERG, A. G., LOWRY, S. P., WADLINGTON, W. B. and KARZON, D. T. (1977) Vaccine-associated poliomyelitis in a child with sex-linked agammaglobulinaemia. *Journal of Pediatrics*, **91**, 408–412

YEATES, D. B., ASPIN, N., LEVISON, H., JONES, M. T. and BRYAN, A. C. (1975) Mucociliary tracheal transport rates in man. *Journal of Applied Physiology*, **39**, 487–495

YULISH, B. S., STERN, R. C. and POLMAR, S. H. (1980) Partial resolution of bone lesions: a child with severe combined immunodeficiency disease and adenosine deaminase deficiency after enzyme-replacement therapy. *American Journal of Diseases of Children*, **134**, 61–63

9
Bronchial responsiveness in children: a clinical view

Michael Silverman and Nicola Wilson

INTRODUCTION

The concept of bronchial responsiveness arose from the observation that the airways of asthmatic subjects were especially likely to respond to irritation by narrowing. The term 'non-specific' responsiveness is sometimes used to imply that the response may be induced by a variety of stimuli in distinction to the response of a sensitized individual to a specific allergen. It is clear that bronchial responsiveness is present to some degree in all individuals. In summary this can be expressed as:

Stimulus + Bronchial responsiveness → Airway obstruction

The extreme degree of responsiveness in asthmatics is distinguished by the term 'hyper-responsiveness'.

A number of trigger stimuli can induce airway narrowing, including pharmacological agents, antigens, viral respiratory tract infections, and physical and chemical agents. Many of these form the basis of the tests for bronchial responsiveness which are described below. Airway obstruction itself may be achieved by several well-recognized pathophysiological processes such as contraction of airway smooth muscle, oedema of bronchial walls and intraluminal mucus secretion, which may affect the small or large airway to differing degrees. Other potentially important responses of the lungs to irritants include glottic narrowing and alteration in the mechanical properties of the peripheral lung tissues. These could also play a part in the response, and may interfere with tests designed to demonstrate changes in obstruction of intrathoracic airways. In normal individuals these responses can be considered as protective responses of the lower respiratory tract. To some degree, therefore, bronchial responsiveness is normal. It is possible that the mechanism of airway obstruction in normal subjects differs from that in asthmatics (Fish *et al.*, 1981; Heaton *et al.*, 1983).

The abnormalities in asthma which lead to bronchial hyper-responsiveness include exaggeration of these normal processes: excessive sensitivity to airway stimuli, imbalance of processes for controlling airway smooth muscle tone and hence airway calibre, and excessive responsiveness of bronchial smooth muscle itself. There are additional pathological processes such as abnormal mediator release by sensitized mast cells or alveolar macrophages (*Figure 9.1*). In chronic asthma, there is an excessive quantity of airway smooth muscle, as well as disordered function; excessive mucus production also occurs. A number of excellent reviews deal with the mechanisms of bronchial responsiveness in some detail (Boushey *et al.*, 1980; Neijens, Duiverman and Kerrebijn, 1983).

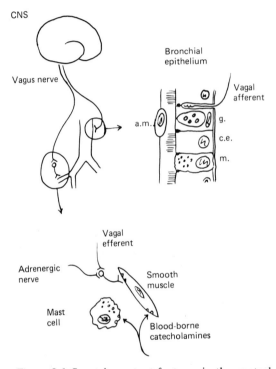

Figure 9.1 Some important features in the control of airway smooth muscle tone.
Key: a.m. alveolar macrophage; g. goblet cell; c.e. ciliated epithelial cell; m. intra-epithelial mast cell

It is possible that homeostatic mechanisms could compensate for minor degrees of responsiveness or for trigger stimuli of low potency, by reducing airway smooth muscle tone. Changes in vagal tone or in β-adrenergic stimulation could do this and might explain the need to exceed a certain threshold before a trigger can produce measurable airway narrowing.

Even though we are only just beginning to unravel possible mechanisms, in order to understand some of the mechanisms involved in obstructive airway disease in general, and in asthma in particular, the general concept of bronchial responsiveness is invaluable in clinical practice. In this review, we will consider in turn the measurement of bronchial responsiveness, its natural history and the applications of bronchial challenge tests in clinical practice.

MEASUREMENT OF RESPONSIVENESS

There are several clinical applications of tests of bronchial responsiveness (*Table 9.1*): the level of bronchial responsiveness calculated from the relationship between a carefully administered stimulus, and the degree of airway obstruction induced. The techniques of challenge and the choice of test to measure the response will be dealt with separately (Benson, 1979; Kerrebijn and Neijens, 1981; Eiser, Kerrebijn and Quanjer, 1983; Woolcock, Yan and Salome, 1983).

Table 9.1 Indications for measurement of bronchial responsiveness

(1) Assessment of child with chronic or recurrent airway disease; diagnosis of asthma
(2) Assessment of degree of responsiveness in asthma
(3) Identification of trigger stimuli in asthma
(4) Evaluation of anti-asthma therapy
(5) Clinical research
(i)   Mechanisms
(ii) Epidemiology
(iii) Drug trials in asthma

The choice of respiratory function test

The purpose of the bronchial challenge test as well as the age of the subjects, will influence the choice of lung function test (Silverman, 1983) used to measure the response. Where changes in response are being monitored in an individual subject, reproducibility is of key importance, whereas in a population survey looking at subjects whose response is expected to be small, sensitivity is of greater value.

In babies, airway resistance can be measured using a whole body plethysmograph and in children under 2 years old the effect of bronchodilators on lung mechanics has been assessed using the jacket plethysmograph (Stokes *et al.*, 1981). The use of flow-volume curves to provide information about intrathoracic airway changes in infants also seems feasible (Taussig *et al.*, 1982). All these methods could be used to measure bronchial responsiveness, but only two studies in this age group have been reported (Benoist, Volanthen and Rufin, 1981; Gutkowski, Nowacka and Migdal, 1983).

The preschool child poses a problem as there is no satisfactory method of measuring airway obstruction. Peak expiratory flow (PEF) can be used in children as young as 2 years old, but the readings are unlikely to be sufficiently reliable under the age of 5.

Over the age of about 7 years, both PEF and forced expiratory volume in one second (FEV_1), are highly reproducible (within-subject coefficient of variation in normal children of 5%) and give similar results (Henry *et al.*, 1982). Unfortunately, the technique of measurement may affect the variable being measured, since deep inspiration and forced expiration may both affect bronchial calibre. The effect is complicated, being different in normal subjects, mild asthmatics and severe asthmatics (Nadel and Tierney, 1961; Orehek, Nicoli, Delpierre *et al.*, 1981). Short-lived bronchodilatation is induced by full inspiration in mild-moderate asthma but repeated forced expiration in severe asthmatics can produce bronchoconstriction lasting for several minutes. In spite of these potential drawbacks, PEF and FEV_1 are the most frequently used measurements in bronchial challenge tests and give reproducible results (Ruffin *et al.*, 1981; Hariparsad *et al.*, 1983).

Plethysmographic measurements of airway resistance or specific conductance overcome the need for maximal respiratory manoeuvres and are tests of greater sensitivity than PEF or FEV_1, but are less reproducible (within-subject coefficient of variation in normal children is about 12%). It is difficult to get children of under 10 years of age to perform consistently in a body plethysmograph. The measurement of total respiratory impedance by the forced oscillation technique requires little subject cooperation and could be used in the younger age group, although the scatter of normal values is wide in the paediatric age group (Silverman, 1983).

Bronchial challenge tests should be interpreted in the light of the particular lung function tests used (Michoud, Ghezzo and Amyot, 1982). Comparisons between different studies or between different tests within individual patients, are not possible unless identical, well-standardized methods are used.

When performing serial measurements there are statistical reasons for taking the mean of several readings (Ullah *et al.*, 1983). However, in children it is probably wise in an effort-dependent test (such as PEF or FEV_1) to take the highest of three readings, as a child's concentration can wander, particularly when repeated tests are being performed.

Types of challenge

Nebulized pharmacological agents (histamine, methacholine, carbachol)

The principle of this form of challenge is to produce a response curve from changes in airway obstruction induced by inhalation of doubling concentrations of a bronchoconstrictor aerosol. The inhalations are continued until the required level of airway obstruction has been obtained or the maximum permitted concentration has been reached.

The important consideration is the choice of jet nebulizer for production of the aerosol. It should produce droplets 1–6 µm in diameter (e.g. Wright nebulizer: mass median diameter 1.2 µm) with narrow distribution (s.d. < 2.0 µm), the optimal size for deposition in the bronchial tree (Muir, 1972). The driving pressure and reservoir volume affect the output so these should be kept constant (Clay *et al.*, 1983; Sterk *et al.*, 1983).

Two methods of inhalation challenge have been well standardized and give similar results (Beaupre and Malo, 1979; Salome, Schoeffel and Woolcock, 1980; Juniper, Frith and Hargreave, 1981).

Tidal breathing method. After allowing time for baseline lung function to stabilize, a control solution of diluent followed by doubling concentrations of the constrictor agent is inhaled, each for a 2-minute period, using a nose clip, either via a facemask or a mouthpiece, using tidal breathing. The response to each concentration is measured serially for 3 min and the inhalations repeated at 5-min intervals until the desired change in lung function is obtained (Cockcroft *et al.*, 1977a). This is a simple procedure in young children (*Figure 9.2*).

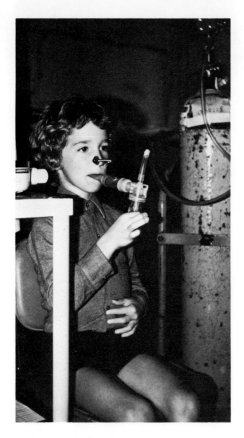

Figure 9.2 Histamine bronchial challenge test

Dosimeter method. A dosimeter is connected to a jet nebulizer so that inhalation triggers the delivery of a set amount of solution. The subject takes five maximal inhalations from functional residual capacity, initially using the diluent control solution and then inhaling doubling concentrations of the constrictor agent. The dosimeter method (Chai *et al.*, 1975) has been used in children (Shapiro *et al.*, 1982), but it requires the ability to perform consistent maximal inhalations, which may prove difficult in young children.

The initial concentration of the bronchoconstrictor agent must be low (e.g. histamine $0.03 \, g \cdot l^{-1}$) where sensitive subjects are being tested. Higher starting concentrations are permissible for less sensitive individuals. There is no refractory period after these pharmacological challenge tests, so that tests may be repeated after short intervals (e.g. 30–60 min), provided that bronchoconstriction has resolved.

Response curves are constructed using a logarithmic or an arithmetical scale for the concentration or cumulative breath units (for dosimeter method) of the constrictor agent. The concentration which produces the required airway response is calculated (*Figure 9.3*) and is known as the provocation concentration (PC) or provocation dose (PD) and represents the 'sensitivity' of the airway. Another point on the curve, the threshold at which the response is first detectable, has been advocated, but it is difficult to determine accurately (Cockcroft, Berscheid and Murdock, 1983a). Some workers stress the importance of measuring the slope of the response curve as a measure of 'reactivity' (degree of response). This index is complicated to measure and its clinical value is obscure (Dehaut *et al.*, 1983; Eiser, Kerrebijn and Quanjer, 1983).

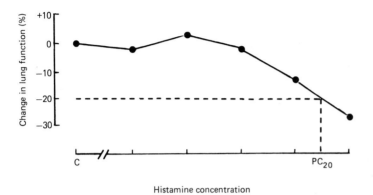

Figure 9.3 Calculation of PC_{20}: the concentration of histamine solution which provokes a 20% change in lung function

The PC is the easiest index to calculate and is the most frequently used measure of responsiveness. The minimum recognizable change in airway obstruction depends on the reproducibility of the lung function test. For PEF or FEV_1 the concentration inducing a 20% fall (PC_{20}) is used and for airway resistance (Raw) or specific airway conductance (sGaw) a 35% change (PC_{35}) is needed.

Inhaled histamine is quickly inactivated so the effect of successive inhalations is not normally considered to be cumulative. Methacholine and carbachol have a longer action (Cartier *et al.*, 1983) and the inhaled concentration can be expressed as cumulative breath units (Chai *et al.*, 1975).

Exercise testing

An exercise test is easily performed in children and for diagnostic purposes a 6-min run up and down stairs or along a corridor is sufficient to induce bronchoconstriction in many asthmatic children, albeit in a poorly reproducible manner. For a more controlled test a treadmill or bicycle ergometer is used. The exercise test has been evaluated and standardized in children using a treadmill (Silverman and Anderson, 1972). A 6-min run at a steady rate of $5-8\,km \cdot h^{-1}$, with a slope of 10–15% will produce a heart rate over 180 beats $\cdot min^{-1}$ and a positive response of more than a 15% fall in PEF or FEV_1 in most asthmatics (Silverman and Anderson, 1972; Burr, Eldridge and Borysiewicz, 1974). Those very sensitive to exercise will need a decrease in the speed or slope to reduce the stimulus. Steady-state bicycle ergometer exercise can be used in place of the treadmill. Indices of lung function are measured repeatedly to obtain a steady baseline and are then repeated at intervals after cessation of exercise, the maximum response occurring 5–8 min later. Lung function is usually back to normal by 30 min (Anderson, McEvoy and

Bianco, 1972; Silverman and Anderson, 1972), but the duration of bronchoconstriction, as in all forms of induced asthma, can be prolonged if a large response is obtained.

The severity of exercise-induced asthma is expressed by the change in PEF or FEV_1 as a percentage of the baseline value. Indices of lability incorporating the rise in PEF or FEV_1 developed during exercise, with the subsequent fall, are confusing.

There are several disadvantages to exercise challenge testing. A refractory period occurs after exercise-induced bronchoconstriction which lasts for an average of 2 h (Edmunds, Tooley and Godfrey, 1978); if the test is repeated during this period a diminished response is seen, so an interval of at least 2 h must be allowed if repeated tests are required. As the temperature and water content of the inspired air affect the response to exercise (McFadden, 1983), an air-conditioned laboratory should be used or the conditions of the inspired air controlled, if tests performed on different occasions are to be compared. The major disadvantage of the exercise test, however, is that only a single stimulus level can easily be tested. Hyperventilation challenge overcomes this problem, allowing a stimulus–response curve to be constructed.

Hyperventilation and cold air challenge

The stimulus of exercise-induced asthma can be explained by heat and water loss in the airway, produced by the increased ventilation of exercise (McFadden, 1983). For a given minute ventilation rate isocapnic hyperventilation induces a similar airway response to exercise (Kilham, Tooley and Silverman, 1979) and this form of challenge has been used in children, although it requires a little more cooperation than an exercise test.

A simple method has been described where minute ventilation is measured during voluntary hyperventilation performed to a target rate, with carbon dioxide added to the inspired air to keep the end-tidal PCO_2 constant (Kilham, Tooley and Silverman, 1979). The stimulus can be standardized as well as being potentiated by using dry air obtained from a source of compressed air (Kivity and Souhrada, 1981) or by using a heat exchanger (Ogilvie, Haresnape and Harris, 1983), so that the inspired air temperature can be reduced to as low as $-20\,°C$ (relative humidity zero) as a means of increasing the stimulus. The size of the stimulus required depends upon the responsiveness of the subject to be tested. Very mild asthmatics or normal subjects will need subfreezing air and/or high ventilation rates to obtain a measurable response whereas moderate or extremely responsive subjects will develop airflow obstruction with room air only.

Lung function is measured before the test to determine a baseline and then again serially for 20 min, after 5-min hyperventilation at a single level ($20 \times FEV_1$) or after 2-min periods of hyperventilation increasing stepwise every 5 min (as in the tidal breathing histamine challenge method), to give a stimulus–response relationship (Wilson *et al.*, 1982). The maximal response occurs a little earlier than with exercise, at 3–5 min. By the use of a stepwise increase in the rate of ventilation, children with very sensitive airways can be safely tested. However, the stimulus–response method, although useful for assessing the protective effect of drugs, is much more time consuming, less popular with the children and unnecessary as a diagnostic test for asthma.

The severity of hyperventilation (or cold-air) induced asthma can be expressed either as the maximum change from baseline after a simple challenge or as the PD_{20}

(PEF or FEV_1) or PD_{35} (sGaw) calculated from a stimulus–response study. As respiratory heat exchange under environmentally controlled conditions is directly proportional to minute ventilation, the minute ventilation is a satisfactory measure of the stimulus. The need for a great degree of subject cooperation is the most critical disadvantage for paediatric application. A refractory period exists after challenge in some children (Wilson *et al.*, 1982).

Other 'non-specific' challenge tests

Inhalation of ultrasonically nebulized distilled water has been shown to induce airflow obstruction in asthmatic but not normal subjects (Anderson, Schoeffel and Finney, 1983). The stimulus is thought to be due to alteration in the osmolality of the airway mucosa, as the effect is seen with both hypertonic and hypotonic, but not isotonic, solutions (Schoeffel, Anderson and Altounyan, 1981). The principle of the technique is to measure the response to inhalation of increasing volumes of distilled water and to note the volume that induces a 20% change in lung function. A frequently encountered problem is distressing cough at the onset of the inhalation which makes continuation of the test difficult in some subjects. If it can be tolerated, the sensation wears off and the advocates of this test claim that it is fast, simple and cheap. Its use in children has not been evaluated.

Many other irritants (sulphur dioxide, ozone) and bronchoconstrictor agents (bradykinin, leukotrienes, prostaglandins) have been used to elicit bronchoconstriction, but mainly in the context of clinical research into mechanisms of bronchial responsiveness, and rarely in children.

Antigen challenge

Antigen challenge has little application in the paediatric age group and should only be performed in specially equipped laboratories. Skin prick tests with serial dilutions of the antigen are performed to determine the most dilute solution which produces a 3-mm wheal at 20 min (Price *et al.*, 1983) and this concentration is used after the control solution, as the starting concentration of allergen for inhalation. Either a tidal breathing method or a dosimeter method can be used to deliver the aerosol. As the response to antigen is less predictable than the response to pharmacological bronchoconstrictor agents the initial inhalation period can be reduced and the monitoring interval between doses increased to 10 min, the time of onset of the maximal response. It is wise to admit subjects to hospital overnight as a late response can occur for up to 8 h and may recur (Davies, Green and Schofield, 1976; Cockroft, Hoeppner and Werner, 1984). The late response (but not the early response) can be prevented by corticosteroid therapy given before the challenge test.

The results of an antigen challenge test are expressed in a similar way to other inhalation challenge tests. The most appropriate lung function test is the FEV_1, although tests of 'small airway' function may be more appropriate to measure the late response (Murray and Ferguson, 1981). It should be remembered that the response to an antigen challenge depends on the individual's 'allergic' hypersensitivity as well as non-specific bronchial responsiveness (Bryant and Burns, 1976a; Cockcroft *et al.*, 1979).

Subject preparation for challenge testing

Drugs used for the treatment of allergic conditions and asthma will modify the response to an inhalation challenge and so they are usually stopped: inhaled β-agonists and sodium cromoglycate for 12 h and long-acting β-agonists, antihistamines and theophylline preparations for 24 h before the test. Inhaled and oral steroids are usually continued although prolonged therapy may alter bronchial responsiveness (Hartley, Charles and Seaton, 1977; Dahl and Johansson, 1982). This will obviously limit the testing of subjects with moderate or severe asthma. Under special circumstances, asthmatic subjects can be tested whilst on treatment.

It is common practice to perform challenge tests in subjects in whom the baseline lung function is >70% predicted. Although desirable this leads to bias towards selection of subjects with stable asthma. Children with poorer lung function can be tested with caution, if a progressively increasing stimulus is used. However, interpretation of results is complicated by reduced baseline lung function.

Reproducibility

Several technical factors already mentioned, such as the temperature and relative humidity of the inspired air during exercise or hyperventilation, nebulizer characteristics and pattern of breathing during an inhalation challenge, and the variability of the lung function test used, will affect the reproducibility of the bronchial challenge. These technical factors should be distinguished from the clinical and physiological factors which can alter bronchial responsiveness in an individual and which will be considered in the next section. Challenge tests repeated over short intervals in normal subjects or in stable asthmatics with normal resting lung function, will reflect the reproducibility of the test procedure independently of clinical or physiological variation (*Table 9.2*). The reproducibility of antigen challenge in children seems to be very poor (Rufin *et al.*, 1984). A state of refractoriness may occur after exercise, isocapnic hyperventilation and nebulized water challenges, so at least 2 h should be allowed before such tests are repeated.

Correlation of responsiveness measured by different methods

Histamine and methacholine inhalation tests usually give very similar results when compared under carefully controlled conditions (Salome, Schoeffel and Woolcock, 1980; Juniper, Frith and Hargreave, 1981; Aquilina, 1983). However, differences have been demonstrated in subgroups of steroid-dependent asthmatic children, suggesting that the underlying mechanisms may vary (Bhagat and Grunstein, 1984). The greater the sensitivity to these agents, the greater the response to exercise (Silverman, 1972; Anderton *et al.*, 1979). Exercise testing may be less sensitive than histamine challenge (Mellis *et al.*, 1978) since exercise employs only a single stimulus level. A closer correlation is seen between methacholine responsiveness and the response to hyperventilation using a stimulus response technique (O'Byrne *et al.*, 1982b; Aquilina, 1983).

The response to allergen challenge is not strictly comparable to other measurements of responsiveness, as individual differences in hypersensitivity to allergen will produce differences in the size of the airway stimulus produced by allergen inhalation, even for a standard dose of allergen (Bryant and Burns, 1976a;

Table 9.2 Reproducibility of tests of bronchial responsiveness

Test	Source	Method	Interval between tests (h)	Number of subjects	Variation* (%)
Histamine	Hariparsad, Wilson, Dixon et al. (1983)	Tidal breathing	1	22	8
	Cockcroft, Killian, Mellon et al. (1977b)		24	22	36
			~4	13	Within 1 dilution
Methacholine	Cockcroft, Killian, Mellon et al. (1977b)	Tidal breathing	~4	7	Within 1 dilution
Exercise	Silverman and Anderson (1972)	Treadmill run 6 min	2	8	31
Hyperventilation	Wilson, Dixon and Silverman (1984a)	Dry air 18°C	2	11	8

* Coefficient of variation (%) unless otherwise stated.

Cockcroft *et al.*, 1979). When this is statistically accounted for the correlation between allergen challenge and tests of 'non-specific' bronchial responsiveness is good (Cockcroft *et al.*, 1979) suggesting that the response to allergen challenge depends both on the degree of allergic hypersensitivity and on the non-specific bronchial responsiveness as measured by histamine inhalation.

PHYSIOLOGICAL AND CLINICAL FACTORS AFFECTING BRONCHIAL RESPONSIVENESS

The longer the interval between tests the greater the variation in bronchial responsiveness (Juniper, Frith and Hargreave, 1982). Given a standard procedure with known confidence limits, any variation beyond these limits must be due to altered subject responsiveness, real or apparent. Several factors are thought to influence bronchial responsiveness.

Baseline pulmonary function

In cross-sectional studies of asthmatic subjects, increased responsiveness is associated with a low baseline lung function. From this evidence it has been argued that a reduced prechallenge airway calibre may produce an apparent rather than a real change in responsiveness due to the exponential relationship between airway resistance and airway radius, when the response to the challenge is measured as a proportional change from baseline (e.g. PC_{20}, post-exercise percentage fall). However, several studies suggest that for an individual subject, bronchial responsiveness is independent of changes in baseline lung function for exercise testing (Silverman and Anderson, 1972), hyperventilation challenge with dry air (Wilson, Dixon and Silverman, 1984a), and histamine challenge (Cartier *et al.*, 1982). Changes in airway calibre induced by drugs also seem to have little effect on 'non-specific' responsiveness (Cockcroft *et al.*, 1977b; Chung and Snashall, 1984).

If a narrower airway alone was responsible for an apparent increase in bronchial responsiveness, then it would be expected that children, with their smaller airway size, would demonstrate a greater degree of responsiveness than adults. Although there are no complete population studies of children and adults which could settle the question, children do seem to have inherently more responsiveness to cold air challenge (Weiss *et al.*, 1984). Thus, although the relationship between the measurement of airflow and airway calibre is complicated, it seems unlikely that a reduction in airway calibre alone is responsible for the finding of increased responsiveness in conditions which produce airway narrowing.

Alterations in airway calibre may, however, alter the penetration and distribution of the trigger stimulus whether it be droplets of a bronchoconstrictor agent or antigen, or cool air. The measurable results of this effect are minimal (Chung and Snashall, 1984), although, as a precaution, it is usually recommended that where comparisons are to be made tests starting from the same baseline should be compared.

Diurnal variation

Bronchial responsiveness has been found to vary throughout the day, being greater at night (de Vries *et al.*, 1962). The reason has not been elucidated.

Recent allergen exposure

Inhalation of a known allergen which produces a late response can increase the sensitivity to inhaled histamine and methacholine in asthmatic subjects for several weeks, depending on the magnitude of the allergen-induced late asthmatic response (*Figure 9.4*; Cockcroft, 1983). The release of inflammatory mediators is

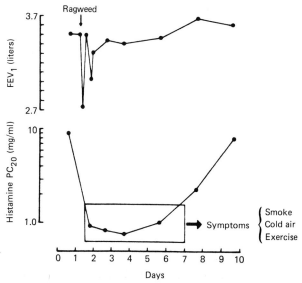

Figure 9.4 Prolonged drop in PC_{20} (increased bronchial responsiveness) after a dual reaction to ragweed pollen extract in one sensitive adult asthmatic. (Reproduced from Cockcroft, 1983, by courtesy of the Editor and Publishers of *Lancet*)

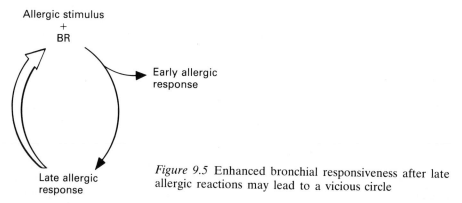

Figure 9.5 Enhanced bronchial responsiveness after late allergic reactions may lead to a vicious circle

probably responsible for the late reaction and the subsequent heightened bronchial responsiveness (Durham *et al.*, 1984). As the airway response to inhaled allergen is determined not only by the individual's immunological sensitivity to that allergen but also by the underlying bronchial responsiveness (Bryant and Burns, 1976a; Cockcroft *et al.*, 1979), it is easy to see how a vicious circle could set up with repeated exposure to an allergen enhancing bronchial responsiveness and resulting in increasingly severe asthma (*Figure 9.5*).

Patients with pollen asthma have been shown to have increased responsiveness during and for some weeks after the pollen season (Boulet *et al.*, 1983), a further illustration of the interaction between allergen and non-specific responsiveness.

Respiratory tract infections

In normal subjects following viral upper respiratory infections, an increase in 'non-specific' bronchial responsiveness (Empey *et al.*, 1976; Hobbins *et al.*, 1982) and hyper-responsiveness to exercise with cold air (Aquilina *et al.*, 1980) has been demonstrated for up to 6 weeks. Although studies have so far not been repeated in asthmatic subjects, children give a very clear history of increasing symptoms of asthma associated with colds and of increased exercise-induced asthma for a period following a cold.

Inhaled irritants

After inhalation of bronchial irritants such as ozone and sulphur dioxide, responsiveness may be increased (Orehek *et al.*, 1976; Golden, Nadel and Boushey, 1978). This has implications for asthmatic subjects living in polluted areas.

Ingested substances

Recently a whole range of ingested substances, including cola drinks, tartrazine and ice (Wilson *et al.*, 1982; Hariparsad *et al.*, 1984; Wilson, Dixon and Silverman, 1984b) as well as milk, eggs or nuts (personal observations, 1984) have been shown

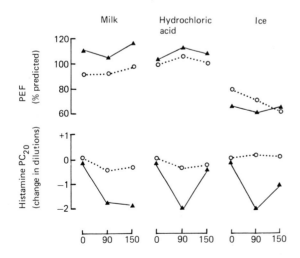

Figure 9.6 Increased bronchial responsiveness induced by food or drink in three children. In each case, the histamine PC_{20} was measured before and after oral challenge with the suspect food substance (▲) or placebo (○) using a blind technique

to increase non-specific bronchial responsiveness in asthmatic children with a history of food sensitivity (*Figure 9.6*). This increase may last for as long as 2.5 h, but is maximal 90 min after ingestion and takes place without alteration in resting pulmonary function in the majority of cases.

Short-term effect of medication on responsiveness

It is necessary to understand the effect of medication on bronchial responsiveness for several reasons. Firstly, administration can affect the results of challenge tests (*Table 9.3*) and, secondly, the efficacy and duration of treatment can be assessed by the use of a bronchial challenge. Pretreatment with drugs has been used extensively as a tool to investigate the mechanism of increased responsiveness but little further insight has yet been gained.

Table 9.3 Short-term modification of tests of bronchial responsiveness by drug treatment before challenge

Drug	Challenge test				
	Histamine	Methacholine	Exercise, hyperventilation, cold air	Allergen	
				Early response	Late response
β-Agonist	++	++	++	++	o
Methylxanthine	+	+	+	±	o
Anticholinergic	+/o	++	+/o	o	o
Cromoglycate	±	±	+	++	+
Corticosteroid	o	o	o*	o*	++
H₁ antagonist	++	o	±	o	o

++ Strong.   o None.
+ Moderate.   * Reduction in responsiveness after several weeks of treatment.
± Slight.   +/o Conflicting reports.

There are problems when investigating protection afforded by a drug which also alters resting airway calibre, as do β-agonists and anticholinergic agents. It is difficult to know how much of the effect is due to bronchodilatation. However, studies with both of these groups of drugs show that the dose required to protect against induced asthma is much greater than that required to cause maximal bronchodilatation (O'Byrne *et al.*, 1982a; Salome *et al.*, 1983). Cromoglycate has little or no effect on baseline lung function but does, to a varying extent, protect against bronchial challenge.

A pharmacological approach presupposes accurate knowledge of the actions of drugs, if it is to lead to further understanding about the mechanism of increased responsiveness. For instance, blockade by cromoglycate was considered to indicate that induced asthma was caused by degranulation of the mast cell. This interpretation is now disputed (Basran *et al.*, 1983).

Long-term variation in responsiveness

Just as clinical asthma is a variable condition, so the underlying increase in bronchial responsiveness, affected by many seasonal and environmental factors, may also change with time. The amount of variation will depend upon the individual under consideration. Those children with the greatest degree of responsiveness have the most potential for change and are also the most susceptible to allergen exposure, viral infections, atmospheric pollutants and food sensitivity. Long-term reproducibility of tests of bronchial responsiveness has mainly been carried out in subjects with mild or stable asthma and, therefore, does not reflect the changes that are seen in those more severely affected. Very sensitive individuals show a higher degree of variability in responsiveness, even from day to day, which cannot be explained in terms of airway narrowing alone (personal observations, 1984).

NATURAL HISTORY

The origins of bronchial responsiveness

Since hyper-responsiveness is such a basic feature of asthma, most work on the origins and natural history of bronchial responsiveness relates to asthma.

It would be useful to know whether infants destined to develop asthma had a more responsive airway than normal children, but there are no prospective studies of bronchial responsiveness in infancy, since the techniques for its measurement are only just becoming available (Benoist *et al.*, 1981; Stokes *et al.*, 1981; Taussig *et al.*, 1982; Gutkowski, Nowacka and Migdal, 1983). Studies of the families of wheezing children suggest that there is a hereditary element to bronchial responsiveness, independent of atopy (Konig and Godfrey, 1973; Sibbald *et al.*, 1980; Townley, 1984).

The parents of children with cystic fibrosis (obligate heterozygotes) have been shown to have increased methacholine responsiveness (Davis, 1984) but not an increased response to exercise (Silverman *et al.*, 1978). This was unrelated to the atopic state.

There are two important clinical associations with the onset of asthma in infancy. Firstly, the link between atopic disease and asthma which persists throughout childhood is such a close association that it becomes increasingly difficult in older children to dissociate bronchial hyper-responsiveness and atopic hypersensitivity. There is circumstantial evidence that cow's milk feeds may predispose to atopic disease, including asthma, in the infants of atopic parents (Burr, 1983), although it should be noted that atopy alone is not necessarily associated with increased bronchial responsiveness (Bryant and Burns, 1976b). The second major inducer of clinical asthma in infancy, independent of atopy (Sims *et al.*, 1981), is viral respiratory tract infection. This is typified by the striking onset of asthma and persistently increased bronchial responsiveness after acute viral bronchiolitis in infancy (Mok and Simpson, 1982; Pullan and Hey, 1982).

The evidence of a familial factor in bronchial responsiveness together with the observations that responsiveness may be induced by powerful environmental factors (allergic and infective) suggests the following scheme:

Inducer + Genetic predisposition → Increased bronchial responsiveness

It seems likely, although unproven, that atopy is the major inducer of bronchial responsiveness in susceptible individuals, and continued exposure to allergens may be responsible for the persistence of a state of heightened bronchial responsiveness in 'typically' atopic childhood asthma (Cockcroft, 1983). The role of recurrent viral infections in the maintenance of hyper-responsiveness in asthmatic children seems clear in clinical practice, but is also unproven.

There has been controversy over the pattern and associations of recurrent postbronchiolitic wheezing. Early studies suggesting that acute viral bronchiolitis was itself an early manifestation of asthma in children of largely atopic background (Rooney and Williams, 1971) were probably erroneous (Sims *et al.,* 1981). Recently, it has clearly been shown that children with postbronchiolitic wheezing do not have 'typical' atopic asthma. As childhood progresses, their symptoms and their bronchial responsiveness (as shown by histamine sensitivity and by exercise tests) seem to decline so that by middle childhood they are largely back to normal (Mok and Simpson, 1982; Pullan and Hey, 1982). In contrast, in the vast majority of atopic childhood asthmatics the more gradual onset of wheeze has a persistent pattern. Recently, a genetic basis for the heterogeneity of childhood asthma has been described (Ronchetti *et al.,* 1984).

Epidemiology during childhood

There are only limited population studies of bronchial responsiveness in childhood (Burr, Eldridge and Borysiewicz, 1974; Kerrebijn, Hoogeveen-Schroot and Van der Wal, 1977; Lee *et al.,* 1983). In adults there appears to be a log-normal distribution of responsiveness, i.e. a unimodal distribution (Cockcroft, Berscheid and Murdock, 1983b). We have no direct data for early childhood but it would be difficult to explain a unimodal distribution of bronchial responsiveness with atopy (population prevalence about 30%) as a major inducer of heightened responsiveness. With a prevalence of asthma of 5–10%, there should be a bimodal distribution, representing the effects of atopy in susceptible individuals leading to bronchial hyper-responsiveness. As yet this is speculative.

Since the prevalence of asthma in Britain and North America appears to change little over the middle years of childhood, it seems likely that the distribution of responsiveness likewise will remain constant over this period. In some parts of the world (e.g. rural West Africa), childhood asthma is uncommon (Abdurrahman and Taqui, 1982). The 'delayed' development of clinical asthma is not due to a low predisposition in the population since adult asthma is prevalent (McFarlane *et al.,* 1979), suggesting an environmental explanation. Longitudinal studies comparing the European and African populations could provide useful information about the relationship between environment and the development of bronchial responsiveness in childhood.

A number of conditions other than asthma have been associated with increased bronchial responsiveness: cystic fibrosis (Mellis and Levison, 1978; Silverman *et al.,* 1978; Davis, 1984), bronchiectasis (Varpela *et al.,* 1978), recurrent croup (Gurwitz, Corey and Levison, 1980; Zach, Erben and Olinsky, 1981), chronic cough (Cloutier and Loughlin, 1981). The total number of such patients is small, so that they would not be expected to show up in a population survey. These children may represent the responsive end of the normal distribution, although the pattern of responsiveness in cystic fibrosis and asthma may be different. In cystic fibrosis, responsiveness increases as lung function deteriorates and may therefore merely reflect decreased airway calibre (Mellis and Levison, 1978); in asthma, there is not a simple relationship between airway calibre and responsiveness.

Decline in responsiveness in asthmatic teenagers

Childhood asthma can remit at any age. Where viral infections alone are responsible for episodes of wheezing and presumably of increased bronchial responsiveness, as in about half of affected preschool children, the remission occurs in younger children, leaving most of them symptom free before puberty (Pullan and Hey, 1982). These children have a moderate degree of bronchial responsiveness (Lee *et al.*, 1983). Those with more hyper-reactive airways respond to many additional triggers including exercise, developing asthma of a more persistent nature. Nevertheless, childhood asthma generally ameliorates during adolescence. The only-term prospective study of bronchial responsiveness in severe childhood asthma during childhood and adolescence used standardized treadmill exercise challenge in a 10–12 year follow-up of 35 chronic asthmatics (Balfour-Lynn, Tooley and Godfrey, 1981). The overall level of responsiveness to exercise changed very little with clinical improvement (as shown by declining need for anti-asthma therapy) until a late stage in the resolution of clinical asthma, represented by the need for no further medication (*Figure 9.7*), when responsiveness declined to virtually normal levels.

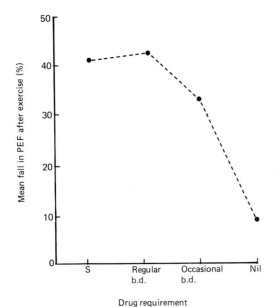

Figure 9.7 Relationship between exercise-induced asthma (EIA) and clinical asthma (as assessed by drug use) in 35 perennial childhood asthmatics, as their asthma ameliorated during puberty. Little change in EIA was apparent until clinical asthma had completely resolved. S = steroids; b.d. = bronchodilators. (From Balfour-Lynn, 1983, personal communication)

The results of this longitudinal study are thus at variance with those cross-sectional studies which have suggested an association between the severity of asthma (judged by drug therapy) and the degree of responsiveness (Juniper, Frith and Hargreave, 1981; Murray, Ferguson and Morrison, 1981). The reason for this apparent contradiction is that, whereas for groups of stable adult asthmatics, those with the most severe disease (and hence those who require most drugs) are likely to be those with the greatest bronchial responsiveness, for teenage children who are outgrowing asthma this relationship does not apply. Cross-sectional studies are misleading when applied to individuals.

The progress of one individual during the teenage years (*Figure 9.8*) shows the relapsing nature of bronchial responsiveness with exposure to a powerful natural inducer. There is other evidence of persisting bronchial responsiveness in some

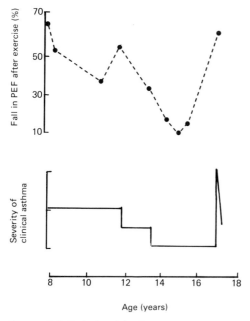

Age (years)

Figure 9.8 Relationship between exercise-induced asthma (EIA) and clinical asthma (arbitrary scale) during and after puberty in a single asthmatic boy. After a 3-year remission, symptoms and EIA recurred on exposure to a potent antigen (cat fur)

young-adult ex-asthmatics (Blackhall, 1970; Martin, Landau and Phelan, 1980) as well as recurrence of clinical symptoms in others, suggesting that adolescence may represent a quiescent phase in the natural history of asthma. Diminished responsiveness in adolescence is not merely due to avoidance of potent inducers since viral infections (albeit with reduced frequency) and allergies (as shown by positive skin prick tests) persist, but may be due to a specific physiological change perhaps hormonally induced.

Increasingly, there is interest in the relationship between increased bronchial responsiveness in childhood and adult chronic obstructive airway disease (Samet, Tager and Speizer, 1983; Phelan, 1984). Although it seems very likely that childhood respiratory symptoms are a precursor of adult chest disease, we do not know whether childhood bronchial hyper-responsiveness is the cause, or even simply an association.

CLINICAL APPLICATIONS OF MEASUREMENTS OF RESPONSIVENESS

Diagnosis of asthma

If asthma were simply the clinical manifestation of the physiological disturbance which we refer to as bronchial responsiveness, then the diagnosis of asthma could be based solely on the measurement of bronchial responsiveness. Indeed, several groups have shown a clear distinction in the level of bronchial responsiveness to a variety of stimuli between normal subjects and patients with definite current asthma as defined by other criteria (Cockcroft *et al.*, 1977a). For histamine responsiveness, the distinction between normal and asthmatic is clearer when the FEV_1 is used as the measure of response, rather than the airway conductance (Michoud, Ghezzo and Amyot, 1982; Dehaut *et al.*, 1983). This is probably because the bronchodilator effect of a deep inspiration preceding the FEV_1 manoeuvre in normal subjects and those with mild asthma fortuitously abolishes a mild response (Orehek *et al.*, 1981).

Within the whole population there is a continuum of bronchial responsiveness, with no clear dividing line between normal individuals and asthmatics (Lee *et al.*, 1983) (*Figure 9.9*). Claims that tests of responsiveness are highly diagnostic are

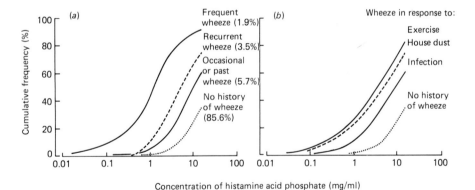

Figure 9.9 Frequency distribution of histamine responsiveness in a population of 7–8-year-old schoolchildren, according to history since school entry. The few children who had a history of wheezing during preschool years (3.3%) were not tested. (Reproduced from Lee *et al.*, 1983, by courtesy of the Editor and Publishers of *British Medical Journal*)

usually based on comparisons between groups of definite asthmatics and normal control subjects (Silverman, 1972; Zach *et al.*, 1984). Moreover, we have seen how even in asthmatics, bronchial responsiveness may vary with time, as most clearly seen in seasonal and occupational asthma. Thus, while it is likely that the detection of increased bronchial responsiveness in symptomatic individuals is indicative of current asthma, the finding of a low level of responsiveness does not exclude the diagnosis, which has to be made on other criteria, including clinical history, bronchodilator responsiveness and variability in diurnal peak flow rate, some of which may change in association with variations in bronchial responsiveness (Ryan *et al.*, 1982).

Where there is a diagnostic quandary, the measurement of bronchial responsiveness should not be thought of as an all-or-none diagnostic test for asthma, but as a means of providing a better understanding of the pathophysiology of lung disease. Increased responsiveness in children who have suffered recurrent croup or infantile bronchiolitis implies that variable airway obstruction could be playing a part in later lung disease. By recognizing this, treatment of symptomatic individuals can be more rationally planned. Similarly in cystic fibrosis and bronchiectasis, tests of bronchial responsiveness should be seen as providing better understanding of the pathophysiology of airway obstruction, and not as a means of adding another diagnostic label. The recognition that in these conditions, airway obstruction can have a variable component, can lead to better treatment.

Measurement of bronchial responsiveness is of least help where it is most needed in the diagnosis of asthma in preschool children who exhibit patterns of illness which are not clearly diagnostic of asthma, such as recurrent night cough or recurrent 'bronchitis'. Although the reversibility of airway obstruction with bronchodilators may, with difficulty, be measured in this age group, no reliable bronchial provocation techniques have been developed.

There is clearly a need for prospective studies in order to determine the role of tests of bronchial responsiveness in the diagnosis of asthma in children. On a more general level, however, there is no doubt that they play a part in the evaluation of any schoolchildren with chronic respiratory disease.

Assessment of severity of asthma

The value of isolated lung function measurements in the management of chronic asthma has often been questioned. They clearly have an 'educational' role, allowing parent, child and doctor to relate the subjective symptoms and physical signs *of the moment* to objective measurements of airway obstruction. Tests of bronchial responsiveness take the process of assessment one stage further, allowing the physician to determine, whatever the prevailing level of airways obstruction, the *potential* severity of an acute attack of asthma. Even children with very sensitive airways (e.g. histamine $PC_{20} < 0.5 \, g \cdot l^{-1}$) may have deceptively normal lung function and few symptoms, especially if they generally take continuous anti-asthma medication. An indication of extreme bronchial responsiveness can provide both a warning of problems ahead and the justification for continued medication.

Because the level of bronchial responsiveness varies from time to time, the converse is unfortunately not true: the finding of a low level of responsiveness is not a guarantee of immunity from asthma in the future (*Figure 9.8*)!

Identification of specific provoking factors

Bronchial challenge can be used to assess the relevance of possible precipitating factors in a child's asthma either by direct challenge with the specific factor (inhaled allergen, exercise) or by seeking an indirect change in bronchial responsiveness after exposure to the suspected agent.

INHALED ALLERGENS

Since a positive IgE-mediated response, as shown by a radioallergosorbent technique (RAST) or skin prick test, does not necessarily imply bronchial sensitivity to a particular allergen, an inhalation challenge can be of practical value. For example, bronchial challenge with animal dander can help elucidate the vexed question of pet sensitivity. It has also been used to identify the select group of subjects in whom hyposensitization therapy *may* be tried (Warner, 1976). In clinical practice, however, inhalant allergen provocation tests are rarely used because they are time consuming, potentially dangerous, poorly standardized and because they may provoke a long-lasting increase in bronchial responsiveness if a dual reaction occurs (*Figure 9.4*; Cockcroft, 1983).

EXERCISE

Exercise is a provoking factor in almost all asthmatic children. It is sometimes valuable to assess the degree of exercise-induced asthma in an individual child. Pretreatment with a drug can allow the physician to determine the degree of protection afforded and to make appropriate adjustments to dosage and therapy.

FOOD

A history of asthma induced by food or drinks is not uncommon in childhood asthma (Wilson and Silverman, 1985). Often a history of food sensitivity cannot be confirmed after double-blind challenge, by measurements of lung function alone (Bock *et al.*, 1978), whereas bronchial responsiveness can be shown to increase dramatically (*Figure 9.6*). By using histamine challenge tests before and after the suspected item has been ingested, we have shown that a wide range of ingested substances can increase bronchial responsiveness under placebo-controlled and often under double-blind conditions (*Figure 9.6*). A decrease of more than one dilution in histamine PC_{20} is considered a significant change. The incriminated substances include cola drinks (Wilson *et al.*, 1982), tartrazine (Hariparsad *et al.*, 1984), egg, peanuts, food cooked in oil, sodium metabisulphite, as well as ice (Wilson, Dixon and Silverman, 1985) and dilute hydrochloric acid (in many asthmatic patients with nocturnal gastro-oesophageal reflux). In only 2 out of 40 positive challenge tests would it have been possible to detect the bronchial effect of the ingested substance by measuring PEF alone (personal observations, 1984). It is most likely that numerous other items in a child's diet can effect bronchial responsiveness in this way.

The measurement of bronchial responsiveness with histamine (or methacholine) should have wide application to the identification of triggers, since it is sufficiently sensitive to permit the assessment of environmentally appropriate doses of suspected agents. Unfortunately, late effects of ingested foods or other triggers cannot easily be recognized because the reproducibility of the histamine PC_{20} declines with time.

ENVIRONMENTAL FACTORS

Occupational asthma may be caused by exposure to potent environmental allergens. The diagnosis can be made by the appropriate specific bronchial challenge or by seeking a change in 'non-specific' responsiveness after exposure. Although children are unlikely to be implicated in industrial hazards, there could be occasion to assess environmental factors (school pets, agricultural agents) in this way. Conversely, demonstration of reduced bronchial responsiveness after avoidance of suspected environmental allergens, has been shown to be useful in children (Murray and Ferguson, 1983).

Drug treatment of asthma

While it is true that in cross-sectional studies the greater the level of bronchial responsiveness the greater the need for anti-asthma therapy, the relationship is too vague to be of help in deciding how to treat an individual patient, except that extreme hyper-responsiveness (e.g. histamine $PC_{20} < 0.25\,g \cdot l^{-1}$) should be a warning to step up the level of treatment. In choosing the appropriate treatment for an individual patient, it is important to realize that drugs which reduce responsiveness cannot be assessed merely by their bronchodilator action. This is most clearly illustrated by the drug sodium cromoglycate which effectively diminishes the early responses to exercise or antigen, but has virtually no bronchodilator effect. Conversely, drugs classified as 'bronchodilators' (β_2-adrenergic and anticholinergic drugs) produce maximum baseline bronchodilatation at doses which are quite inadequate to protect against a powerful bronchoconstrictor stimulus (O'Byrne *et al.*, 1982a; Salome *et al.*, 1983). Hence bronchial responsiveness tests are needed to assess anti-asthma drugs both for individual patients and in the more general context of drug trials. Short-term laboratory tests provide only a barely significant predictor of the long-term outcome of treatment in chronic childhood asthma (Silverman *et al.*, 1972). The duration of action of a drug can be assessed by carrying out a series of challenge tests in the few hours after dosing (Bar-Yishay *et al.*, 1983), the interval between tests depending on any carry-over effect (e.g. refractoriness) between one test and another.

There are several problems in measuring drug-induced changes in responsiveness: the dose of a drug required to abolish the response to a challenge may depend not only on the physiological mechanisms involved in the response, but also on the degree of responsiveness of the individual patient and on the potency of the challenge stimulus (*Table 9.4*). The importance of all these variables has been

Table 9.4 Drugs and bronchial responsiveness: problems of interpretation

Problem	Effect
Altered baseline lung function	Probably has little effect on measured responsiveness
Variations in responsiveness within or between individuals	Efficacy of drug may vary with responsiveness; in general only mild asthmatics are tested
Level of stimulus applied	Effective drug doses may be quite different for weak and potent stimuli
Drug dose used	There is no single effective dose; single-dose studies provide little useful information

demonstrated in studies of the effects of sympathomimetic (O'Byrne *et al.*, 1982a; Salome *et al.*, 1983) or anticholinergic (Wilson, Dixon and Silverman, 1984) agents on hyperventilation asthma.

Assessing the efficacy of treatment

If bronchial hyper-responsiveness is fundamental in asthma, then the aims of treatment may be seen not only as the removal of symptomatic airway obstruction but the reduction of bronchial responsiveness itself. Insufficient long-term studies have been performed to know whether this is feasible, but in seasonal asthma, double-blind treatment with sodium cromoglycate during the pollen season has been claimed to reduce seasonally enhanced bronchial responsiveness (Cole and Simpson, 1982). Treatment of chronic perennial childhood asthmatics with sodium cromoglycate, corticosteroids and bronchodilators has not lead to persistent changes in bronchial responsiveness despite good control of asthmatic symptoms (Silverman, 1972; Silverman *et al.*, 1972; Balfour-Lynn, Tooley and Godfrey, 1981). Fluctuations in bronchial responsiveness in severe perennial asthma make it difficult to interpret changes in responsiveness to particular treatment regimes in individual patients.

Research into mechanisms of asthma

The ability of a particular group of drugs to modify tests of bronchial responsiveness is often used as evidence that a certain mechanism is involved in the process of increased responsiveness. Anticholinergic agents have most frequently been used in this way, in an attempt to incriminate a vagal reflex, particularly in exercise-induced asthma, using exercise (Hartley and Davies, 1980), cold air challenge (Griffin *et al.*, 1982) or hyperventilation (Wilson *et al.*, 1982). The results have often been conflicting mainly because of variation in the type of challenge and mode of administration as well as several other factors (*Table 9.4*).

Modulation of the response to inhaled histamine by different drugs has also been used to suggest that α-receptor activity (Barnes, Wilson and Vickers, 1981), altered calcium flux (Williams *et al.*, 1981) and increased prostaglandin release (Walters, 1981) may play a part in the mechanism of increased bronchial responsiveness. The ability of inhaled cromoglycate to blunt or abolish the response to a variety of forms of induced asthma was, until recently, considered evidence of mast cell involvement, but as there is now growing evidence that there are many other theoretical means by which cromoglycate may act (Basran *et al.*, 1983), this conclusion is no longer justified.

The period of relative refractoriness which follows some forms of bronchial challenge has intrigued several groups. The possibility that it represented partial exhaustion of 'mediators' of bronchoconstriction has been partly borne out (Wilson *et al.*, 1982). Cross-refractoriness between different challenge procedures suggest common pathways which it would be profitable to explore (Weiler-Ravell and Godfrey, 1981).

The pharmacological approach to the study of the underlying mechanisms of bronchial responsiveness has suggested several possibilities but as yet no unifying concept. Further work in this field may give the answer.

CONCLUSIONS AND FUTURE DEVELOPMENTS

The role of bronchial responsiveness in the pathogenesis of childhood respiratory disease is becoming clearer. The recognition that there is no sharp dividing line between normal and abnormal responsiveness may at first seem disappointing, particularly to those who view bronchial challenge tests as diagnostic procedures for asthma. Its consequence is that we can begin to see how differences between individuals can provide a basis for understanding the variations in patterns of both acute and chronic illness.

Laboratory tests of bronchial responsiveness measure only acute changes in response, usually to a single stimulus. The brevity of response and the ease with which airway obstruction reverses with β-agonists is taken to imply that its basis is airway smooth muscle contraction. While this sort of model can only explain to a very limited extent the pathophysiology of severe chronic asthma, we have suggested that useful clinical information can be gained from bronchial challenge tests.

Standardized bronchial challenge tests for adult use can be applied to older children (Eiser, Kerrebijn and Quanjer, 1983), but there is no generally recognized procedure for challenge tests in infants and preschool children. Progress in understanding the pathogenesis of respiratory disease in childhood will await the development of these techniques. The origins of adult chronic obstructive airway disease may have their origin in childhood. Evidence in adults suggests that bronchial responsiveness may be implicated, lending urgency to prospective studies of at-risk populations, from early infancy. If a causal relationship were found between increased bronchial responsiveness in infancy and adult lung disease, then its prevention would be a major public health concern.

Airway disease of infancy and early childhood is poorly classified and treated because of the limited techniques available for investigation, so that the role of bronchial responsiveness is undefined. Even when responsiveness does appear to be enhanced, for instance in the energetic toddler who develops exercise-induced wheeze, drugs which are useful in older subjects often seem ineffective (Milner and Henry, 1982; Silverman, 1984).

If the central problem in asthma is bronchial hyper-responsiveness, then it would be appropriate not merely to avoid trigger factors (Murray and Ferguson, 1983) or to improve airway obstruction with bronchodilators, but to tackle the responsiveness itself (Cole and Simpson, 1982). This may already be possible in individuals whose asthma is induced by a single major stimulus (e.g. pollen-sensitive seasonal asthma). However, regular inhaled corticosteroids or sodium cromoglycate do not seem to affect the natural history of bronchial responsiveness in uncontrolled observations of chronic perennial childhood asthma (Balfour-Lynn, Tooley and Godfrey, 1981). It is probable that research into the cellular mechanisms of bronchial hyper-responsiveness will lead to treatment designed to block its induction at a more fundamental level. When this is achieved, it may really be possible to alter the natural history of bronchial responsiveness in children, bringing benefits which could well be lifelong.

Acknowledgements

We thank our technicians, Helen Vickers and Caroline Dixon, for loyal help and the Asthma Research Council and Boehringer Ingelheim (UK) for their continued financial support.

References

The references which we have quoted do not imply precedence. We have chosen the most recent suitable evidence.

ABDURRAHMAN, M. and TAQUI, A. M. (1982) Childhood asthma in northern Nigeria. *Clinical Allergy*, **12**, 379–384

ANDERSON, S. D., MCEVOY, J. D. S. and BIANCO, S. (1972) Changes in lung volumes and airways resistance following exercise in asthmatic subjects. *American Review of Respiratory Disease*, **106**, 30–37

ANDERSON, S. D., SCHOEFFEL, R. E. and FINNEY, M. (1983) Evaluation of ultrasonically nebulised solutions for provocation testing in patients with asthma. *Thorax*, **38**, 284–291

ANDERTON, R. C., CUFF, M. T., FRITH, P. A., COCKCROFT, D. W., MORSE, J. L., JONES, N. L. *et al.* (1979) Bronchial responsiveness to inhaled histamine and exercise. *Journal of Allergy and Clinical Immunology*, **63**, 315–320

AQUILINA, A. T. (1983) Comparison of airway reactivity induced by histamine, methacholine and isocapnic hyperventilation in normal and asthmatic subjects. *Thorax*, **38**, 766–770

AQUILINA, A. T., HALL, W. J., DOUGLAS, R. G. and UTELL, M. J. (1980) Airway reactivity in subjects with viral upper respiratory tract infections: the effects of exercise and cold air. *American Review of Respiratory Disease*, **122**, 3–10

BALFOUR-LYNN, L., TOOLEY, M. and GODFREY, S. (1981) Relationship of exercise-induced asthma to clinical asthma in childhood. *Archives of Disease in Childhood*, **56**, 450–454

BAR-YISHAY, E., GUR, I., LEVY, M., VOLOZNI, D. and GODFREY, S. (1983) Duration of action of sodium cromoglycate in exercise-induced asthma: comparison of two formulations. *Archives of Disease in Childhood*, **58**, 624–627

BARNES, P. J., WILSON, N. M. and VICKERS, H. (1981) Prazosin, an alpha$_1$-adrenoceptor antagonist, partially inhibits exercise-induced asthma. *Journal of Allergy and Clinical Immunology*, **68**, 411–415

BASRAN, G. S., PAGE, C. P., PAUL, W. and MORLEY, J. (1983) Cromoglycate (DSCG) inhibits response to platelet activating factor (PAF- acether) in man: an alternative mode of action for DSCG in asthma. *European Journal of Pharmacology*, **86**, 143–144

BEAUPRE, A. and MALO, J. J. (1979) Comparison of histamine bronchial challenges with Wright nebuliser and the dosimeter. *Clinical Allergy*, **9**, 575–583

BENOIST, M. R., VOLANTHEN, M. C., RUFIN, P. and JEAN, R. (1981) Apports des tests de provocation bronchique chez le nourrisson. *Respiration*, **42** (suppl. 1) 51–52

BENSON, M. K. (1979) Bronchial provocation tests. *British Journal of Clinical Pharmacology*, **8**, 417–424

BHAGAT, R. G. and GRUNSTEIN, M. M. (1984) Comparison of responsiveness to methacholine, histamine and exercise in subgroups of asthmatic children. *American Review of Respiratory Disease*, **129**, 221–224

BLACKHALL, M. I. (1970) Ventilatory function in subjects with childhood asthma who have become symptom free. *Archives of Disease in Childhood*, **45**, 363–366

BOCK, S. A., WAI LING, L., RENNIGO, L. K. and MAY, C. D. (1978) Studies of hypersensitivity reactions to foods in infants and children. *Journal of Allergy and Clinical Immunology*, **62**, 327–334

BOULET, I-P., CARTIER, M., THOMSON, N. C., ROBERTS, R. S., TECH, M. *et al.* (1983) Asthma and increases in non-allergic bronchial responsiveness from seasonal pollen exposure. *Journal of Allergy and Clinical Immunology*, **71**, 399–406

BOUSHEY, H. A., HOLTZMAN, M. J., SHELLER, J. R. and NADEL, J. A. (1980) Bronchial hyper-reactivity. *American Review of Respiratory Diseases*, **121**, 389–413

BRYANT, D. H. and BURNS, M. W. (1976a) Bronchial histamine reactivity: its relationship to the reactivity of the bronchi to allergens. *Clinical Allergy*, **6**, 523–532

BRYANT, D. H. and BURNS, M. W. (1976b) The relationship between bronchial histamine reactivity and atopic status. *Clinical Allergy*, **6**, 373–381

BURR, M. L. (1983) Does infant feeding affect the risk of allergy. *Archives of Disease in Childhood*, **53**, 561–565

BURR, M. L., ELDRIDGE, B. A. and BORYSIEWICZ, L. K. (1974) Peak expiratory flow rates before and after exercise in schoolchildren. *Archives of Disease in Childhood*, **49**, 923–926

CARTIER, A., MALO, J-L., BEGIN, P., SESTIER, M. and MARTIN, R. R. (1983) Time course of the bronchoconstriction induced by inhaled histamine and methacholine. *Journal of Applied Physiology*, **54**, 821–826

CARTIER, A., THOMSON, N. C., FRITH, P. A., ROBERTS, R. and HARGREAVE, F. E. (1982) Allergen-induced increase in bronchial responsiveness to histamine: relationship to the late asthmatic response and change in airway calibre. *Journal of Allergy and Clinical Immunology*, **70**, 170–177

CHAI, H., FARR, R. S., FROEHLICH, L. A., MATHISON, D. A., MCLEAN, J. A. et al. (1975) Standardisation of bronchial inhalation challenge procedures. *Journal of Allergy and Clinical Immunology*, **56,** 323 327

CHUNG, K. F. and SNASHALL, P. D. (1984) Effect of prior bronchoconstriction on the airway response to histamine in normal subjects. *Thorax*, **39,** 40–45

CLAY, M. M., PAVIA, D., NEWMAN, S. P., LENNARD-JONES, T. and CLARKE, S. W. (1983) Assessment of jet nebulisers for lung aerosol therapy. *Lancet*, **2,** 592–594

CLOUTIER, M. M. and LOUGHLIN, G. M. (1981) Chronic cough in children: a manifestation of airway hyper-reactivity. *Pediatrics*, **67,** 6–12

COCKCROFT, D. W. (1983) Mechanism of perennial allergic asthma. *Lancet*, **ii,** 253–256

COCKCROFT, D. W., BERSCHEID, B. A. and MURDOCK, K. Y. (1983a) Measurement of responsiveness to inhaled histamine using FEV_1: comparison of PC_{20} and threshold. *Thorax*, **38,** 523–526

COCKCROFT, D. W., BERSCHEID, B. A. and MURDOCK, K. Y. (1983b) Unimodal distribution of bronchial responsiveness to inhaled histamine in a random population. *Chest*, **83,** 751–754

COCKCROFT, D. W., HOEPPNER, V. H. and WERNER, G. D. (1984) Recurrent nocturnal asthma after bronchoprovocation with western Red Cedar sawdust: association with acute increase in non-allergic bronchial responsiveness. *Clinical Allergy*, **14,** 61–68

COCKCROFT, D. W., KILLIAN, D. N., MELLON, J. J. A. and HARGREAVE, F. E. (1977a) Bronchial reactivity to inhaled histamine: a method and a clinical survey. *Clinical Allergy*, **7,** 235–243

COCKCROFT, D. W., KILLIAN, D. N., MELLON, J. J. A. and HARGREAVE, F. E. (1977b) Protective effect of drugs on histamine-induced asthma. *Thorax*, **32,** 429–437

COCKCROFT, D. W., RUFFIN, R. E., FRITH, P. A., CARTIER, A., JUNIPER, E. F., DOLOVITCH, J. et al. (1979) Determinants of allergen-induced asthma: dose of allergens, circulating IgE antibody concentration, and bronchial responsiveness to inhaled histamine. *American Review of Respiratory Disease*, **120,** 1053–1058

COLE, M. and SIMPSON, W. T. (1982) Bronchial hyper-reactivity and the effect of sodium cromoglycate. *Modern Problems in Paediatrics*, **21,** 104–112

DAHL, R. and JOHANSSON, S. A. (1982) Importance of duration of treatment with inhaled budesonide on the immediate and late bronchial reaction. *European Journal of Respiratory Disease*, Suppl. 122, 167–175

DAVIES, R. J., GREEN, M. and SCHOFIELD, N. M. C. (1976) Recurrent nocturnal asthma after exposure to grain dust. *American Review of Respiratory Diseases*, **114,** 1011–1019

DAVIS, P. B. (1984) Autonomic and airway activity in obligate heterozygotes for cystic fibrosis. *American Review of Respiratory Disease*, **129,** 911–914

DE VRIES, K., GOEI, J. T., BOOJ-NOORD, H. and ORIE, N. G. M. (1962) Changes during 24 hours in the lung function and hyper-reactivity of the bronchial tree in asthmatic and bronchitic patients. *International Archives of Allergy*, **20,** 93–101

DEHAUT, P., RACHIELE, A., MARTIN, R. R. and MALO, J-L. (1983) Histamine dose–response curves in asthma: reproducibility and sensitivity of different indices to assess response. *Thorax*, **38,** 516–522

DURHAM, S. R., LEE, T. H., SHAW, R. J. et al. (1984) Immunological studies in allergen-induced late-phase asthmatic reactions. *Journal of Allergy and Clinical Immunology*, **74,** 49–60

EDMUNDS, A. T., TOOLEY, M. and GODFREY, S. (1978) The refractory period following exercise induced asthma, its duration, and its relation to the severity of exercise. *American Review of Respiratory Disease*, **117,** 247–254

EISER, N. M., KERREBIJN, K. F. and QUANJER, P. H. (1983) Guidelines for standardisation of bronchial challenges with (non-specific) bronchoconstricting agents. *Bulletin European de Physiopathologie Respiratoire*, **9,** 495–514

EMPEY, D. W., LAITINEN, L. A., JACOBS, L., GOLD, W. M. and NADEL, S. A. (1976) Mechanisms of bronchial hyper-reactivity in normal subjects after upper respiratory tract infection. *American Review of Respiratory Disease*, **113,** 131–139

FISH, J. E., ITKIN, M. G., ADKINSON, N. F. and PETERMAN, V. I. (1981) Indomethacin modification of immediate-type immunologic airway responses in allergic asthmatic and non-asthmatic subjects. *American Review of Respiratory Disease*, **123,** 609–614

GOLDEN, J. A., NADEL, J. A. and BOUSHEY, H. A. (1978) Bronchial hyper-irritability in healthy subjects after exposure to ozone. *American Review of Respiratory Disease*, **118,** 287–294

GRIFFIN, M. P., FUNG, K. F., INGRAM, R. H. and MCFADDEN, E. R. (1982) Dose response effects of atropine on thermal stimulus–response relationships in asthma. *Journal of Applied Physiology*, **53,** 1576–1582

GURWITZ, D., COREY, M. and LEVISON, H. (1980) Pulmonary function and bronchial reactivity in children after croup. *American Review of Respiratory Disease*, **122,** 95–99

GUTKOWSKI, P., NOWACKA, K. and MIGDAL, M. (1983) Bronchial reactivity in babies studied by inhalation provocation tests. *Bulletin, European de Physiopathologie Respiratoire*, **19,** 5p

HARIPARSAD, D., WILSON, N., DIXON, C. and SILVERMAN, M. (1983) Reproducibility of histamine challenge tests in asthmatic children. *Thorax,* **38,** 258–260

HARIPARSAD, D., WILSON, N., DIXON, C. and SILVERMAN, M. (1984) Oral tartrazine in childhood asthma: effect on bronchial reactivity. *Clinical Allergy,* **14,** 81–85

HARTLEY, J. P. R., CHARLES, T. J. and SEATON, A. (1977) Betamethasone valerate inhalation and exercise-induced asthma in adults. *British Journal of Diseases of the Chest,* **71,** 253–258

HARTLEY, J. P. R. and DAVIES, B. H. (1980) Cholinergic blockade in the prevention of exercise -induced asthma. *Thorax,* **35,** 680–685

HEATON, R. W., HENDERSON, A. F., GRAY, B. J. and COSTELLO, J. F. (1983) The bronchial response to cold air challenge: evidence for different mechanisms in normal and asthmatic subjects. *Thorax,* **38,** 506–511

HENRY, R. L., MELLIS, C. M., SOUTH, R. T. and SIMPSON, S. J. (1982) Comparison of peak expiratory flow rate and forced expiratory volume in one second in histamine challenge studies in children. *British Journal of Diseases of the Chest,* **76,** 167–170

HOBBINS, T. E., HUGHES, T. P., RENNELS, M. B., MURPHY, B. R. and LEVINE, M. M. (1982) Bronchial reactivity in experimental infections with influenza virus. *Journal of Infectious Diseases,* **146,** 468–471

JUNIPER, E. F., FRITH, P. A. and HARGREAVE, F. E. (1981) Airway responsiveness to histamine and methacholine: relationship to minimum treatment to control symptoms of asthma. *Thorax,* **36,** 575–579

JUNIPER, E. F., FRITH, P. A. and HARGREAVE, F. E. (1982) Long-term stability of bronchial responsiveness to histamine. *Thorax,* **37,** 288–291

KERREBIJN, K. F., HOOGEVEEN-SCHROOT, H. C. A. and VAN DER WAL, M. C. (1977) Chronic non-specific respiratory disease in children, a five-year follow-up study. *Acta Paediatrica Scandinavica,* Suppl. 261,

KERREBIJN, K. F. and NEIJENS, H. J. (1981) Measurement of bronchial responsiveness in children. *Progress in Respiratory Research,* **17,** 143–154

KILHAM, M., TOOLEY, M. and SILVERMAN, M. (1979) Running, walking and hyperventilation causing asthma in children. *Thorax,* **34,** 582–586

KIVITY, S. and SOUHRADA, J. F. (1981) A new diagnostic test to assess airway reactivity in asthmatics. *Clinical Respiratory Physiology,* **17,** 243–254

KONIG, P. and GODFREY, S. (1973) Exercise induced bronchial lability and atopic status of families of infants with wheezy bronchitis. *Archives of Disease in Childhood,* **48,** 942–946

LEE, D. A., WINSLOW, N. R., SPEIGHT, A. N. D. and HEY, E. N. (1983) Prevalence and spectrum of asthma in childhood. *British Medical Journal,* **286,** 1256–1258

McFADDEN, E. R. (1983) Respiratory heat and water exchange: physiological and clinical implications. *Journal of Applied Physiology,* **54,** 331–336

McFARLANE, J. T., BACHELOR, M., RIDYARD, J. B. and BALL, P. A. J. (1979) Asthma IgE and environment in northern Nigeria. *Clinical Allergy,* **9,** 333–337

MARTIN, A. J., LANDAU, L. I. and PHELAN, P. D. (1980) Lung function in young adults who had asthma in childhood. *American Review of Respiratory Disease,* **122,** 609–616

MELLIS, C. M., KATTAN, M., KEANS, T. G. and LEVISON, H. (1978) Comparative study of histamine and exercise challenges in asthmatic children. *American Review of Respiratory Disease,* **117,** 911–915

MELLIS, C. M. and LEVISON, H. (1978) Bronchial reactivity in cystic fibrosis. *Pediatrics,* **61,** 446–450

MICHOUD, M. C., GHEZZO, H. and AMYOT, R. (1982) A comparison of pulmonary function tests used for bronchial challenges. *Bulletin European de Physiopathologie Respiratoire,* **18,** 609–621

MILNER, A. D. and HENRY, R. L. (1982) Acute airways obstruction in children under five. *Thorax,* **37,** 641–645

MOK, S. Y. Q. and SIMPSON, H. (1982) Outcome of acute lower respiratory tract infection in infants: preliminary report of seven-year follow-up study. *British Medical Journal,* **285,** 333–337

MUIR, D. C. F. (Ed.) (1972) *Clinical Aspects of Inhaled Particles.* pp. 1–20. Philadelphia: Davis

MURRAY, A. B. and FERGUSON, A. C. (1981) Comparison of spirometric measurements in allergen bronchial challenge testing. *Clinical Allergy,* **11,** 87–93

MURRAY, A. B. and FERGUSON, A. C. (1983) Dust free bedrooms in the treatment of asthmatic children with house dust or house dust mite allergy: a controlled trial. *Pediatrics,* **71,** 418–422

MURRAY, A. B., FERGUSON, A. C. and MORRISON, B. (1981) Airway responsiveness to histamine as a test for overall severity of asthma in children. *Journal of Allergy and Clinical Immunology,* **68,** 119–124

NADEL, J. A. and TIERNEY, D. F. (1961) Effects of a previous deep inspiration on airway resistance in man. *Journal of Applied Physiology,* **16,** 717–719

NEIJENS, H. J., DUIVERMAN, E. J. and KERREBIJN, K. F. (1983) Bronchial responsiveness in children. *Pediatrics Clinics of North America,* **30,** 829–846

O'BYRNE, P. M., MORRIS, M., ROBERTS, P. and HARGREAVE, F. E. (1982a) Inhibition of bronchial response to respiratory heat exchange by increasing doses of terbutaline sulphate. *Thorax,* **37,** 913–917

O'BYRNE, P. M., RYAN, G., MORRIS, M., MCCORMACK, D., JONES, N. L., NORSE, J. L. C. *et al.* (1982b) Asthma induced by cold air and its relation to non-specific bronchial responsiveness to methacholine. *American Review of Respiratory Disease*, **125**, 281–285

OGILVIE, C. A., HARESNAPE, A. M. and HARRIS, E. A. (1983) Apparatus for bronchial challenge with cold air. *Medical and Biological Engineering and Computing*, **21**, 235–238

OREHEK, J., MESSARI, J. P., GAYRARD, P., GRINAND, C. and CHARPIN, J. (1976) Effects of short term, low level nitrogen dioxide exposure on bronchial sensitivity of asthmatic patients. *Journal of Clinical Investigations*, **57**, 301–310

OREHEK, J., NICOLI, M. M., DELPIERRE, N. S. and BEAUPRE, A. (1981) Influence of previous deep inspiration on the spirometric measurement of provoked bronchoconstriction in asthma. *American Review of Respiratory Diseases*, **123**, 269–272

PHELAN, P. D. (1984) Does adult chronic obstructive lung disease really begin in childhood? *British Journal of Diseases of the Chest*, **78**, 1–9

PRICE, J. F., TURNER, M. W., WARNER, J. O. and SOOTHILL, J. F. (1983) Immunological studies in asthmatic children undergoing antigen provocation in the skin, lung and nose. *Clinical Allergy*, **13**, 419–426

PULLAN, C. R. and HEY, E. N. (1982) Wheezing, asthma and pulmonary dysfunction 10 years after infection with respiratory syncital virus in infancy. *British Medical Journal*, **284**, 1665–1669

RONCHETTI, R., LUCARINI, N., LUCARELLI, P. *et al.* (1984) A genetic basis for heterogeneity of asthma syndrome in pediatric ages: adenosine deaminase phenotypes. *Journal of Allergy and Clinical Immunology*, **74**, 81–84

ROONEY, J. C. and WILLIAMS, H. E. (1971) The relationship between proved viral bronchiolitis and subsequent wheezing. *Journal of Pediatrics*, **79**, 744–747

RUFFIN, R. E., ALPERS, J. H., CROCKETT, A. J. and HAMILTON, R. (1981) Repeated histamine inhalation tests in asthmatic patients. *Journal of Allergy and Clinical Immunology*, **67**, 285–289

RUFIN, P., BENOIST, M. R., SCHEINMANN, P. and POPE, J. (1984) A study on the reproducibility of specific bronchial provocation testing in children. *Clinical Allergy*, **14**, 387–397

RYAN, C., LATIMER, K. M., DOLOVITCH, J. and HARGREAVES, F. E. (1982) Bronchial responsiveness to histamine: relationship to diurnal variation of peak flow rate: improvement after bronchodilator and airway calibre. *Thorax*, **37**, 423–429

SALOME, C. M., SCHOEFFEL, R. E. and WOOLCOCK, A. J. (1980) Comparison of bronchial reactivity to histamine and methacholine in asthmatics. *Clinical Allergy*, **10**, 541–546

SALOME, C. M., SCHOEFFEL, R. E., YAN, K. and WOOLCOCK, A. J. (1983) Effect of aerosol fenoterol on the severity of bronchial hyper-reactivity in patients with asthma. *Thorax*, **38**, 854–858

SAMET, J. A., TAGER, I. B. and SPEIZER, F. E. (1983) The relationship between respiratory illness in childhood and chronic airflow obstruction in adulthood. *American Review of Respiratory Disease*, **127**, 508–523

SCHOEFFEL, R. E., ANDERSON, S. D. and ALTOUNYAN, R. E. C. (1981) Bronchial hyper-reactivity in response to inhalation of ultrasonically nebulised solutions of distilled water and saline, *British Medical Journal*, **283**, 1285–1287

SHAPIRO, G. G., FURUKAWA, C. T., PIERSON, W. E. and BIERMAN, C. W. (1982) Methacholine bronchial challenge in children. *Journal of Allergy and Clinical Immunology*, **69**, 365–369

SIBBALD, B., HORN, M. E. C., BRAIN, E. A. and GREGG, I. (1980) Genetic factors in childhood asthma. *Thorax*, **35**, 671–674

SILVERMAN, M. (1972) Exercise studies in asthmatic children. University of Cambridge: MD Thesis

SILVERMAN, M. (1983) Respiratory function testing in infancy and childhood. In *Measurement in Clinical Respiratory Physiology*. Eds G. Lazlo and M. F. Sudlow. pp. 293–328. London: Medical Physics Series, Academic Press

SILVERMAN, M. (1984) Bronchodilators for wheezy infants? *Archives of Disease in Childhood*, **59**, 84–87

SILVERMAN, M. and ANDERSON, S. D. (1972) Standardisation of exercise tests in asthmatic children. *Archives of Disease in Childhood*, **47**, 882–889

SILVERMAN, M., CONNOLLY, N. M., BALFOUR-LYNN, L. and GODFREY, S. (1972) Long term trial of disodium cromoglycate and isoprenaline in children with asthma. *British Medical Journal*, **3**, 378–381

SILVERMAN, M., HOBBS, F. D. R., GORDON, I. R. S. and CARSWELL, F. (1978) Cystic fibrosis, atopy and airways lability. *Archives of Disease in Childhood*, **53**, 873–877

SIMS, D. G., GARDNER, P. S., WEIGHTMAN, D., TURNER, M. W. and SOOTHILL, J. F. (1981) Atopy does not predispose to RSV bronchiolitis or prebronchiolitic wheezing. *British Medical Journal*, **282**, 2086–2088

STERK, P. J., PLOMP, A., CROBACH, M. J. S. S., VAN DE VATE, J. F. and QUANJER, P. H. (1983) The peripheral properties of a jet nebuliser and their relevance for the histamine provocation test. *Bulletin European de Physiopathologie Respiratoire*, **19**, 27–36

STOKES, G. M., MILNER, A. D., JOHNSON, F., HODGES, I. G. C. and GROGGINS, R. C. (1981) Measurement of work of breathing in infancy. *Pediatric Research,* **15,** 22–27

TAUSSIG, L. M., LANDAU, L. I., GODFREY, S. and ARAD, I. (1982) Determinants of forced expiratory flows in newborn infants. *Journal of Applied Physiology,* **53,** 1220–1227

TOWNLEY, R. (1984) Methacholine inhalation challenge as a potential genetic marker. *Respiration,* **46** (S1), 62

ULLAH, M. I., CUDDIHY, V., SAUNDERS, K. B. and ADDIS, G. J. (1983) How many blows really make and FEV_1, FVC or PEFR? *Thorax,* **38,** 113–118

VARPELA, E., LAITINEN, L. A., KESKINEN, H. and KORHOLA, O. (1978) Asthma, allergy and bronchial hyper-reactivity to histamine in patients with bronchiectasis. *Clinical Allergy,* **8,** 273–280

WALTERS, E. H. (1981) Prostaglandins and the control of airway responses to histamine in normal and asthmatic subjects. *Thorax,* **38,** 188–194

WARNER, J. O. (1976) Significance of late reactions after bronchial challenge with house dust mite. *Archives of Diseases in Childhood,* **51,** 905–911

WEILER-RAVELL, D. and GODFREY, S. (1981) Do exercise- and antigen-induced asthma utilise the same pathways. *Journal of Allergy,* **67,** 391 397

WEISS, S. T., TAGER, I. B., WEISS, S. W., MUNOZ, A., SPEIZER, F. E. and INGRAM, R. H. (1984) Airways responsiveness in a population sample of adults and children. *American Review of Respiratory Disease,* **129,** 898–902

WILLIAMS, D. O., BARNES, P. J., VICKERS, H. P. and RUDOLF, M. (1981) Effect of nifedipine on bronchomotor tone and histamine reactivity in asthma. *British Medical Journal,* **283,** 348

WILSON, N., BARNES, P. J., VICKERS, H. and SILVERMAN, M. (1982) Hyperventilation-induced asthma: evidence for two mechanisms. *Thorax,* **37,** 657–662

WILSON, N., DIXON, C. and SILVERMAN, M. (1984) Bronchial responsiveness to hyperventilation in children with asthma: response to ipratropium bromide. *Thorax,* **39,** 588–593

WILSON, N., DIXON, C. and SILVERMAN, M. (1985) Increased bronchial responsiveness caused by ingestion of ice. *European Journal of Respiratory Diseases,* **66,** 25–30

WILSON, N. and SILVERMAN, M. (1985) The diagnosis of food sensitivity in asthmatic children. *Journal of the Royal Society of Medicine,* (in press)

WILSON, N., VICKERS, H., TAYLOR, G. and SILVERMAN, M. (1982) Objective test for food sensitivity in asthmatic children: increased bronchial reactivity after cola drinks. *British Medical Journal,* **284,** 1226–1228

WOOLCOCK, A. J., YAN, K. and SALOME, C. (1983) Methods for assessing bronchial reactivity. *European Journal of Respiratory Diseases,* **64** (Suppl 128), 181–194

ZACH, M., ERBEN, A. and OLINSKY, A. (1981) Croup, recurrent croup and airways hyper-reactivity. *Archives of Disease in Childhood,* **56,** 336–341

ZACH, M., POLGAR, G., KUMP, H. and KROISEL, L. (1984) Cold air challenge of airway hyperreactivity in children: practical application and theoretical aspects. *Pediatric Research,* **18,** 469–478

10
Allergy and infection in cystic fibrosis
Robert W. Wilmott*

INTRODUCTION

Cystic fibrosis (CF) is a multisystem disease affecting exocrine gland function. Although not clearly described until the late 1930s (Fanconi, 1936; Andersen, 1938), it is now recognized as the most common lethal recessively inherited disorder that affects Caucasian people (Wood, Boat and Doershuk, 1976).

The clinical features of CF have been extensively reviewed (Wood, Boat and Doershuk, 1976; Talamo, Rosenstein and Berninger, 1983). Chronic pulmonary infection and progressive small airway obstruction account for most of the morbidity and mortality of CF and eventually most patients die from progressive lung disease. The unusual susceptibility to pulmonary infection is associated with hyperplasia of the mucus-secreting cells in the bronchial tree, although the lungs are histologically normal at birth (Reid, 1980). The characteristic lesion is a purulent bronchitis which eventually results in bronchiectasis, peribronchial fibrosis and airway obstruction. In turn, this leads to progressive deterioration in lung function with airflow limitation and gas trapping. Later pulmonary complications in CF include recurrent haemoptysis (Di Sant'Agnese and Davis, 1979) and spontaneous pneumothorax (Lifshitz et al., 1968). Respiratory failure and cor pulmonale are the eventual cause of death in most children with CF (Wood, Boat and Doershuk, 1976).

Factors that appear to influence the lung disease include chronic infection, especially infection with *Pseudomonas aeruginosa* (Hoiby et al., 1977) and allergy (Warner et al., 1976); the role of each in the rate of disease progression will be discussed.

PSEUDOMONAS AERUGINOSA INFECTION IN CYSTIC FIBROSIS

Chronic infection with *P. aeruginosa* in CF is associated with a poor clinical course and high titres of pseudomonas precipitins have been correlated with a poor prognosis (Hoiby et al., 1977). The concept that *P. aeruginosa* is a pathogen in patients with CF has however, not always been accepted (Di Sant'Agnese and

*Formerly Robert W. Pitcher-Wilmott.

190

Talamo, 1967). There are few data from longitudinal studies to resolve this question of *P. aeruginosa* pathogenicity, although it was recently shown in a Danish CF centre that initiation of regular antibiotic therapy directed at *P. aeruginosa* was associated with better survival rates compared to historical controls (Szaff, Hoiby and Flensborg, 1983).

The majority of *P. aeruginosa* isolates in CF are distinctive for the production of a copious extracellular slime material that has been characterized as a polysaccharide similar in structure to alginic acid (Linker and Jones, 1966; Doggett, Harrison and Carter, 1971). These *P. aeruginosa* isolates have smooth 'mucoid' colonies, and are easily isolated on conventional media. Mucoid *P. aeruginosa* accounts for only 0.8–2.1% of clinical pseudomonas isolates in general (Doggett, Harrison and Carter, 1971), but in CF up to 80% of all *P. aeruginosa* isolates have this characteristic (Doggett *et al.*, 1966; Reynolds *et al.*, 1975). Although the significance of this finding is unclear, there are several observations which suggest that this material may inhibit host defence mechanisms. The alginate inhibits *in vitro* opsonization for polymorphonuclear neutrophils of mucoid *P. aeruginosa* strains by rabbit serum (Schwartzman and Boring, 1971), and significantly higher concentrations of antiserum are required to achieve a greater than 10-fold reduction in bacterial concentration of mucoid strains compared to their non-mucoid revertants (Baltimore and Mitchell, 1980). Thus the alginate appears to act as an inhibitor of opsonization. In addition, it inhibits the diffusion of aminoglycoside antibiotics (Slack and Nichols, 1981), and may provide a mechanical barrier to the action of antibodies and antibiotics (Lam *et al.*, 1980). However, in a guinea-pig model there was no evidence that alginate synthesis protected *P. aeruginosa* against antibiotics or antibodies when it was instilled into the bronchial tree (Blackwood and Pennington, 1981).

Recent studies have shown that chronic colonization by *P. aeruginosa* in CF is associated with changes in the organism which becomes serum sensitive, loses its O serotype antigen, and becomes polyagglutinable (Hancock *et al.*, 1983; Penketh *et al.*, 1983). These characteristics are unrelated to the synthesis of alginate and more closely related to the chronicity of infection.

BRONCHIAL LABILITY IN CYSTIC FIBROSIS

Normal adults may have increased bronchial lability for several months after an upper respiratory tract infection (Empey *et al.*, 1976). A similar mechanism may operate in CF. A study from Toronto investigated 113 CF patients by bronchial provocation testing with histamine and methacholine (Mitchell *et al.*, 1978). Using methacholine, increased bronchial lability was found in 51% (compared to 98% in asthma), but only 20% reacted to histamine. Other studies, using varying doses, have found positive responses to histamine in as many as 68% (Haluszka and Scislicki, 1975), or as few as 24% (Mellis and Levison, 1978). A significant proportion of CF patients with almost normal pulmonary function had increased bronchial lability in one study (Van Asperen *et al.*, 1981), although other studies have shown that increased bronchial lability correlates with poor baseline pulmonary function (Mellis and Levison, 1978; Holzer, Olinsky and Phelan, 1981).

CF patients as a group are not as labile as asthmatics (Mitchell *et al.*, 1978). They respond differently to exercise with the predominant response being an abnormal rise in peak expiratory flow rate (Day and Mearns, 1973; Price *et al.*, 1979; Holzer, Olinsky and Phelan, 1981).

Variability in response complicates the interpretation of both bronchial provocation and exercise challenge tests. When a group of patients was tested 4 times in 6 months, 44% gave a variable response to histamine and 56% to exercise (Holzer, Olinsky and Phelan, 1981). This variation was unrelated to pulmonary infections or changes in pulmonary function, although positive responses were more common in those with advanced pulmonary disease.

ALLERGY IN CYSTIC FIBROSIS

Initial clinical studies described a small number of patients who had coexistent CF and allergic diseases such as asthma and hayfever.

Van Metre *et al.* (1960) performed a clinical review of 135 CF patients for symptoms of atopic allergy. Nineteen patients had evidence of hayfever, nasal polyps, eczema, urticaria or positive skin test reactions. The clinical significance and the prevalence of atopic allergy in the 135 patients was unclear as only the 19 'allergic patients' were skin tested and 8 of them had clinical evidence suggesting respiratory tract allergy. Seven of these 8 had nasal polyps which were not associated with allergies in a later study of CF children (Drake Lee and Pitcher-Wilmott, 1982). Asthma was not accepted as evidence of an allergic respiratory disorder although 12 of the 'allergic group' and 51 of the 'non-allergic' group had such a history. Kulczycki *et al.* surveyed 266 CF patients to determine the prevalence of respiratory allergy (Kulczycki, Mueller and Shwachman, 1961). Detailed allergy questionnaires were completed and allergy skin tests were performed on 51 patients who had allergic symptoms. In an attempt to control for selection, skin tests were performed on 4 CF patients with a negative history for allergy and there were no reactions. It was concluded that 16.6% of the CF patients had asthma, allergic rhinitis, latent allergies (positive skin tests and a history of allergy without current symptoms) or a combination of these criteria. Evidence of allergy may have been missed in the patients who were not skin tested and it is difficult to assess the significance of the findings in the group with 'latent allergies' as many normal people have positive skin tests without symptoms.

Rachelefsky *et al.* (1974) evaluated 63 CF patients for the presence of respiratory allergy using allergy questionnaires, physical examinations and allergy skin tests. Fifteen of the patients had hayfever or asthma that correlated with positive skin tests. The diagnosis of asthma was supported in 9 of 13 tested by a significant improvement in FEV_1 after treatment with isoprenaline or adrenaline. The entire 'allergic group' and 9 of the 'non-allergic group' were skin tested with 60 environmental allergens; all of the former group were positive whereas all of the latter were negative. Since skin tests and bronchodilator tests were not given to all patients, it is difficult to evaluate the prevalence of allergy in these 63 patients.

The prevalence of atopic allergy in CF depends on the criteria chosen. Although wheezing is commonly associated with asthma, CF patients often wheeze because of infection. When asked directly for a history of recurrent wheezing, 53% of CF children reported the symptom (Unpublished data, 1981). However, only 12% had a history of exercise-induced bronchospasm and 7% of pollen asthma. Seasonal allergic rhinitis was reported by 20% and infantile eczema by 10%. Thus wheezing alone was reported much more frequently than other allergic symptoms and it appears that the incidence of classical symptoms of allergy in CF is similar to that in unselected schoolchildren.

Nasal polyps in cystic fibrosis

Nasal polyps are a well-described complication of CF. The prevalence varies with age and the overall prevalence in a series of 605 patients was 26% (Stern *et al.*, 1982). In normal adults, nasal polyps are associated with nasal allergies and aspirin-sensitive asthma, but whether they have an allergic aetiology in CF is uncertain. The clinical histories, allergy skin test results and IgE levels of 20 CF children with nasal polyps were compared with those from 97 CF controls (Drake Lee and Pitcher-Wilmott, 1982). There was no association between the presence of polyps, and either allergic symptoms, positive skin tests, or increased serum IgE levels. We proposed that nasal polyps in CF are not an allergic disease and that they might be an expression of the primary gene defect or of chronic sinus infection. The former theory is supported by the demonstration of increased rates of mucus secretion by respiratory epithelium from CF patients, including samples of polyp material (Frates, Kaizu and Last, 1983). The demonstration of this abnormality agrees with the suggestion that dilated mucous glands in the nasal mucosa obstruct venous and lymphatic drainage causing stromal oedema of the nasal mucous membrane which eventually prolapses and forms a polyp (Rulon, Brown and Logan, 1963). As many CF adults have a history of nasal polyps that developed in childhood, it has been suggested that they may confer a survival advantage (Stern *et al.*, 1982). This idea is supported by our observation that nasal polyps in CF were significantly associated with milder clinical disease (Drake Lee and Pitcher-Wilmott, 1982), yet the basis for this favourable association is unknown. As the incidence of nasal polyps is lower in CF after adolescence (Stern *et al.*, 1982), the explanation is not that polyps are simply found more frequently in older patients.

Allergy skin tests in cystic fibrosis

A high prevalence of positive skin prick test reactions to common allergens, particularly to *Aspergillus fumigatus*, has been reported. Mearns, Longbottom and Batten (1967) reported positive prick tests with *A. fumigatus* in 33 of 86 patients investigated. McCarthy, Pepys and Batten (1969) similarly investigated 37 CF patients and found immediate skin test reactions to *A. fumigatus* in 18 and late skin test reactions (4–6 h reactions) in 16. A more comprehensive study of 43 patients aged 2–34 years who were prick tested with a control and 23 allergens revealed that 70% had at least one positive skin test reaction, 28% had multiple reactions and 58% reacted to *A. fumigatus*. (Warren *et al.*, 1975)

A study of 123 children from the Hospital for Sick Children, London used 12 allergens which included 2 moulds. Fifty-nine per cent had immediate skin test reactions with a wheal measuring more than 3 mm, or flare greater than 5 mm diameter, 20 min after testing. The commonest reaction was to *A. fumigatus* which was positive in 56% of the children (Warner *et al.*, 1976). Many other studies have reported similar data (Allan *et al.*, 1975; Counahan and Mearns, 1975; Warren *et al.*, 1975; Barron *et al.*, 1977; Silverman *et al.*, 1978; Carswell, Oliver and

Silverman, 1979a; Nelson, Callerame and Schwartz, 1979; Ormerod *et al.*, 1980; Tacier-Eugster, Wuthrich and Meyer, 1980; Van Asperen, Mellis and South, 1980; Clarke, Hampshire and Hannant, 1981; Holzer, Olinsky and Phelan, 1981; Reen *et al.*, 1981).

A common feature to all the studies of allergy skin testing in CF is an increased overall prevalence of positive prick tests due to the high prevalence of sensitivity to *A. fumigatus* which is higher than that of age-matched controls, whereas the prevalence of sensitivity to non-mould allergens is similar. *Table 10.1* shows the results in 104 CF patients that we recently investigated (Pitcher-Wilmott *et al.*,

Table 10.1 Frequency of positive skin tests in 104 cystic fibrosis patients

	Percentage positive			
Allergen	All cases	Pseudomonas negative cases	Pseudomonas* positive cases	P. value†
A. fumigatus	35	25	53	<0.01
Rye grass pollen	30	22	44	<0.05
Timothy grass pollen	26	21	36	NS
House dust extract	24	21	31	NS
D. pteronyssinus	16	12	25	NS
Cat fur	15	12	22	NS
Alternaria alternata	15	12	22	NS
Whole milk	14	10	19	NS
A. niger	11	7	17	NS
Cladosporium herbarum	9	7	11	NS
Feathers	8	4	14	NS
Dog hair	8	3	17	<0.05
Whole egg	8	7	8	NS

* *Pseudomonas* were grown consistently from the sputum of 35% ($n = 36$) of the patients.
† By χ^2 on absolute numbers.

1982). Possible explanations of these findings include increased permeability of respiratory mucous membranes (Leskowitz, Salvaggio and Schwartz, 1972), abnormal IgA protection of mucosal surfaces (Taylor *et al.*, 1973), retention of small allergen particles because of gas trapping (Warner *et al.*, 1976) and a form of allergic bronchopulmonary aspergillosis (Nelson, Callerame and Schwartz, 1979). A recent study of 49 patients from whom mucoid *P. aeruginosa* had been isolated showed that 31 of 42 had positive immediate prick tests with 21 patients reacting to *A. fumigatus* (Clarke, Hampshire and Hannant, 1981). This observation prompted the theory that the abundance of bacterial and fungal antigens in the respiratory tract of CF patients may lead to enhanced IgE responses to common inhaled allergens due to an adjuvant effect. This theory is supported by our observation that CF patients chronically colonized with *P. aeruginosa* had positive skin test reactions to 1 or more of 13 allergens significantly more frequently than *P. aeruginosa*-negative patients (*Table 10.2*). This association was most marked for *A. fumigatus*, but it was also found with rye grass and dog hair (*Table 10.1; Figure 10.1*).

Table 10.2 Skin prick test results in relationship to chronic pulmonary pseudomonas colonization in 104 CF patients

	*Skin test positive**	*Skin test negative*
Chronically colonized by *P. aeruginosa*	28	8
Not colonized by *P. aeruginosa*	30	38
	$P<0.05$ by χ^2	

* To one or more of the 13 test allergens.

   The positive skin test reactions in CF appear to be mediated by mast-cell-bound IgE and not by any other immune mechanism. Positive radioallergosorbent tests (RAST) to *A. fumigatus* were reported in 15 of 21 patients with positive skin tests to it in the study by Warren *et al.* (1975) and similarly positive reactions were found to grass pollen and *Dermatophagoides pteronyssinus* in appropriate subjects. These results were confirmed subsequently in two studies of children by our group

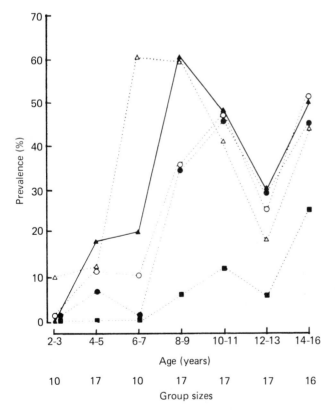

Figure 10.1 Prevalences by age of pseudomonas colonization (solid line) and positive skin prick tests (broken lines) in 104 cystic fibrosis patients. (△) *Aspergillus fumigatus*; (○) rye grass pollen; (●) timothy grass pollen; (■) dog hair

(Turner *et al.*, 1978; Pitcher-Wilmott *et al.*, 1982) and by other investigators (Carswell, Oliver and Silverman, 1979a).

Total serum IgE levels have been measured in several series of CF patients (Turner *et al.*, 1978; Nelson, Callerame and Schwartz, 1979; Pitcher-Wilmott *et al.*, 1982) and levels are increased for age in patients with positive skin tests (Turner *et al.*, 1978), allergic bronchopulmonary aspergillosis (Nelson, Callerame and Schwarz, 1979) and those with many recent chest infections (Turner *et al.*, 1978). Total IgG$_4$ levels are also increased in CF compared to normal (Shakib *et al.*, 1976; Carswell, Oliver and Silverman, 1979b). However, there is little evidence to implicate IgG$_4$ reaginic antibodies in the production of disease (Turner *et al.*, 1978), although they may have an important pathogenetic role in inhibiting the opsonization of *P. aeruginosa* for phagocytosis by pulmonary alveolar macrophages (Moss *et al.*, 1982).

Reproducibility of allergy tests in cystic fibrosis

Allergy skin tests seem to be a reliable marker of IgE sensitization in CF. In patients tested 6 months after the 1974 study (Warner, 1977), the pattern was similar to the first test in 69%. Some of the remainder had gained reactions whilst others had lost them. A more recent study assessed patients every 6 weeks during a 6-month period. The reproducibility was greater with only 24% showing variability (Holzer, Olinsky and Phelan, 1981). This level of reproducibility, whilst not complete, is high enough for skin tests to be used in clinical studies of allergy in CF.

The clinical relevance of positive allergy skin tests in cystic fibrosis

CF patients with positive skin tests have worse lung function (Warner *et al.*, 1976; Silverman *et al.*, 1978), higher hospital admission rates (Warner *et al.*, 1976), worse chest radiograph scores (Warner *et al.*, 1976; Silverman *et al.*, 1978) and lower Taussig–Kattwinkel clinical scores (Nelson, Callerame and Schwartz, 1979) than non-allergic CF patients. This difference was most marked in patients who reacted to *A. fumigatus* (Silverman *et al.*, 1978). These observations, and the increased IgE levels in patients with more frequent respiratory infections, led us to investigate the hypothesis that allergic reactions damage the lungs of CF patients. We used clinical and laboratory criteria to diagnose allergy and to study the relevance of allergy and other selected factors on pulmonary function data from 104 CF children who were currently attending our clinic. Longitudinal data from 54 of these patients were analysed similarly (Pitcher-Wilmott *et al.*, 1982). The question of the role of allergy in CF lung disease is directly relevant to therapy, since pulmonary symptoms of type I allergy may respond to treatment with inhaled cromoglycate, inhaled steroids, or systemic steroids. The CF patients with positive reactions to one or more allergens had significantly worse forced expiratory flow rates (FEF$_{25}$), residual volume to total lung capacity ratios, chest radiograph scores and hospital admission rates (*Table 10.3*). Thus, these data supported our hypothesis, but it was noted that the patients with one or more positive skin test reactions were older than the skin test negative patients (*Table 10.3*) and were more likely to have chronic pulmonary infection with *P. aeruginosa* (*Table 10.2*) but not with *Staphylococcus aureus*. When the data were grouped by *P. aeruginosa* colonization, patients who

Table 10.3 Lung function, chest radiograph score, hospital admission rate, pseudomonas colonization and age in 104 CF children according to skin test results

	Skin test negative	Skin test positive to any allergen	P
FEF$_{25}$ (% predicted) (mean ± s.e.)	65 ± 7	44 ± 4	<0.01*
RV/TLC (%) (mean ± s.e.)	40 ± 2	47 ± 2	<0.05*
Chest radiograph score (mean ± s.e.) (median)	6.0 ± 0.6 5.4	10.0 ± 0.6 9.6	<0.0001†
Admissions/year (mean ± s.e.) (median)	0.17 ± 0.08 0.08	0.91 ± 0.22 0.23	<0.02†
Age (years) (mean ± s.e.)	8.25 ± 0.62	10.40 ± 0.47	<0.01*
N	46	58	

* By Student's *t* test.   FEF$_{25}$ = foreced expiratory flow at 25% vital capacity.
† By Mann–Whitney U test.   RV/TLC = residual volume/total lung capacity.

were colonized had significantly worse pulmonary function, chest radiograph scores, and hospital admission rates than patients free from such infection (*Table 10.4*). Thus, age, allergy, and pseudomonas infection appeared to be associated with worse pulmonary function. Analysis of variance was used to sort out which of these associations was most significant.

The relative contributions of age, positive skin prick test reactions, and chronic *P. aeruginosa* colonization to severity of pulmonary disease were determined by multiple regression analysis using a stepwise elimination procedure. As allergy to *A. fumigatus* might have been the most significant correlate of poor lung function the skin test results (*Table 10.1*) were entered in four categories: (*a*) patients sensitive to one of the four mould allergens; (*b*) patients sensitive to one of the non-mould allergens; (*c*) patients sensitive to both mould and other allergens; (*d*) patients with no positive skin tests to any of the allergens. We also investigated the significance of other selected factors such as staphylococcal colonization and duration of respiratory complaints.

The factor most strongly correlated with severity of pulmonary disease in CF was chronic pulmonary colonization with *P. aeruginosa* (*Table 10.5*). Positive skin test reactions were only weakly, and insignificantly, associated with severity of lung disease. The effect of chronic staphylococcal colonization was also insignificant. There were only two other variables significantly associated with severity of lung disease in the analysis and these were age, which was a significant covariate with FEF$_{25}$ (*P*<0.01) and duration of respiratory symptoms which was a significant covariate with peak expiratory flow rate (*P*<0.05). Hospital admission rate and chest radiograph score were not analysed in this manner because they were not normally distributed.

Table 10.4 Lung function, chest radiograph score and hospital admission rate in 36 CF patients chronically colonized with *P. aeruginosa* (CF + PA) and 68 CF patients without such infection (CF − PA)

	CF − PA	CF + PA	P
VC (% predicted) (mean ± s.e.)	85 ± 2	68 ± 3	<0.001*
TGV (% predicted) (mean ± s.e.)	128 ± 3	154 ± 7	<0.005*
PEF (% predicted) (mean ± s.e.)	97 ± 2	79 ± 4	<0.001*
FEF$_{25}$ (% predicted) (mean ± s.e.)	68 ± 5	32 ± 4	<0.001*
RV/TLC (%) (mean ± s.e.)	39 ± 2	53 ± 2	<0.001*
Chest radiograph score (mean ± s.e.) (median)	6.3 ± 0.4 6.1	12.1 ± 0.9 11.3	<0.0001†
Hospital admissions/year (mean ± s.e.) (median)	0.06 ± 0.03 0.03	1.57 ± 0.31 0.81	<0.001†

* By Student's *t* test.
† By Mann–Whitney U test.

VC = vital capacity.
TGV = thoracic gas volume.
PEF = peak expiratory flow rate.
FEF$_{25}$ = forced expiratory flow at 25% vital capacity.
RV/TLC = residual volume/total lung capacity.

IgE concentrations, positive RAST tests (to *A. fumigatus*, rye grass or *D. pteronyssinus*) and whether or not patients had a history of asthma or hayfever were analysed similarly. The effects of chronic *P. aeruginosa* colonization and significant covariates were controlled as before. None of these laboratory or clinical variables were significantly related to pulmonary function (*Table 10.5*).

Results from an earlier study were available for 52 of the 104 patients (Warner *et al.*, 1976). Analysis of variance on changes in chest radiograph score, hospital admission rate, peak expiratory flow rate and vital capacity was performed over 5 years. Changes in radiograph scores and admission rates could be analysed as they were normally distributed. The only significant factor correlating with progression of pulmonary disease in analysis of variance was *P. aeruginosa* colonization. Acquisition of positive skin test reactions and *Staph. aureus* colonization were not significantly related to progression of lung disease when the change in *P. aeruginosa* status was allowed for (*Table 10.6*).

These results do not support the hypothesis that allergic CF patients have worse pulmonary disease nor do they support the earlier report of milder clinical disease in CF patients with asthma or hayfever (Rachelefsky *et al.*, 1974). The data show that, of the factors examined, chronic *P. aeruginosa* colonization is most closely associated with the degree of pulmonary disease and that the effect of allergy is small. Although pulmonary function is significantly worse in those patients with

Table 10.5 Associations (variance ratios – F) of selected variables on lung function in analysis of variance

Dependent variables	Independent variables							
	Pseudomonas colonization	*Staphylococcal colonization*	*Age*	*Duration of respiratory symptoms*	*Skin test positivity*	*Log$_{10}$ IgE*	*Positive RAST*	*Respiratory allergic disease*
FEF$_{25}$	29.3‡	1.54	7.22†	0.77	1.34	0.11	0.63	1.03
RV/TLC	22.9‡	0.19	0.02	0.61	0.52	0.82	2.21	0.05
TGV	13.0‡	2.53	1.88	0.20	1.92	0.39	3.67	0.17
VC	19.3‡	0.63	1.74	1.19	0.80	0.00	0.46	0.59
PEF	11.3‡	1.00	0.01	5.03*	0.37	0.45	0.16	0.64

Values for *P. aeruginosa* and *Staph. aureus* colonization, age, duration of respiratory symptoms and skin tests were obtained during analysis of variance and sequential elimination. Those for FEF$_{25}$ and PEF are corrected for significant independent variables. Values for serum IgE (logged to normalize), positive RAST tests and allergic disease are those calculated when these variables were added to the significant parsimonious effects model (*see text*).

* $P < 0.05$
† $P < 0.01$
‡ $P < 0.001$

FEF$_{25}$ = forced expiratory flow at 25% vital capacity.
PEF = peak expiratory flow rate.
RV/TLC = residual volume/total lung capacity.
TGV = thoracic gas volume.
VC = vital capacity.

Table 10.6 Variance ratios (F) in analysis of variance on changes in severity in CF patients over 5 years

Dependent variables	Independent variables			
	Change in pseudomonas colonization	*Change in staphylococcal colonization*	*Change in skin test reactivity*	*Age*
Change in chest radiograph score	5.55*	0.38	1.61	0.49
Change in hospital admission rate	7.20*	0.37	1.38	1.01
Change in VC	3.66*	0.36	1.11	0.39
Change in PEF	3.28*	0.07	0.56	1.09

For significant independent variables final F values are shown.
Other F values are those during sequential removal in stepwise analysis.
* $P <0.01$.   VC = vital capacity.
                         PEF = peak expiratory flow rate.

positive skin prick test reactions, this association is insignificant when the data are adjusted for the effects of *P. aeruginosa*. This discrepancy suggests that the apparent effect of skin test reactions in this and other studies results from their significant association with chronic *P. aeruginosa* infection. The 35% prevalence of chronic *P. aeruginosa* infection observed in our patients is lower than that seen at some other CF centres (Doggett *et al.*, 1966). This allowed the effect of *P. aeruginosa* to be separated from that of allergy skin tests in the analysis of variance. The analysis of both the current (cross-sectional) data and the longitudinal data supports the view that the association of chronic *P. aeruginosa* colonization with poor pulmonary function is a cause and effect relationship (Hoiby *et al.*, 1977).

P. aeruginosa is a well-recognized pathogen which may cause lung disease by proteases, exotoxins or other inflammatory substances (Marks, 1981). It is also possible that the IgE response to *P. aeruginosa* in CF is important (Moss, Hsu and Lewiston, 1981). A local reaction between *P. aeruginosa* and mast-cell-bound anti-*P. aeruginosa* IgE could result in the release of mediators such as histamine, leukotrienes and platelet-activating factor. The effect of *P. aeruginosa* in analysis of variance was independent of the effect of positive skin test reactions and, also, independent of other markers of allergy. We did not investigate the possible role of anti-*P. aeruginosa* IgE, but the significance of these antibodies is questioned by the lack of clinical improvement when chronically colonized CF patients were treated with inhaled beclomethasone in a double-blind trial (Schiotz *et al.*, 1983).

A possible explanation for the high prevalence of *A. fumigatus* sensitization in CF, and its association with chronic *P. aeruginosa* infection, is antigenic cross-reactivity. However, aspergillus antibody isolated from CF subjects was not blocked by *P. aeruginosa* antigens in a sensitive primary binding assay (Bardana *et al.*, 1975). In another study using rabbit antisera, there was no evidence for cross-reactivity by immunofluorescence, double diffusion or immunoelectrophoresis (Pitcher-Wilmott, 1984). These results provide no support for the theory that cross-reactivity with *P. aeruginosa* is the explanation for *A. fumigatus* sensitivity in CF.

EFFECTS OF *PSEUDOMONAS* AND ALLERGY ON SURVIVAL

The prevalence of *P. aeruginosa* colonization declined between 10–11 years and 12–13 years of age (*Figure 10.1*) (Pitcher-Wilmott *et al.*, 1982), although no patients ever cleared *P. aeruginosa* infection once it had become chronic. Possible explanations include a negative effect of *P. aeruginosa* colonization on survival rates. This possibility was, therefore, investigated with actuarial analysis which allowed investigation of the effects of *P. aeruginosa* and hypersensitivity reactions, without introducing the selection bias associated with cross-sectional analysis of current, surviving populations.

Data were obtained from the hospital records of 117 CF children tested in 1974 for our first allergy study (Warner *et al.*, 1976). The SURVIVAL programme of the Statistical Package for the Social Sciences (Nie *et al.*, 1975) was used to compute life tables by the actuarial method of Berkson and Gage (1950). This method allowed the analysis of survival rates by subgroups and significance testing for differences in survival rates between those subgroups with the non-parametric rank sum method described by Lee and Desu (1972).

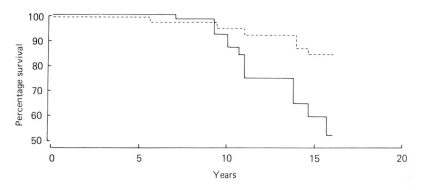

Figure 10.2 Survival rates in 117 CF children according to pseudomonas colonization in 1974. Separate lines are shown for those who were colonized (solid) and those who were negative (broken). (Desu comparison statistic, $\chi^2 = 4.838$; $P<0.05$)

Pulmonary colonization with *P. aeruginosa* in 1974 was strongly associated with a worse survival rate (*Figure 10.2*). In the 31 patients colonized with *P. aeruginosa* in 1974, survival at 16 years was 53% (s.e. 11.3%) compared to 84% (s.e. 6.4%) in those who were not colonized ($\chi^2 = 4.838$; $P<0.05$ by Desu rank sum test). There was no significant difference in survival rates to 16 years of age, when the curve for those patients with one or more positive skin test reactions in 1974 was compared with that for patients with negative skin tests in that study (*Figure 10.3*).

To examine whether there was evidence of interaction between chronic *P. aeruginosa* colonization and immediate hypersensitivity reactions, the patients were analysed using a two-way classification by skin tests and *P. aeruginosa* which created 4 groups. This analysis was done to test whether positive skin test reactions make the effect of *P. aeruginosa* significantly better or worse. The skin-test-positive, *P. aeruginosa*-colonized patients had the poorest survival rates, but there

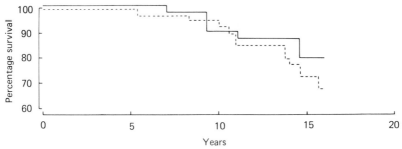

Figure 10.3 Survival rates in 117 CF children according to immediate skin test results in 1974. Separate lines are shown for one or more positive tests (broken) and those with negative tests (solid). The Desu statistic was not significant ($\chi^2 = 0.25$)

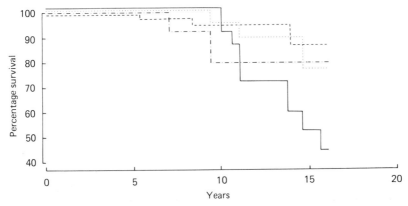

Figure 10.4 Survival rates in 117 CF children grouped according to allergy skin test results and pseudomonas colonization in 1974. ($\cdots\cdots$) pseudomonas negative, skin test negative, $N = 51$; ($-----$) pseudomonas negative, skin test positive, $N = 35$; ($-\cdot-\cdot-$) pseudomonas positive, skin test negative, $N = 14$; ($\underline{\hspace{1cm}}$) pseudomonas positive, skin test positive, $N = 17$. Overall Desu comparison, $\chi^2 = 5.440$, $P<0.05$

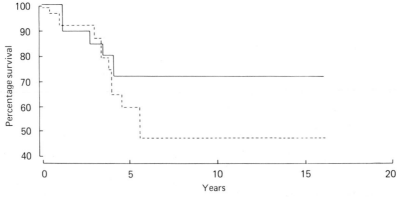

Figure 10.5 Actuarial analysis of survival periods from age of chronic pseudomonas colonization until death in 60 CF patients who had allergy skin tests in 1974. Separate lines are shown for those with positive reactions to one or more of 12 allergens (broken) and those patients with negative skin tests (solid). The Desu rank sum test was not significant

was no statistically significant difference between this curve and that of *P. aeruginosa*-positive, skin-test-negative children (*Figure 10.4*). We also investigated the question of interaction with allergy by entering the children at the time of *P. aeruginosa* colonization. However, only 60 patients were available for analysis if all patients colonized by 1979 were studied. There was no significant difference in survival rates according to the results of skin prick tests in 1974 (*Figure 10.5*).

These results of survival analysis demonstrate that having positive allergy skin tests does not have a significant effect, whereas *P. aeruginosa* colonization is strongly associated with poor survival. As lung disease accounts for most mortality in this disorder (Wood, Boat and Doershuk, 1976), the analysis confirms the conclusions drawn from the analysis of pulmonary function tests, chest radiograph scores and hospital admission rates (Pitcher-Wilmott *et al.*, 1982).

TREATMENT OF ALLERGY IN CYSTIC FIBROSIS

There appears to be no rationale for treatment of allergy in the CF patients who have positive allergy skin tests but who are asymptomatic on exposure to the putative allergens. The allergic symptoms seen in CF children are usually asthma or allergic rhinitis.

Asthma

Asthma in the CF child may be treated in the conventional way with bronchodilators, mast-cell-stabilizing agents or steroids, either inhaled or systemic. The use of bronchodilators has been studied in random samples of CF children and positive responses have been reported with salbutamol (Kattan *et al.*, 1980; Ormerod *et al.*, 1980), atropine and isoproterenol (Larsen *et al.*, 1979), ipratroprium bromide (Ormerod *et al.*, 1980) and theophylline (Larsen *et al.*, 1980). Positive bronchodilator responses in random samples of CF children have been correlated with IgE level and they occur more frequently in those with positive allergy skin tests (Ormerod *et al.*, 1980). In some studies, 30% of CF children have shown significant improvement after inhaled bronchodilators, but whether all such patients should receive bronchodilator therapy has not been resolved by controlled therapeutic trials. Before the results of such trials are available, bronchodilators should be used cautiously because decreased flow rates have been reported following their use in CF (Landau and Phelan, 1973). The explanation of this paradox is thought to be increased compressibility of the large airways when smooth muscle tone is reduced by bronchodilatation (Landau and Phelan, 1973; Kattan *et al.*, 1980).

The use of the mast-cell-stabilizing drug disodium cromoglycate (Intal) is well established in children with allergic or exercise-induced asthma, and it appears to be equally effective in patients with both asthma and CF. However, the use of the powdered form of this drug is not recommended as CF patients may have heightened reactivity to bronchial irritants (Mellis and Levison, 1978), and this sometimes results in troublesome coughing or wheezing after treatment with inhaled powders. Inhalation of cromoglycate solution is usually tolerated better than the powder. Whether this treatment is effective in managing mediator release from infection or other triggers has not been explored.

The value of systemic or inhaled steroids in CF has been the subject of controversy. There is no controlled double-blind study of corticosteroids, yet initial results in an open study appear promising (Lewiston and Moss, 1982). Whether the improvement was related to inhibition of immunological reactions in the lungs, or some other effect, is uncertain. The child with status asthmaticus and CF should be treated with systemic steroids in the conventional way. Inhaled steroids, such as beclomethasone, are useful in the treatment of asthma and may be useful in CF patients with asthma, as they may allow systemic steroids to be avoided. Although a double-blind study of inhaled beclomethasone showed no benefit in alleviating the effect of chronic *P. aeruginosa* infection, its use in asthma complicating CF was not addressed (Schiotz *et al.*, 1983).

Allergic rhinitis

Many CF patients complain of nasal congestion which is due to allergic rhinitis in some and nasal polyps in others. Allergic rhinitis should be treated with decongestants that do not thicken or dry out secretions. Antihistamines are best avoided but pseudoephedrine is sometimes useful. More severe cases of allergic rhinitis may respond well to topical treatment with cromoglycate powder or a steroid spray such as beclomethasone (Beconase). If the nasal allergy is related to seasonal pollen exposure, immunotherapy should be considered, although most patients can be managed with other medical treatments.

Nasal polyps

Nasal polyps can be treated medically with steroid nasal sprays, systemic steroids or antihistamines but, although these treatments may help symptomatically, their long-term results are usually disappointing (Stern *et al.*, 1982). These authors noted that spontaneous and permanent resolution of nasal polyps may occur in as many as 31% of patients and that, for those with severe symptoms, simple polypectomy is usually sufficient, although recurrences are seen in 54% of patients.

ASPERGILLOSIS IN CYSTIC FIBROSIS

The clinical features of allergic bronchopulmonary aspergillosis (ABPA) include (1) intermittent airflow obstruction, (2) pulmonary infiltrates, (3) eosinophilia of blood or sputum, (4) positive *A. fumigatus* skin tests (immediate or dual), (5) *A. fumigatus* precipitins, (6) increased serum IgE concentration, (7) proximal bronchiectasis, and (8) increased levels of IgE and IgG antibodies to *A. fumigatus* (McCarthy and Pepys, 1971; Rosenberg *et al.*, 1977). Common radiographic findings include transient infiltrates, massive atelectasis, toothpaste shadows, gloved finger shadows, tram lines, cystic lesions and honeycombing. Expectoration of brown plugs is sometimes reported and examination of the sputum may reveal the presence of fungal hyphae (*Figure 10.6*), whilst its culture can lead to isolation of the mould. That there may be a significant role for allergy in the progression of CF lung disease is suggested by the diagnosis of ABPA in a substantial proportion of CF patients at some CF centres (Nelson, Callerame and Schwartz, 1979; Laufer

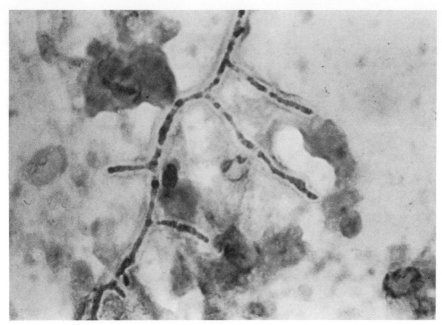

Figure 10.6 Hyphae of *Aspergillus fumigatus* demonstrated in the sputum of a 9-year-old cystic fibrosis girl whose presenting complaint was allergic bronchopulmonary aspergillosis

et al., 1983; unpublished data, T. Murphy, Children's Hospital National Medical Center, Washington, DC, USA).

ABPA was first diagnosed in 3 asthma patients in England by Hinson, Moon and Plummer in 1952. It was subsequently diagnosed in 2 CF children by Mearns, Young and Batten (1965) who observed transient pulmonary infiltrates, peripheral blood eosinophilia, *A. fumigatus* precipitins, a positive *A. fumigatus* skin test and isolation of *A. fumigatus* from the sputum.

Although initially recognized as a complication of asthma that was rarely seen outside the United Kingdom, there has been increasing recognition of this disorder in CF. Forty-six patients were studied prospectively in Rochester, New York, USA and *A. fumigatus* was cultured from the sputum of 57% of those who expectorated with sputum hyphae seen in 95% of those with positive cultures. Five patients fulfilled the criteria for ABPA, which in a 2-year period had an incidence of 11% (Nelson, Callerame and Schwartz, 1979). The incidence of ABPA appears to be lower in most other CF centres, although many patients have positive skin tests to the mould as discussed. A small cluster of cases was recently reported from Birmingham, England (Brueton *et al.*, 1980), and sporadic cases have been seen at the Hospital for Sick Children, London (unpublished data, R. Dinwiddie and D. J. Matthew). When all sputum specimens from 165 patients at the Hospital for Sick Children, London, were examined every 2 months for 1 year, only 9 isolations of *A. fumigatus* were reported (unpublished data, 1981). Only one of these developed ABPA by standard criteria (McCarthy and Pepys, 1971). Positive *A. fumigatus* precipitins can be demonstrated in 31% of CF patients (Mearns, Longbottom and Batten, 1967), and 5 out of 20 patients with antibodies had *A. fumigatus* demonstrated in the sputum. The significance of the high rates of sensitization to the mould, and the cause of the varying incidence of ABPA in CF are unclear. There appears to be no association with the use of mist tents (Nelson, Callerame and Schwartz, 1979) or with the use of handheld nebulizers (unpublished data, 1981). Geographical variations in incidence may relate to exposure to old buildings, damp basements, or agriculture. The apparent incidence is also affected by whether or not the diagnosis of ABPA is actively sought. However, the *A. fumigatus* spore is ubiquitous and the high prevalence of positive skin test reactions suggests high rates of exposure. Selective filtration of spores by the respiratory tract has been proposed as a significant factor in the pulmonary mycoses of man (Austwick, 1966). The small airway disease of CF and asthma may facilitate deposition of the mould spores or colonization of the mucosal surface, perhaps because of the tenacious mucus found in these diseases (Ricketti *et al.*, 1983).

Laboratory tests

A high index of clinical suspicion is needed to diagnose ABPA in CF where the syndrome may be incomplete and where many of the symptoms are common to the underlying disease. CF patients may present with increasing dyspnoea, wheezing, or coughing and the chest radiograph usually shows new infiltrates or atelectasis. However, it is possible for ABPA to be associated with a normal chest radiograph (Rosenberg *et al.*, 1977), although tomography or bronchography usually demonstrate abnormalities.

Laboratory tests which may support the diagnosis of ABPA include examination of the sputum for hyphae or eosinophils, total serum IgE level and specific IgE to *A. fumigatus*. The serum IgE is usually greatly increased in ABPA, although much of the increase is not directed against the organism (Patterson, Rosenberg and Roberts, 1977). Serial measurement of serum IgE is useful in monitoring disease activity as a clinical flare-up is usually heralded by an increase in its level. Other useful clues are peripheral eosinophilia and persistent isolation of *A. fumigatus* from the sputum.

Treatment

There appears to be little value in treating ABPA with antifungal agents such as nystatin or amphotericin B. Initial therapy may include a trial of bronchodilators, which can be combined with nebulized cromoglycate. Systemic steroids are indicated if there is no improvement with these treatments. Prednisone is the treatment of choice (Ricketti *et al.*, 1983) and usually produces improvement in clinical symptoms with radiographic resolution, decrease in IgE level and a decrease in the incidence of positive sputum cultures for *A. fumigatus* (Rosenberg *et al.*, 1978). The use of prednisone is well established although its mechanism of action is unclear (Safirstein *et al.*, 1973). The usual dose is $0.5\,\mathrm{mg}\cdot\mathrm{kg}^{-1}\cdot\mathrm{d}^{-1}$ given daily for 2 weeks and then the same dose is given on alternate days for 3–6 months. The prednisone should then be slowly withdrawn while the serum IgE and chest radiograph are monitored for evidence of a recrudescence (Ricketti *et al.*, 1983). Sometimes higher initial dosages (1–$2\,\mathrm{mg}\cdot\mathrm{kg}^{-1}\cdot\mathrm{d}^{-1}$) are used to achieve remission. Monthly serum IgE levels are helpful in the long-term follow-up of ABPA and a

2-fold increase in level should be evaluated with a chest radiograph. Annual chest radiographs and pulmonary function tests are helpful in the evaluation of both ABPA and CF. Immunotherapy for ABPA can lead to severe systemic reactions and there is no place for such treatment. Inhaled steroids also appear to be ineffective. As exacerbations of ABPA usually occur at times of the year when spore counts are increased (Radin *et al.*, 1983), it is reasonable to advise CF patients who have had ABPA to avoid exposure to barns, mouldy basements, compost heaps and stored grain which have very high spore counts (Slavin and Winzenberger, 1977).

SUMMARY

The incidence, significance, pathogenesis and treatment of allergy and aspergillosis in cystic fibrosis have been discussed. There is little evidence that the high prevalence of positive allergy skin tests in cystic fibrosis is associated with a hypersensitivity disease complicating the primary pulmonary disorder which is caused by excessive bronchial secretions and recurrent infection. There are two important questions concerning these reactions: are they clinically significant and why do they occur? The former question is partly resolved by the data presented, although well-controlled studies of intervention would help to resolve it further. The cause of these reactions, which occur particularly in relationship to the mould *Aspergillus fumigatus*, is unknown and various theories are discussed.

Allergic bronchopulmonary aspergillosis is an important complication of cystic fibrosis which may cause progression of the obstructive lung disease. Allergic bronchopulmonary aspergillosis has been reported from several cystic fibrosis centres and seems to vary in prevalence according to climate, housing or geographical location. A high index of clinical suspicion is needed to diagnose this disease in CF and its clinical presentation, investigation and treatment are reviewed.

Further studies on the efficacy of corticosteroids, the role of *Pseudomonas aeruginosa* and the pathogenesis of hypersensitivity reactions in cystic fibrosis are indicated.

Acknowledgements

Steven D. Douglas MD, Burton Zweiman MD, Gerald B. Kolski MD, and Janet Fithian kindly reviewed the manuscript and gave constructive criticism.

References

ALLAN, J. D., MOSS, A. D., WALLWORK, J. C. and McFARLANE, H. (1975) Immediate hypersensitivity in patients with cystic fibrosis. *Clinical Allergy*, **5**, 255–261

ANDERSEN, D. H. (1938) Cystic fibrosis of the pancreas and its relation to celiac disease: a clinical and pathological study. *American Journal of Diseases of Children*, **56**, 344–399

AUSTWICK, P. K. C. (1966) The role of spores in the allergies and mycoses of man and animals. In *Proceedings of the Eighteenth Symposium of the Colston Research Society*, ed. M. F. Madelin, pp. 321–338, London: Butterworths

BALTIMORE, R. S. and MITCHELL, M. (1980) Immunologic investigations of mucoid strains of *Pseudomonas aeruginosa*: comparison of susceptibility to opsonic antibody in mucoid and non-mucoid strains. *Journal of Infectious Disease*, **141**, 238–247

BARDANA, E. J., SOBTI, K. L., CIANCIULLI, F. D. and NOONAN, M. J. (1975) Aspergillus antibody in patients with cystic fibrosis. *American Journal of Diseases in Children*, **129**, 1164–1167

BARRON, R., COTTON, E., LARSEN, G. and BROOKS, J. (1977) The prevalence of atopy in cystic fibrosis. *CF Club Abstracts*, **23**

BERKSON, J. and GAGE, R. (1950) Calculation of survival rates for cancer. *Proceedings of the Mayo Clinic*, **25**, 270–286

BLACKWOOD, L. L. and PENNINGTON, J. E. (1981) Influence of mucoid coating on clearance of *Pseudomonas aeruginosa* from lungs. *Infection and Immunity*, **32**, 443–448

BRUETON, M. J., ORMEROD, L. P., SHAH, K. J. and ANDERSON, C. M. (1980) Allergic bronchopulmonary aspergillosis complicating cystic fibrosis in childhood. *Archives of Disease in Childhood*, **55**, 348–353

CARSWELL, F., OLIVER, J. and SILVERMAN, M. (1979a) Allergy in cystic fibrosis. *Clinical and Experimental Immunology*, **35**, 141–146

CARSWELL, F., OLIVER, J. and SILVERMAN, M. (1979b) The cystic fibrosis gene, IgE and IgG4. *Monographs in Paediatrics*, **10**, 144–147

CLARKE, C. W., HAMPSHIRE, P. and HANNANT, C. (1981) Positive immediate skin tests in cystic fibrosis: a possible role for Pseudomonas infection. *British Journal of Diseases of the Chest*, **75**, 15–21

COUNAHAN, R. and MEARNS, M. B. (1975) Prevalence of atopy and exercise-induced bronchial lability in relatives of patients with cystic fibrosis. *Archives of Disease in Childhood*, **50**, 477–481

DAY, G. and MEARNS, M. B. (1973) Bronchial lability in cystic fibrosis. *Archives of Disease in Childhood*, **48**, 355–359

DI SANT'AGNESE, P. A. and DAVIS, P. B. (1979) Cystic fibrosis in adults. *American Journal of Medicine*, **66**, 121–132

DI SANT'AGNESE, P. A. and TALAMO, R. C. (1967) Pathogenesis and physiopathology of cystic fibrosis of the pancreas. *New England Journal of Medicine*, **277**, 1399–1408

DOGGETT, R. G., HARRISON, G. M. and CARTER, R. E. (1971) Mucoid *Pseudomonas aeruginosa* in patients with chronic illness. *Lancet*, **i**, 236–237

DOGGETT, R. G., HARRISON, G. M., STILLWELL, R. N. and WALLIS, E. S. (1966) An atypical *Pseudomonas aeruginosa* associated with cystic fibrosis of the pancreas. *Journal of Pediatrics*, **68**, 215–221

DRAKE LEE, A. B. and PITCHER-WILMOTT, R. W. (1982) The clinical and laboratory correlates of nasal polyps in cystic fibrosis. *International Journal of Pediatric Otorhinolaryngology*, **4**, 209–214

EMPEY, D. W., LAITINEN, L. A., JACOBS, L., GOLD, W. M. and NADEL, J. A. (1976) Mechanisms of bronchial hyper-reactivity in normal subjects after upper respiratory tract infection. *American Review of Respiratory Disease*, **113**, 131–139

FANCONI, G., UEHLINGER, E. and KNAUER, C. (1936) Celiac syndrome with congenital cystic pancreatic fibromatosis and bronchiectasis. *Wiener klinische Wochenschrift*, **86**, 753–756

FRATES, R. C., KAIZU, T. T. and LAST, J. A. (1983) Mucus glycoproteins secreted by respiratory epithelial tissue from cystic fibrosis patients. *Pediatric Research*, **17**, 30–34

HALUSZKA, J. and SCISLICKI, A. (1975) Bronchial lability in children suffering from some diseases of the bronchi. *Respiration*, **32**, 217–226

HANCOCK, R. E. W., MUTHARIA, L. M., CHAN, L., DARVEAU, R. P., SPEERT, D. P. and PIER, G. B. (1983) *Pseudomonas aeruginosa* isolates from patients with cystic fibrosis: A class of serum-sensitive, nontypable strains deficient in lipopolysaccharide O side chains. *Infection and Immunity*, **42**, 170–177

HINSON, K. F. W., MOON, A. J. and PLUMMER, N. S. (1952) Bronchopulmonary aspergillosis. *Thorax*, **7**, 317–333

HOIBY, N., FLENSBORG, E. W., BECK, B., FRIIS, B., JACOBSEN, S. V. and JACOBSEN, L. (1977) *Pseudomonas aeruginosa* infection in cystic fibrosis. Diagnostic and prognostic significance of *Pseudomonas aeruginosa* precipitins determined by means of crossed immunoelectrophoresis. *Scandinavian Journal of Respiratory Disease*, **58**, 65–79

HOLZER, F. J., OLINSKY, A. and PHELAN, P. D. (1981) Variability of airways hyper-reactivity and allergy in cystic fibrosis. *Archives of Disease in Childhood*, **56**, 455–459

KATTAN, M., MANSELL, A., LEVISON, H., COREY, M. and KRASTINS, I. R. B. (1980) Response to aerosol salbutamol, SCH 1000, and placebo in cystic fibrosis. *Thorax*, **35**, 531–535

KULCZYCKI, L. L., MUELLER, H. and SHWACHMAN, H. (1961) Respiratory allergy in patients with cystic fibrosis. *Journal of the American Medical Association*, **175**, 358–364

LAM, J., CHAN, K., LAM, L. and COSTERTON, J. W. (1980) Production of mucoid microcolonies by *Pseudomonas aeruginosa* within infected lungs in cystic fibrosis. *Infection and Immunity*, **28**, 546–556

LANDAU, L. I. and PHELAN, P. D. (1973) The variable effect of a bronchodilating agent on pulmonary function in cystic fibrosis. *Journal of Pediatrics*, **82**, 863–868

LARSEN, G. L., BARRON, R. J., COTTON, E. K. and BROOKS, J. G. (1979) A comparative study of inhaled atropine sulphate and isoproterenol hydrochloride in cystic fibrosis. *American Review of Respiratory Disease,* **119**, 399–407

LARSEN, G. L., BARRON, R. J., LANDAY, R. L., COTTON, E. K., GONZALEZ, M. A. and BROOKS, J. G. (1980) Intravenous aminophylline in patients with cystic fibrosis: pharmacokinetics and effect on pulmonary function. *American Journal of Diseases of Children,* **134**, 1143–1148

LAUFER, P., BRUNS, W. T., FINK, J. N., UNGER, G. F., COLBY, H. H., GREENBERGER, P. A. *et al.* (1983) Allergic bronchopulmonary aspergillosis in cystic fibrosis. *CF Club Abstracts,* **24**, 129

LEE, E. T. and DESU, M. M. (1972) A computer program for comparing K samples with right-censored data. *Computer Programs in Biomedicine,* **2**, 315–321

LESKOWITZ, S., SALVAGGIO, J. E. and SCHWARTZ, H. E. (1972) An hypothesis for the development of atopic allergy in man. *Clinical Allergy,* **2**, 237–246

LEWISTON, N. J. and MOSS, R. B. (1982) Circulating immune complexes decrease during corticosteroid therapy in cystic fibrosis. *Pediatric Research,* **4**, 354A

LIFSCHITZ, M. I., BOWMAN, F. O., DENNING, C. R. and WYLIE, R. H. (1968) Pneumothorax as a complication of cystic fibrosis. *American Journal of Diseases of Children,* **116**, 633–640

LINKER, A. and JONES, R. S. (1966) A new polysaccharide resembling alginic acid isolated from Pseudomonas. *Journal of Biological Chemistry,* **245**, 3845–3851

McCARTHY, D. S. and PEPYS, J. (1971) Allergic broncho-pulmonary aspergillosis. Clinical immunology: (1) clinical features. *Clinical Allergy,* **1**, 261–286

McCARTHY, D. S., PEPYS, J. and BATTEN, J. C. (1969) Hypersensitivity to fungi in cystic fibrosis. *Fifth International Cystic Fibrosis Conference. London: Cystic Fibrosis Research Trust*

MARKS, M. I. (1981) The pathogenesis and treatment of pulmonary infections in patients with cystic fibrosis. *Journal of Pediatrics,* **98**, 173–179

MEARNS, M. B., LONGBOTTOM, J. and BATTEN, J. C. (1967) Precipitating antibodies to *Aspergillus fumigatus* in cystic fibrosis. *Lancet,* **i**, 538–539

MEARNS, M. B., YOUNG, W. and BATTEN, J. C. (1965) Transient pulmonary infiltrations in cystic fibrosis due to allergic aspergillosis. *Thorax,* **20**, 385–392

MELLIS, C. M. and LEVISON, H. (1978) Bronchial reactivity in cystic fibrosis. *Pediatrics,* **61**, 446–450

MITCHELL, I., COREY, M., WOENNE, R., KRASTINS, I. R. B. and LEVISON, H. (1978) Bronchial hyperreactivity in cystic fibrosis and asthma. *Journal of Pediatrics,* **93**, 744–748

MOSS, R. B., YAO-PI HSU, M. S., LEAHY, M. and HALPERN, G. (1982) IgG4 antibody to *Pseudomonas aeruginosa* in cystic fibrosis. *CF Club Abstracts,* **23**, 13

MOSS, R. B., YAO-PI HSU, M. S. and LEWISTON, N. J. (1981) 125I-C1q-binding and specific antibodies as indicators of pulmonary disease activity in cystic fibrosis. *Journal of Pediatrics,* **99**, 215–222

NELSON, L. A., CALLERAME, M. L. and SCHWARTZ, R. H. (1979) Aspergillosis and atopy in cystic fibrosis. *American Review of Respiratory Disease,* **120**, 863–873

NIE, N. H., HADLAI HULL, C., JENKINS, J. G., STEINBRENNER, K. and BERT, D. H. (1975) *Statistical Package for the Social Sciences,* 2nd ed. New York: McGraw Hill

ORMEROD, L. P., THOMSON, R. A., ANDERSON, C. M. and STABLEFORTH, D. E. (1980) Reversible airway obstruction in cystic fibrosis. *Thorax,* **36**, 768–772

PATTERSON, R., ROSENBERG, M. and ROBERTS, M. (1977) Evidence that *Aspergillus fumigatus* growing in the airway of man can be a potent stimulus of specific and nonspecific IgE formation. *American Journal of Medicine,* **63**, 257–266

PENKETH, A., PITT, T., ROBERTS, D., HODSON, M. and BATTEN, J. C. (1983) The relationship of phenotype changes in *Pseudomonas aeruginosa* to the clinical condition of patients with cystic fibrosis. *American Review of Respiratory Disease,* **127**, 605–608

PITCHER-WILMOTT, R. W. (1984) Allergy and the lung disease of cystic fibrosis. London University: MD Thesis

PITCHER-WILMOTT, R. W., LEVINSKY, R. J., GORDON, I., TURNER, M. W. and MATTHEW, D. J. (1982) Pseudomonas infection, allergy and cystic fibrosis. *Archives of Disease in Childhood,* **57**, 582–586

PRICE, J. F., WELLER, P. H., HARPER, S. A. and MATTHEW, D. J. (1979) Response to bronchial provocation and exercise in children with cystic fibrosis. *Clinical Allergy,* **9**, 563–570

RACHELEFSKY, G. S., OSHER, A., DOOLEY, R. E., ANK, B. and STIEHM, E. R. (1974) Co-existent respiratory allergy and cystic fibrosis. *American Journal of Diseases of Children,* **128**, 355–359

RADIN, R. C., GREENBERGER, P. A., PATTERSON, R. and GHORY, A. (1983) Mold counts and exacerbations of allergic bronchopulmonary aspergillosis. *Clinical Allergy,* **13**, 271–275

REEN, D. J., CARSON, J., MAGUIRE, O., FITZGERALD, M. X. and TEMPANY, E. (1981) Atopy and cystic fibrosis: A study of CF sibling pairs and their families. *Clinical Allergy,* **11**, 571–577

REID, L. (1980) Cardiopulmonary pathology. In *Perspectives in Cystic Fibrosis* (Proceedings of the 8th international cystic fibrosis congress), ed. J. M. Sturgess, pp. 198–214. Toronto: Canadian Cystic Fibrosis Foundation

REYNOLDS, H. Y., LEVINE, A. S., WOOD, R. E., ZIERDT, C. H., DALE, D. C. and PENNINGTON, J. E. (1975) Pseudomonas infections: persisting problems and current research to find new therapies. *Annals of Internal Medicine,* **82,** 819–831

RICKETTI, A. J., GREENBERGER, P. A., MINTZER, R. A. and PATTERSON, R. (1983) Allergic bronchopulmonary aspergillosis. *Archives of Internal Medicine,* **143,** 1553–1557

ROSENBERG, M., MINTZER, R., AARONSON, D. W. and PATTERSON, R. (1977) Allergic bronchopulmonary aspergillosis in three patients with normal chest X-ray films. *Chest,* **72,** 597–600

ROSENBERG, M., PATTERSON, R., ROBERTS, M. and WANG, J. (1978) The assessment of immunologic and clinical changes occurring during corticosteroid therapy for allergic bronchopulmonary aspergillosis. *American Journal of Medicine,* **64,** 599–606

RULON, J. T., BROWN, H. A. and LOGAN, G. B. (1963) Nasal polyps and cystic fibrosis of the pancreas. *Archives of Otolaryngology,* **78,** 192–199

SAFIRSTEIN, B. H., D'SOUZA, M. F., SIMON, G., TAI, E. H-C. and PEPYS, J. (1973) Five-year follow-up of allergic bronchopulmonary aspergillosis. *American Review of Respiratory Disease,* **108,** 450–459

SCHIOTZ, P. O., JORGENSEN, M., FLENSBORG, E. W., FAERO, O., HUSBY, S., HOIBY, N. *et al.* (1983) Chronic *Pseudomonas aeruginosa* lung infection in cystic fibrosis: A longitudinal study of immune complex activity and inflammatory responses in sputum sol-phase of cystic fibrosis patients with chronic *Pseudomonas aeruginosa* lung infections. Influence of local steroid treatment. *Acta Paediatrica Scandinavica,* **72,** 283–287

SCHWARTZMAN, S. and BORING, J. R. (1971) III. Antiphagocytic effect of slime from a mucoid strain of *Pseudomonas aeruginosa. Infection and Immunity,* **3,** 762–767

SHAKIB, F., STANWORTH, D. R., SMALLEY, C. A. and BROWN, G. A. (1976) Elevated serum IgG4 levels in cystic fibrosis patients. *Clinical Allergy,* **6,** 237–240

SILVERMAN, M., HOBBS, F. D. R., GORDON, I. R. S. and CARSWELL, F. (1978) Cystic fibrosis, atopy and airways lability. *Archives of Disease in Childhood,* **53,** 873–877

SLACK, M. P. E. and NICHOLS, W. W. (1981) The penetration of antibiotics through sodium alginate and through the exopolysaccharide of a mucoid strain of *Pseudomonas aeruginosa. Lancet,* **ii,** 502–503

SLAVIN, R. and WINZENBERGER, P. (1977) Epidemiologic aspects of allergic aspergillosis. *Annals of Allergy,* **38,** 215–218

STERN, R. C., BOAT, T. F., WOOD, R. E., MATTHEWS, L. W. and DOERSHUK, C. F. (1982) Treatment and prognosis of nasal polyps in cystic fibrosis. *American Journal of Diseases of Children,* **136,** 1067–1070

SZAFF, M., HOIBY, N. and FLENSBORG, E. W. (1983) Frequent antibiotic-therapy improves survival of cystic fibrosis patients with chronic *Pseudomonas aeruginosa* infections. *Acta Paediatrica Scandinavica,* **72,** 651–657

TACIER-EUGSTER, H., WUTHRICH, B. and MEYER, H. (1980) Atopic allergy, serum IgE and RAST-specific IgE antibodies in patients with cystic fibrosis. *Helvetica Paediatrica Acta,* **35,** 31–37

TALAMO, R. C., ROSENSTEIN, B. J. and BERNINGER, R. W. (1983) Cystic fibrosis. In *The Metabolic Basis of Inherited Disease,* eds J. B. Stanbury, J. B. Wyngaarden, D. S. Fredrickson, J. L. Goldstein and M. S. Brown, pp. 1889–1917. New York: McGraw-Hill

TAYLOR, B., NORMAN, A. P., ORGEL, H. A., STOKES, C. R., TURNER, M. W. and SOOTHILL, J. F. (1973) Transient IgA deficiency and pathogenesis of infantile atopy. *Lancet,* **ii,** 111–113

TURNER, M. W., WARNER, J. O., STOKES, C. R. and NORMAN, A. P. (1978) Immunological studies in cystic fibrosis. *Archives of Disease in Childhood,* **53,** 631–638

VAN ASPEREN, P., MELLIS, C. M. and SOUTH, R. T. (1980) Respiratory allergy in cystic fibrosis. *Australian Paediatric Journal,* **16,** 53–56

VAN ASPEREN, P., MELLIS, C. M., SOUTH, R. T. and SIMPSON, S. J. (1981) Bronchial reactivity in cystic fibrosis with normal pulmonary function. *American Journal of Diseases of Children,* **135,** 815–819

VAN METRE, T. E., COOKE, R. E., GIBSON, L. E. and WINKENWERDER, W. L. (1960) Evidence of allergy in patients with cystic fibrosis of the pancreas. *Journal of Allergy,* **31,** 141–150

WARNER, J. O. (1977) The variability of skin test hypersensitivity reactions in cystic fibrosis and asthma. *Clinical Allergy,* **7,** 385–389

WARNER, J. O., TAYLOR, B. W., NORMAN, A. P. and SOOTHILL, J. F. (1976) Association of cystic fibrosis with allergy. *Archives of Disease in Childhood,* **51,** 507–511

WARREN, C. P. W., TAI, E., BATTEN, J. C., HUTCHCROFT, B. J. and PEPYS, J. (1975) Cystic fibrosis-immunological reactions to *A. fumigatus* and common allergens. *Clinical Allergy,* **1,** 1–12

WOOD, R. E., BOAT, T. F. and DOERSHUK, C. F. (1976) Cystic fibrosis: state of the art. *American Review of Respiratory Disease,* **113,** 833–878

11
Outcome of respiratory disease in childhood
Hamish Simpson and Jacqueline Y. Q. Mok

INTRODUCTION

A link between respiratory illnesses in childhood and chronic bronchitis in the adult has been suspected for some years (Oswald, Harold and Martin, 1953; Reid, 1969). As evidence for and against this hypothesis has accumulated the possible relation of childhood respiratory illness to subsequent chronic airflow obstruction (CAO), a term which embraces chronic bronchitis, emphysema and irreversible obstructive lung disease (Thurlbeck, 1976), has become the subject of recent review (Samet, Tager and Speizer, 1983). Convincing data which document progressive disease starting as isolated or recurrent lower respiratory tract infection in infancy or early childhood and culminating in clinically apparent CAO in mid-adult life, after years of freedom from symptoms, are not presently available. Indeed, the logistics of planning and time scale of conducting the longitudinal studies which might provide a definitive answer, make it unlikely that they will ever be conducted. Circumstantial evidence is derived mainly from epidemiological investigations of social and environmental factors which contribute to both the development and outcome of respiratory illnesses in children, from follow-up studies of groups of children with previous lower respiratory infections documented according to clinical diagnosis or aetiological agent(s) responsible for infection, and from observations on the natural history of CAO in adults.

The idea that insult to the lungs in early childhood may have a bearing on subsequent lung function and susceptibility to disease becomes more plausible when one considers that the lung is still growing and developing when such insults usually occur. Lung growth is incomplete at birth and during the first decade there is a 10-fold increase in the number of lung alveoli (Dunnill, 1962). Development of the airway is completed *in utero*, but during the early years of life peripheral airway conductance is low. The marked increase which occurs after the age of 5 has been attributed to an increase in diameter of the small peripheral airway (Hogg *et al.*, 1970). Closing volume, the volume at which the peripheral airway begins to close during expiration is also higher in young children (Mansell, Bryan and Levison, 1972). These observations, together with those of Polgar and Weng (1979) on the functional development of the respiratory system, support the notion that the developing lung is vulnerable to injury. The pattern of injury may be determined by

211

the stage of lung development at which injury occurs (Reid, 1977; Inselman and Mellins, 1981).

The pathophysiology most widely proposed (Macklem, 1973) and which would be consistent with the clinical sequence described, holds that the structure and function of the small peripheral airway are affected first (Niewoehner, Kleinerman and Rice, 1974; Cosio *et al.*, 1978) with progression after a long asymptomatic period to extensive airway abnormalities and emphysema (Thurlbeck, 1979). This sequence has not been confirmed directly, but may be the most significant pathological progression from health to established disease. However, a variety of environmental insults may compromise the growth of lung function during childhood so that full growth potential is not realized in early adult life. Conceivably the main impact is on alveolar development. The inevitable functional decline which follows during adult life would then result in symptomatic 'disease' at an earlier stage than would otherwise have been expected if lung growth had been optimal (Samet, Tager and Speizer, 1983).

The present chapter does not attempt to examine the evidence to support a particular pathological hypothesis. Some of the epidemiological investigations of social and environmental factors which contribute to the development of respiratory illnesses in childhood and potentiate their immediate and long-term effects are reviewed, and the outcome for groups of children with documented index respiratory illnesses and for illness caused by specific aetiological agents described. Many studies do not extend beyond late childhood or early adult life, so that ultimate outcome is not known. The conditions reviewed may have varying natural 'pathological' end-points sometimes modified by additional environmental insults, such as cigarette smoke. They have in common a propensity to increase liability to recurrent respiratory symptoms and impair ventilatory function during childhood, probably by affecting lung growth and development. The scene is then set for early natural decline in lung function, or accelerated decline with subsequent infection or environmental hazard. The evidence from adult studies implicates two factors, cigarette smoking and α_1-anti-trypsin deficiency (Morse, 1978) as causally related to the development of CAO in the adult. The deleterious effects of these factors on the normally developed lung might well be exaggerated in the lung where growth and development has been compromised by childhood respiratory illness.

The natural history of chronic bronchitis and emphysema in the adult has been the subject of reviews by Fletcher *et al.* (1976) and Speizer and Tager (1979). Only key studies which relate adult respiratory status and childhood respiratory illness will be discussed.

SOCIAL AND ENVIRONMENTAL FACTORS

Social and environmental factors have been studied in relation to the susceptibility of infants and children to acute lower respiratory tract illnesses and their sequelae, the occurrence of recurrent or chronic respiratory symptoms in children with no previous history of acute respiratory illness, abnormalities of lung function in apparently healthy children with or without antecedent respiratory symptoms, and the pathogenesis of chronic obstructive lung disease in adults. A host of inter-relating factors operate throughout infancy and childhood whose individual contributions to morbidity are extremely difficult to assess. These include social status, urban or rural residence, housing conditions, family size, respiratory symptoms in other family members, and atmospheric pollution including passive and active smoking.

Air pollution, social and family factors

Colley and Holland (1967) studied the effects of social and family factors and air pollution on respiratory disease in over 2000 families from 2 areas in a north-west London suburb. All infants born within a 2-year period were selected and reviewed annually for 5 years. An attack of bronchitis or pneumonia in a sibling, especially during the first year of life of the index infant, was the most important determinant of respiratory illness in young children. Respiratory illness increased with the number of siblings and the age of the eldest – being most prevalent when the latter were of school age. Tests of ventilatory function soon after birth in a sample of index cases were comparable in the subgroups of infants suffering chest illnesses and those remaining well during the subsequent 5 years (Colley *et al.*, 1976). However, at the age of one year, crying (peak expiratory flow rate, PEFR) was significantly lower in infants who had suffered from bronchitis or pneumonia in the first year of life.

In a later study of 6–10-year-old primary school children in areas representative of a wide range of urban and rural environments in England and Wales, Colley and Reid (1970) found a pronounced social class gradient in the prevalence of recurrent respiratory tract infections and chronic cough. In addition, children with chronic cough were more likely to have suffered previous bronchitis or pneumonia. Air pollution did not influence the prevalence of upper respiratory tract infections, but was a significant contributory factor to lower respiratory illnesses in children from social classes IV and V.

Yarnell and St Leger (1977) examined the influence of housing conditions by comparing the occurrence of respiratory illnesses in children from traditional valley houses with that in children from modern council estates in South Wales. Upper respiratory tract infections were more common in children from modern council estates, the children from valley houses being relatively free of such illnesses. The forced expiratory volume in 0.75 s ($FEV_{0.75}$) and the forced vital capacity (FVC) performed in a random sample were lower in children from council houses. The authors attributed these findings to differences in the type of heating employed. Estate houses were centrally heated whereas traditional valley houses had coal fires.

Wahdan (1963) compared children from an industrial town (Sheffield) with those living in a rural environment (Vale of Glamorgan) and found that upper respiratory tract infection, recurrent or persistent cough, and attacks of bronchitis and pneumonia were more common in children from the polluted industrial area. The peak expiratory flow rate (PEFR) and $FEV_{1.0}$ were significantly lower in these children. When the family structure was examined, 'overcrowding' (defined as more than two persons per room) was associated with an increase in chest illnesses especially if there was a bronchitic person in the family. A preschool child in the home increased still further the likelihood of recurrent colds and sore throats. Although type of dwelling, area of residence, and level of atmospheric pollution tend to be inter-related, there are now several reports on the effects of pollution *per se*. Toyama (1964) showed that acute exposure to pollutants in the air temporarily affected respiratory function in children, with improvement when the level of pollution dropped. Stebbings and Fogleman (1977) presented similar findings in non-asthmatic white school children exposed acutely to air pollution in Pittsburg. Forced vital capacity (FVC) was reduced in 10–15% of children, but increased subsequently by 20% on average (as judged from trends in the regression curves for FVC) when the pollution had subsided.

The effect of prolonged exposure to varying degrees of air pollution was assessed by Douglas and Waller (1966) in a group of 15-year-old children with documented information on respiratory illnesses and exposure to air pollution from birth. Only families who remained at the same address or who had moved to areas of comparable pollution were included. Social class distribution was similar in areas with differing levels of pollution, but lower respiratory tract infection was more common and more severe in children from the more polluted areas. Respiratory function was not assessed in this study.

Lunn, Knowelden and Handyside (1967) studied primary schoolchildren from 4 areas in Sheffield with contrasting pollution levels. Children from the most polluted areas had more respiratory illnesses and significantly lower values for $FEV_{0.75}$ and FVC. Impairment of ventilatory function was greatest in children with previous lower respiratory tract infections. Four years later, after clean air measures had been introduced, no differences were noted in the prevalence of respiratory illnesses in children from these areas (Lunn, Knowelden and Roe, 1970). This suggests that clean air measures were effective even though only 68% of the original sample was available for subsequent review.

Similar conclusions on the effects of air pollution on the respiratory tract have been drawn from studies in Europe and North America. Zapletal *et al.* (1973) assessed respiratory function in school children from a heavily polluted industrial city in Czechoslovakia. The $FEV_{1.0}$ and FVC values were within the predicted normal ranges for height and sex. However, more sensitive tests for respiratory function in children with $FEV_{1.0}$ values near the lower end of the normal range showed a significant reduction in the maximum mid-expiratory flow rate (MMEFR). Static lung volumes and elastic properties of the lungs were within normal limits. It was concluded that air pollutants caused changes in airway function revealed only by sensitive tests of ventilatory function. The findings for this group were compared with those in children from an area of lower pollution (Zapletal *et al.*, 1977). The groups were similar in respect of housing, socioeconomic status, dietary habits, and family smoking practices. No differences were observed in the occurrence of upper respiratory problems, but the prevalence of pneumonia was twice as great in children from the more polluted areas. Likewise, abnormalities of lung function were more common. During the subsequent 2 years, the number of children with significant airflow limitation at low lung volume (reduction in maximum airflow at 25% vital capacity ($V25$) in the polluted area was double that of controls in the non-polluted areas. In North America, Sharratt and Cerny (1979) examined pulmonary function in children from two cities with contrasting levels of air pollution. The children selected were comparable in age, height, weight and socioeconomic status. Respiratory illnesses were more frequent in those from the more heavily polluted area; their parents and siblings also suffered more chest illness. Despite its careful design, this study illustrates some of the difficulties of separating the effects of atmospheric pollution from potentially significant intra-family variables.

Passive and active smoking

Norman-Taylor and Dickinson (1972) drew attention to the adverse effects of 'passive' smoking in a study of more than 1000 infant schoolchildren and their families. Thirty-three and a half per cent of non-smoking families had children with respiratory symptoms, compared with 44.5% of heavy smoking families. Similarly, Colley, Holland and Corkhill (1974) showed that parents' smoking habits and phlegm production contributed significantly to recurrent cough in 6–14-year-old children. This was true within a given social class and in families of similar size. The vulnerability of the infant to the effects of inhaled cigarette smoke was further demonstrated in a longitudinal study of over 2000 infants assessed annually for 5 years (Colley, Holland and Corkhill, 1974). Comparison of parents' replies to postal questionnaires and general practitioner records showed broad agreement between respective accounts of illness. In the first year of life, the prevalence of bronchitis and pneumonia was highest when both parents smoked and lowest when they were non-smokers. In subsequent years there was no clear association between parents' smoking habits and chest illnesses in children, but during the first 5 years of life, the occurrence of pneumonia or bronchitis was influenced by parents' respiratory symptoms irrespective of smoking habits. The higher incidence of lower respiratory illnesses in infants whose parents smoked could not be accounted for by social class, family size or weight of the infants.

In a study of white families from three towns in the USA, Schilling *et al.* (1977) were unable to demonstrate a significant relationship between respiratory symptoms in children and those of their parents. They concluded also that parental smoking had no effect on the frequency and severity of respiratory symptoms or lung function. These findings, which appear to contradict UK experience, might be explained by the age at which the children were studied. All were over 7 and probably less likely to be exposed to their parents' chest symptoms or cigarette smoke to the same extent as infants and younger children. In another American study, Lebowitz and Burrows (1976) found that social status, family size or age of children were not significantly related to the effect of parental smoking on children's respiratory symptoms. No differences were noted in the respiratory symptoms of children when either or both parents smoked. 'Children' in this study were subjects under 15 years of age, and no further breakdown of age is given. This study did confirm that respiratory symptoms in children were directly influenced by those in adults.

Several other American studies using analyses of cross-sectional data have suggested that maternal cigarette smoking does influence lung function in children (Tager *et al.*, 1979; Weiss *et al.*, 1980; Hasselblad, 1981). Tager *et al.* (1983) have subsequently reported a longitudinal study of the effects of maternal smoking on pulmonary function in children. A cohort of children and adolescents were observed prospectively for 7 years. The authors concluded that maternal cigarette smoking significantly lowered the expected average increase in FEV_1, and may adversely affect the development of pulmonary function in children.

Passive smoking also appears to influence medical referrals of infants and young children. In a study of hospital admissions, Harlap and Davies (1974) reported increased morbidity in infants from homes where mothers smoked. Bronchitis and pneumonia were significantly more common (as were injuries and poisonings) in such infants. This increase in hospital admission for chest illnesses was most marked in the winter months, perhaps because infants spent more time indoors with increased likelihood of exposure to cigarette smoke. More recently, Fergusson, Horwood and Shannon (1980) followed a cohort of infants from the age of one and found that the risk of medical attendance for lower respiratory illness more than doubled when both parents smoked. This increase was more closely related to maternal than paternal smoking.

Bland *et al.* (1978) studied the relation of active smoking and respiratory illness in first year secondary school children. Smoking was more common in boys than girls and increased in both sexes if their parents smoked. Morning cough was more common in smokers and increased in severity with the number of cigarettes smoked. The development of symptoms was related to the smoking habits of both children and their parents. Tager *et al.* (1979) assessed respiratory function in a random sample of 5–9-year-old children whose personal and parental smoking habits were known. The MMEFR was highest in children who had never smoked and came from non-smoking families. Lung function was influenced by active smoking whether or not parents smoked. Likewise, lung function was impaired in non-smoking children whose parents smoked even though respiratory symptoms were no more common in this group.

Apart from its effect on respiratory status, parental smoking also affects the growth of children (Rona *et al.*, 1981). Using data from the National Study of Health and Growth these investigators found a strong inverse relationship between children's heights and the number of smokers in the home, not accounted for by maternal smoking during pregnancy or by respiratory symptoms impairing growth.

CHILDHOOD RESPIRATORY ILLNESS AND SUBSEQUENT PROBLEMS IN ADULT LIFE

The social and environmental factors discussed operate throughout childhood and influence the outcome for children suffering lower respiratory tract illnesses in infancy and early childhood. However, there is increasing evidence that such illnesses have an independent effect on outcome. In an investigation of the effects of environmental and personal factors on ventilatory function in approximately 11 000 schoolchildren from 4 different areas in Kent at ages 5, 11, and 14, Holland *et al.* (1969) found that PEFR was lowest in children from the area of worst pollution and in those children with a previous history of respiratory illnesses. Social class and family size exerted less influence on respiratory function. Bland, Holland and Elliott (1974) reviewed about 40% of these children at age 11 and found that those with a history of respiratory illness had more respiratory symptoms and a lower PEFR than those who had escaped such illnesses. The inclusion of asthmatic children in this study could have explained the reduction in PEFR. A smaller proportion (12%) of the original sample was examined at ages 5, 11, and 14 by Holland, Bailey and Bland (1978) who found that children with bronchitis in the first 5 years of life were more prone to bronchitis at the age of 11 and to more severe colds, coughs, wheeze and phlegm production at 11 and 14. As the numbers in the final study were too few to be representative of the original sample, definitive conclusions could not be drawn. In another follow-up study designed to assess the effects of social and environmental factors, Leeder *et al.* (1976) found that children with a history of bronchitis or pneumonia had lower values for PEFR than those who had escaped such illnesses. This effect was most significant when respiratory illness had occurred before the age of 2. Recurrent illness had a greater influence than single episodes of respiratory ill-health. Parental social class, respiratory symptoms and smoking habits had no effect on PEFR.

In a study of a random sample of schoolchildren in Sydney, Woolcock *et al.* (1977) emphasized the contribution of early childhood bronchitis to impairment of ventilatory function as children grew older. Both bronchitis and asthma contributed to airflow limitation (maximum airflow at 50% vital capacity, *V*-50) confirmed during 3 consecutive annual check-ups. Lung function diminished further when children started to smoke.

The longer-term consequences of childhood respiratory illnesses have been highlighted by the findings of Colley, Douglas and Reid (1973) in a cohort of infants born in the last week of March 1946 and followed up to the age of 20. Health visitors interviewed parents when the children were aged 2 and documented episodes of respiratory disease occurring before that age. At the age of 20, the occurrence of chronic winter cough was related both to smoking and early childhood chest illnesses. The social class of the father and air pollution had only minor effects.

Kiernan *et al.* (1976) studied 54% of this cohort 5 years later. Current smoking habits and an early childhood chest illness continued to be the main determinants of chronic cough. A reduction in respiratory symptoms was reported in those who had stopped smoking, but the effects of childhood respiratory illnesses were still clearly seen.

Similar conclusions have been reached by Burrows, Knudson and Lebowitz (1977) in a study of random sample of white non-Mexican American adults over the age of 20. Respiratory illnesses before the age of 16 and current smoking habits were the subject of enquiry by means of self-administered questionnaires to 2626 adults. Maximum expiratory flow–volume curves were then obtained and analysed. An increased prevalence of cough and sputum was observed in subjects who reported 'childhood respiratory trouble' irrespective of their smoking history. Ventilatory function declined with age more rapidly in smokers with 'childhood respiratory trouble' than in smokers without previous chest illness. Among non-smokers, ventilatory function declined with age more rapidly in those who reported childhood respiratory illnesses than in those who had remained free of chest problems. These observations held when numbers were adjusted to exclude subjects with probable asthma. No further details are given of the nature of the chest illnesses from which these subjects suffered. Moreover, the study was subject to recall of childhood events which might have preferentially recalled childhood illnesses thereby introducing a bias. Despite these qualifications, the results of this investigation are consistent with the view that childhood respiratory illnesses predispose to chest diseases in adult life. Recent editorials have considered the evidence for this association, with varying degrees of scepticism (Streider, 1974; Burrows and Taussig, 1980; Holland, 1982; Phelan, 1984).

Wheezy bronchitis and asthma

Several Australian studies describe the natural history of asthma in childhood and early adult life. Williams and McNicol (1969) reported a survey of 7-year-old Melbourne schoolchildren from whom 3 groups were selected for longitudinal evaluation – 182 with wheezy bronchitis (when wheeze occurred only in association with respiratory infection), 113 with asthma, and 106 control children. An additional 83 children with severe asthma were subsequently added (McNicol and Williams, 1973). Their progress was reviewed, including assessment of ventilatory function and bronchial reactivity at 10, 14 and 21 years of age. The severity of wheezing diminished between 14 and 21 years of age (Martin *et al.*, 1980). Ventilatory function was comparable in the control group and the index group with no episodes of wheeze in the preceding 3 years. Bronchial reactivity was increased in children with a history of wheeziness irrespective of the continuing severity of symptoms. Pulmonary function abnormalities documented at 14 years of age persisted at 21 years of age in children with the most severe clinical symptoms (Martin *et al.*, 1980). The extent to which childhood lower respiratory infections might have contributed to outcome was not assessed. Williams and McNicol (1969) had been unable to demonstrate differences between groups of children with wheezy bronchitis and asthma, though both differed from controls with respect to atopic features, and respiratory function status. Phelan (1984) argues that asthma (including wheezy bronchitis) in childhood is a more likely antecedent of CAO than childhood respiratory infection. However, childhood respiratory infection frequently precipitates episodes of wheeze ('asthma') (Henderson *et al.*, 1979) making it impossible to separate 'infective' and 'asthmatic' components. This compels us to return to the unresolved difficulty – how best to define 'bronchitis' and 'asthma' in childhood?

OUTCOME FOR BRONCHIOLITIS AND PNEUMONIA IN INFANCY – RESPIRATORY SYNCYTIAL VIRUS INFECTIONS

Studies of the outcome for bronchiolitis and pneumonia in infancy cannot be discussed in isolation from the outcome for respiratory syncytial virus (RSV) infections of the lower respiratory tract. RSV is the most important respiratory pathogen in infancy in developed countries, and in hospital-based studies it may be isolated or identified by immunofluorescent techniques in some 70% of cases of acute bronchiolitis and 30% cases of pneumonia in the first year of life (Clarke *et al.*, 1978). Bronchiolitis is the commonest lower respiratory illness caused by this virus and, although many infants appear to recover uneventfully, there is growing suspicion that the immediate and long-term outlook is not entirely benign.

Following acute bronchiolitis, many infants recover clinically within 1–2 weeks. Phelan, Williams and Freeman (1968) reported normal lung function within 3 months of an attack whereas Wohl, Stigol and Mead (1969) reported an increase in the overall resistance to airflow by the forced oscillation technique some weeks following apparent recovery from bronchiolitis. Persistent functional abnormality in the early weeks or months following bronchiolitis was confirmed by Stokes *et al.* (1981) in a study of 22 infants. In a subsequent report of 93 children admitted to hospital with acute bronchiolitis, Henry *et al.* (1983) found that 77% had hyperinflated lungs in the immediate convalescent period which persisted in 43% 3 months later. After 1 year, 60% had abnormalities of lung function.

Longer-term follow-up studies of infants with bronchiolitis give conflicting results. Inadequate information on the agents responsible, varying criteria for the selection of index cases, absence of comparison groups, and differing periods of follow-up contribute to this uncertainty. Rooney and Williams (1971) reviewed 62 of 100 children admitted to hospital in the first 18 months of life with proven RS virus infection, 2–7 years later. Fifty-six per cent had wheezed recurrently, 43% on more than 5 occasions. Seventy-two per cent of wheezy children gave a positive family history of atopy, compared with 18% of non-wheezing children. No information was given on wheezing prior to index infections.

Beckerman, Taussig and Sieber (1978) reported a prospective study of 7 children who had bronchiolitis in infancy, but remained symptom free 3–6 years later. Lung function abnormalities maximum airflow ↓ (Vmax) FRC and exercise-induced bronchospasm) occurred independent of any allergic tendency. However, the numbers in the study were small, and only two children performed the exercise test.

Sims *et al.* (1978) reviewed 35 children 8 years after previous RS virus bronchiolitis in infancy and compared the findings with controls matched for age, sex and social class, but with no previous hospital admissions for respiratory illness in infancy. Although half of the index group wheezed subsequently, symptoms were not severe and had usually resolved by the age of 8. Only 1 child in the control group wheezed. The bronchiolitis group had lower resting PEF rates and greater bronchial lability following a non-standardized exercise test. The prevalence of atopic features in children and their first degree relatives was similar in the two groups. However, the families of those with bronchiolitis were larger and their parents smoked more in the first year of the child's life. The authors concluded that environmental factors were more important than respiratory tract infection in determining the outcome. From the same centre, Pullan and Hey (1982) reported the outcome for 130 children 10 years following RSV lower respiratory tract infection in infancy. They did not have an excess of atopic features when compared with 111 control children, but had more wheeze (42% index children, 19% controls), cough (9% index, 2% controls) and upper respiratory infections (22% index, 4.5% controls). Bronchial reactivity by histamine challenge or exercise testing was 3 times as common in index children. Ventilatory function was also reduced significantly. As in the preceding study, index children had more siblings and their parents, especially mothers, smoked more during the children's first year of life (68% mothers of index children compared with 46% of mothers of control children). The relative effects of infection and environmental factors could not be separated.

Comparable findings on bronchial reactivity following bronchiolitis have been reported by Gurwitz, Mindorff and Levison (1981). Forty-eight children were assessed some years following their index illness, and 57% were found to have bronchial reactivity on challenge with methacholine. A significant correlation was found between a positive methacholine response and a history of recurrent bronchiolitis. Positive responders also had impaired ventilatory function. Fourteen children gave a history of wheezing, but few were on long-term treatment for asthma. The finding that 33% of first-degree relatives of positive methacholine responders also had a positive response, suggested a genetic predisposition to airway reactivity and 'susceptibility' to bronchiolitis.

Mok and Simpson (1982) reported a 7-year follow-up study of 200 children admitted to hospital for acute lower respiratory tract infection in infancy and their matched controls. The index group comprised 100 cases where RS virus had been responsible for the index illness and 100 in whom this virus had not been found. Matched controls were of the same sex and age (to within 3 months), and from the same class in the same school as index cases. Social indices, such as class distribution and family size, were less favourable in the index group but housing standards and maternal smoking habits were similar. Subsequent respiratory symptoms (cough, wheeze, nasal discharge, and hearing difficulties) were significantly increased in index cases, as was absence from school and family doctor consultation for respiratory illness. Established 'bronchitis' and 'asthma', impairment of ventilatory function and bronchial reactivity (in response to a standardized exercise test) were also more common. No differences were found in clinical characteristics or outcome between RS virus positive and RS virus negative subgroups of index cases.

In a subsequent report (Mok and Simpson, 1984b), outcome was assessed in relation to the index diagnosis (bronchitis, bronchiolitis, pneumonia). All three clinical subgroups fared less well than corresponding case controls, the differences being greatest for bronchiolitis. The relation of atopic status and bronchial reactivity was also studied (Mok and Simpson, 1984a). Subdivision of the index group of infants into atopic and non-atopic subgroups did not separate bronchial reactive and non-reactive cases; conversely, subdivision of the index group on the basis of bronchial reactivity did not effect separation of atopic and non-atopic cases. These observations suggested that atopic status and bronchial reactivity were not closely related. The separation of index subgroups on the basis of bronchial reactivity proved more helpful than the more widely used atopic/non-atopic classification in separating children with recurrent cough and/or wheeze into 'bronchitic' and 'asthmatic' subgroups – the former defined by recurrent cough and the latter by recurrent wheeze on at least 4 occasions in the year prior to review (i.e. at age 6 to 7). The question whether bronchial reactivity predated infection or resulted from it could not be answered. The authors argued that the latter sequence was more likely. There have been few long-term follow-up studies of infants who remained symptom free following acute bronchiolitis. Kattan *et al.* (1977) showed that lung function abnormalities may persist following apparent clinical recovery from bronchiolitis in infancy. Respiratory function tests were performed on 23 children who remained symptom free and gave no history of asthma some 10 years following bronchiolitis. Most had evidence of hyperinflation (increase in residual volume/total lung capacity, i.e. $\uparrow$ RV/TLC), hypoxaemia, and airflow limitation at low lung volume (decrease in flow at iso-volume or $\downarrow$ *VisoV*; decrease in maximum airflow at 60% total lung capacity, $\downarrow$ V60). One-third of the children had all 3 abnormalities indicating residual parenchymal or airway lesions. More sensitive tests of lung function suggested that the small airway was affected (Kattan, Levison and Bryan, 1978). The small number of cases studied and the lack of a comparison group suggest that these findings should be interpreted with caution. Mok and Simpson (1984a) failed to demonstrate differences in ventilatory function between children who remained symptom free following lower respiratory tract infections (predominantly bronchiolitis) 7 years previously and carefully matched case controls. Any link between bronchiolitis in infancy and CAO in the adult remains speculative.

Respiratory infection, wheeze and atopy

Earlier studies of the subsequent course of infants with 'bronchiolitis' have concentrated on the prevalence of 'recurrent wheeze' or 'asthma' and their relation to a personal or family history of atopic disorders. Selection of index cases poses difficulties, partly because of the confused terminology applied to illnesses characterized by wheeziness in infants and young children. The diagnoses 'bronchiolitis', 'wheezy bronchitis' and 'asthmatoid bronchitis' are made on a clinical basis so that distinction (in the pathological sense) between 'bronchiolitis' and 'bronchitis' is not clearcut. Moreover, 'asthma' can seldom be diagnosed with confidence under the age of 18 months, though review of the histories of older children with unequivocal asthma often makes it clear that asthmatic symptoms had started in the first year of life.

The table summarizes the results of some early follow-up studies of 'bronchiolitis' and 'asthmatic bronchitis'. Several suggest that a significant proportion of infants with the clinical picture 'bronchiolitis' are experiencing a first attack of asthma. Most emphasize the subsequent occurrence of recurrent wheeziness or established asthma, often years later, and observe that wheezing or allergic features during index illnesses appear to predict a subsequent tendency to wheeze and 'allergic' symptoms. Whether pre-existing allergy predisposes to clinically severe bronchiolitis remains unanswered. In many of these studies virological findings during index illness (when given) have not been correlated with subsequent events. They suggest, in general, that bronchiolitis, especially in the absence of personal or family history of atopy, carries a good prognosis.

There have been few subsequent studies designed specifically to assess the role of atopy in the pathogenesis of bronchiolitis and wheezing following it. Cogswell, Halliday and Alexander (1982) studied 92 infants each of whom had one parent with asthma or hay fever from birth to 1 year of age. During this time respiratory symptoms, eczema and respiratory viral infections were all reported. At a year, atopic and non-atopic subgroups were defined, the former comprising infants who developed eczema or positive skin-patch responses to cutaneous allergens. The number of respiratory infections in the 2 groups was similar as were the nature and number of viruses isolated during infection. Wheezing was observed in 6 children during respiratory infections. Six were 'atopic' in the first year, and by 3 years 1 of the remaining 6 had developed eczema, and 5 an increase in total serum IgE. It was concluded that atopic predisposition was an important determinant of *wheezing* during viral respiratory infections. Laing *et al.* (1982) found an excess of atopy in infants admitted to hospital with bronchiolitis, compared with controls with non-respiratory illnesses, implying that atopic infants were more liable to develop severe infection and merit hospital admission. Both studies support views expressed previously (see *Table 11.1*).

Sims *et al.* (1981) studied 26 8-year-old children who had had RS virus bronchiolitis in infancy and their paired controls in an attempt to assess the role of immunodeficiency and atopy in the pathogenesis of RSV bronchiolitis and wheezing following it. There were no differences between patients and controls in the prevalence of atopy assessed by skin prick tests, eosinophil counts, yeast opsinization defect, C2 deficiency, and immunoglobulin concentrations of IgE antibody to common allergens. Exercise-induced bronchial lability, higher in patients than controls, did not correlate significantly with eosinophil counts or IgE concentrations. The authors concluded that atopy did not predispose to RSV bronchiolitis or postbronchiolitic wheezing. The studies of Pullan and Hey (1982) and Mok and Simpson (1982) support this conclusion.

Respiratory infection and bronchial reactivity

Recent interest has centred on the occurrence of bronchial reactivity following lower respiratory tract infections, particularly those caused by RS virus. In a follow-up study of 46 infants with 'obstructive bronchitis' almost 8 years later,

Table 11.1 Early studies of bronchiolitis, allergy and subsequent wheeziness

Author(s)	Cases	Number	Follow-up period	Conclusions
Boeson, 1953	'Asthmatic bronchitis'	162	6–11 y	Index illness 1 y 6% asthma Index illness 1–3 y 25% asthma Index illness 3 y 43% asthma
Witting, Cranford and Glaser, 1959	'Bronchiolitis'	100	1–7 y	32% asthma 49% respiratory allergies
Freeman and Todd, 1962	'Viral respiratory illnesses'	230	5–42 months	Wheezing during index illness predicted subsequent asthmatic bronchitis or allergy
Eisen and Bacal, 1963	'Bronchiolitis – single attack'	63	4–14 months	25% asthma, 21% 'wheezy bronchitis'
Hyde and Saed, 1966	'Bronchiolitis'	100	6–20 months	31% 'wheezers' of whom almost half wheezed before index illness
Zweiman, Schoenwetter and Hildeth, 1966; Zweiman, Schoenwetter, Pappano et al., 1971	'Bronchiolitis'	24	3–5 y	Approx. 50% recurrent wheezers; wheezing related to personal or family history of allergy; allergic features prominent in recurrent wheezers; wheezing usually associated with respiratory infection
Simon and Jordan, 1969	'Bronchiolitis'	66	–	RS−ve bronchiolitis predisposed to asthma; RS+ve bronchiolitis did not
Foucard, Berg, Johansson et al., 1971	'Wheeze associated respiratory illness'	72	–	IgE increased in patients with 'allergic' features; positive viral serology not related to IgE levels
Polmar, Robinson and Minnefor, 1972	'Bronchiolitis' and controls	33	–	IgE increased in 'sporadic' but not 'epidemic' bronchiolitic cases

Scislicki *et al.* (1978) concluded that bronchial reactivity (not allergy) during index illnesses predicted subsequent asthma. These observations have been extended by Gurwitz, Mindorff and Levison (1981), Pullan and Hey (1982) and Mok and Simpson (1982, 1984a). These studies place more emphasis on bronchial reactivity than atopy but do not clarify whether reactivity is the determinant of outcome in RS virus lower respiratory infections or whether it occurs as a sequel to infection. Frick, German and Mills (1979) postulated that virus infections induce bronchial reactivity in atopic infants, perhaps by causing abnormal lymphocyte responses and the release of chemical mediators which influence airway calibre (Welliver, Kaul and Ogra, 1979).

Bronchial reactivity has also been observed in respiratory disorders which are not thought to have an allergic basis. It has been reported in cystic fibrosis (Mellis and Levison, 1978), croup (Laughlin and Taussig, 1979; Gurwitz, Corey and Levinson, 1980; Zak, Erben and Olinsky, 1981), following surgery for tracheo-oesophageal fistula (Milligan and Levison, 1979; Couriel *et al.*, 1982), post-foreign body inhalation (Givan *et al.*, 1981) and near-drowning (Laughlin and Eiger, 1982). It seems likely, therefore, that a host of insults other than infection contribute to the production of bronchial reactivity. The natural history of bronchial reactivity and its relation to the pathogenesis of CAO is not known, but it may be a risk factor for its development. Britt *et al.* (1980) studied the sons of subjects with chronic obstructive lung disease and found that those with reactive bronchi had a more rapid decline in lung function than those without bronchial reactivity.

SPECIFIC AETIOLOGICAL AGENTS

There have been few follow-up studies of acute lower respiratory infections in children relating outcome to specific causative agents other than respiratory syncytial virus (RSV). Adenoviruses usually cause mild respiratory illnesses in children, but severe, and sometimes fatal, pneumonia has been reported (Chany *et al.*, 1958; Becroft, 1971). Long-term sequelae in survivors have also been reported. Gold *et al.* (1969) described chronic pulmonary disease (bronchiectasis, interstitial fibrosis and hyperlucent lung) in 53% of children following severe adenoviral chest illnesses. Adenovirus types 1, 3, and 4 were implicated in subjects examined between 1 month and 5 years following index illnesses. Adenovirus type 21 may also cause serious lung problems. In a study of children 1 month to 3.5 years following index illnesses, 65% had chronic respiratory symptoms and radiological evidence of bronchiectasis or other lung changes. These follow-up studies were of indigenous populations in whom poor housing and malnutrition almost certainly contributed to the unfavourable outcome. In a Finnish study comparing 43 children with pneumonia caused by adenovirus type 7 with a group of children with pneumonia due to other agents, Simila, Ylikorkala and Wasz-Hockert (1971) found that the clinical course of adenovirus type 7 pneumonia was especially severe. After 2.5 years, postal enquiry revealed that children with adenovirus pneumonia were treated more often in hospital for chest infections. Four of 9 who attended for review showed residual abnormalities on X-ray. In a more recent study, 12 of 22 children with previous adenovirus infection (Lanning, Simila and Linna, 1980) showed residual changes on X-ray 10 years later.

None of these reports give data on respiratory function status; from the clinical descriptions of outcome, functional impairment would seem likely.

Harrison (1982) studied 40 infants for up to 5 years (mean 26 months) following hospital admission for bronchiolitis or pneumonia in the first 6 months of life. *Chlamydia trachomatis* infection was diagnosed by retrospective serological investigation in 10 infants. On follow-up, patients with *Chlamydia trachomatis* respiratory infection had significantly more reported chronic cough and abnormalities of lung function (functional residual capacity, FRC) than those where infection was due to other agents, or where no agent was found. They had more cough and wheeze than a group of 71 age-matched normal infants. Lourdes *et al.* (1977) reported chronic pulmonary sequelae in 3 children following influenza virus infection at 5, 24 and 42 months of age. Varying degrees of interstitial fibrosis, bronchial and bronchiolar damage, and interstitial inflammatory infiltrates were found on lung biopsy. Pulmonary function tests were abnormal, with deterioration following exercise. The follow-up periods for both studies were too short to allow comment on longer-term outcome for infection caused by these organisms.

In many countries, pertussis is still a major cause of mortality and morbidity in young children. In the UK, Lees (1950) studied 150 consecutive cases severe enough to be admitted to hospital. Sixty-four (43%) had radiological evidence of atelectasis during the acute phase. All were symptom free or had a normal chest X-ray within a year. Similar encouraging results were reported by Fawcett and Parry (1957) in a review of children hospitalized for pertussis or measles. During the acute illness, abnormalities in chest X-ray were more likely in children with measles, especially those over the age of 1 year. At follow-up 1–6 years later, 87 (4.6%) of the original 1894 children had residual radiological changes. Respiratory symptoms persisted in 34, all of whom had abnormalities on chest X-ray. Jernelius (1964) studied a group of children 7–10 years following pertussis with pulmonary complications. None had further pneumonia, but 25% had recurrent cough for up to 3 years following the acute illness. Chest X-rays were normal, but static lung volumes were slightly lower than predicted. However, in a case control study to assess pulmonary and neurological outcome in 75 infants with pertussis, White, Finberg and Tramer (1964) found no evidence of chronic pulmonary disease in patients or controls after 9 years. To some extent these findings are at variance with the results of earlier follow-up studies of Perry and King (1940) who documented an association between bronchiectasis and previously inadequately treated measles or whooping cough. In a recent hospital-based retrospective study of 116 cases (mainly adult) of bronchiectasis, presumed causes were pneumonia (28%), pertussis (10%), tuberculosis (5%), 'bronchitis' and 'bronchiolitis' (5%), measles (3%) and other causes (5%) (Ellis *et al.*, 1981). These associations were not observed in the remaining 44%.

Kjellman (1968) found that ventilatory function was impaired in the acute phase of mycoplasma chest infections in children. Following apparent clinical recovery 1–3 months later, functional abnormalities sometimes persisted. Mok, Waugh and Simpson (1979) compared the respiratory status of 50 children (1 to 10 years, median 3) following admission to hospital for *Mycoplasma pneumoniae* respiratory illnesses, with a healthy control group of children. Simple tests of ventilatory function were similar in both groups. However, flow–volume curves obtained breathing and then helium/oxygen revealed residual dysfunction shown by an impaired response to breathing He/O_2. Permanent lung damage following *M. pneumoniae* infection has also been documented (Stokes *et al.*, 1978).

There have been few long-term studies of outcome for bacterial pneumonia in infancy except for primary staphylococcal pneumonia. This condition still carried a high mortality rate, but the long-term outlook for survivors is generally favourable. Binder *et al.* (1961) reported recurrent pneumonia in 22 of 92 patients recalled for study and 17 had residual radiological abnormalities. The interval between diagnosis and follow-up assessment is not stated. Huxtable, Tucker and Wedgewood (1964) contacted all 22 survivors of staphylococcal pneumonia about 4 years later. They had thrived satisfactorily and none had chronic cough or diminished exercise tolerance. Similar findings have been reported by Ceruti, Contreras and Neira (1971) in a study of 36 children 2–4 years after staphylococcal pneumonia. Only one had recurrent respiratory symptoms, but 13 had minor changes on chest X-ray – in one due to bronchiectasis. Arterial blood gas tensions were normal at rest and on exertion in 25 children investigated. No abnormalities of ventilatory function were detected in 12 children studied. The short period of follow-up and paucity of data on respiratory function status indicate that long-term outcome for staphylococcal pneumonia in childhood is uncertain.

OTHER FACTORS INFLUENCING RESPIRATORY ILLNESSES

Obesity

Hutchinson-Smith (1970) demonstrated an association between lower respiratory infection in infants and obesity in a prospective study of 200 infants during the first year of life. The early introduction of solid feeds (at <9 weeks of age) was associated with more frequent chest infections and an increased tendency to obesity. Infants less than 2.5 kg at birth were also more prone to chest infection. Those exclusively breast-fed gained weight less rapidly than partially breast-fed or artificially fed infants, and were less vulnerable to severe infections.

Feeding practices

Other studies have suggested that human milk has a protective effect and helps reduce the incidence of respiratory infection in infants. In a hospital-based study of infants with RS virus infection, Downham *et al.* (1976) found that breast-feeding was significantly less common than in a control group without respiratory illnesses. To elucidate the mechanism of this possible protection, human milk was examined for RS virus neutralizing activity. The detection of specific IgA or IgG in most of the specimens examined led to the hypothesis that breast-feeding contributed to the acquisition of local immunity in the respiratory tract, perhaps by the aspiration of milk containing specific IgA. The results might equally have been explained on the basis of social class. However, the suggestion that breast-feeding confers protection is supported by anecdotal evidence (Evans-Jones *et al.*, 1978) of the very low incidence of breast-fed babies admitted to hospital with acute bronchitis. In a prospective study from birth, Watkins, Leeder and Corkhill (1979) found that breast-fed babies had fewer episodes of bronchitis or pneumonia than those who were bottle-fed. This held true when other factors (family size, birth order, and maternal smoking habits) were taken into account. Cunningham (1979) reported similar findings in a study of infants seen regularly during the first year of life. Protection from significant respiratory or gastrointestinal illness was greatest in the early months of life and increased with the duration of breast feeding. This effect was independent of the social and environmental factors studied. In a subsequent study, Fallot, Boyd and Oski (1980) compared the prevalence of exclusive breast-feeding in community and hospitalized infants under 3 months of age. The incidence of breast-feeding was significantly lower in hospitalized patients. Upper respiratory infection, bronchiolitis and pneumonia occurred predominantly in exclusively bottle-fed babies. The authors advocate breast-feeding as a means of reducing the number of infants admitted to hospital.

Further evidence of the positive effects of breast-feeding comes from the prospective studies of Chandra (1979) in 3 separate communities. In an Indian rural community, breast-fed infants had significantly less cough, otitis or pneumonia than artificially fed matched controls. In an urban population in Canada breast-feeding was also associated with a decrease in colds and otitis media. A further beneficial effect of breast-feeding was also demonstrated in newborn siblings of children known to suffer from atopic disorders. A decrease in the incidence of eczema and recurrent wheeziness was observed together with a reduction in serum IgE and cow's milk antibodies.

Immaturity

Premature birth, without neonatal respiratory complications, influences susceptibility to chest infections. Douglas and Mogford (1953) and Drillien (1959) reported a high incidence of respiratory illnesses in premature infants outside the newborn period. Coates *et al.* (1977) studied the pulmonary function of 14 children born at about 33 weeks of gestation and weighing approximately 2000 g at birth. Seven had had respiratory distress syndrome of the newborn and 7 had escaped neonatal lung problems. The respiratory function of each subgroup was then compared with that of 7 normal children born at term and without subsequent pulmonary disease. The 3 groups were comparable in respect of lung volumes, MMEFR and PEF. However, functional abnormalities were revealed by flow–volume curves obtained breathing air and an O_2/He mixture. Children born prematurely had lower expiratory flow rates in air than full-term infants. The volume of iso-flow was highest in the preterm group with RDS, intermediate in 'normal' preterm children and lowest in those born at term.

The Wilson–Mikity syndrome (1960) affects premature infants and is thought to result from delayed and uneven alveolar development. Coates *et al.* (1977) assessed pulmonary function status of 5 surviving children with this condition, none of whom had received ventilatory support, 8–10 years later. Flow–volume variables were compared with those of 6 apparently normal premature children and 8 healthy children born at term. The lowest expiratory flow rates were observed in survivors of the Wilson–Mikity syndrome, and next in preterm infants without respiratory distress. No information was given of the possible influence of intrauterine growth retardation on subsequent lung function status.

Idiopathic respiratory distress syndrome (IRDS)

The effects of immaturity on lung growth and function are exaggerated by the occurrence of IRDS and the need for high inspired oxygen concentrations and mechanical ventilation (Northway, Rosan and Porter, 1967). Among survivors of

IRDS, Lewis (1968) reported that 11 (18%) of 63 were admitted to hospital subsequently with lower respiratory infection; in another series Shepard *et al.* (1968) found that 30% developed bronchiolitis or pneumonia. Outerbridge, Nobrady and Beaudry (1972) reported similar findings in a follow-up study of 53 infants with normal chest X-rays prior to discharge from hospital. Eleven (21%) were admitted to hospital later with severe lower respiratory infection, of whom 8 had persistent radiological changes. The follow-up period was short (26 months), and the prospects for eventual recovery uncertain. Johnson *et al.* (1974) studied infants treated by mechanical ventilation in the newborn period. Five to 6 years later those with a diagnosis of bronchopulmonary dysplasia in the newborn period had had recurrent chest infections and persisting abnormalities on chest X-ray. Harrod *et al.* (1974) studied 22 survivors of IRDS treated by intermittent positive pressure ventilation (IPPV) in the newborn period 1–5 years later. Only 2 had respiratory infections after the age of 1. Chest X-ray abnormalities, observed in two-thirds of cases were related to the duration of oxygen therapy. Of 16 apparently well children over 2, 8 had right ventricular hypertrophy, 10 had arterial hypoxaemia, and 15 an increased alveolar/arterial oxygen tension difference breathing 100% oxygen.

Ahlström (1973) studied 24 survivors of severe neonatal respiratory distress during the first year of life. The infants treated by continuous positive airway pressure (CPAP) alone had normal lung mechanics. IPPV-treated infants had a decrease in dynamic compliance and conductance, especially if treatment had been prolonged. However, the latter were, on average, 3 weeks more preterm than the CPAP group. Pressure–flow loops were abnormal in most infants indicating airflow obstruction, irrespective of original diagnosis or treatment.

The relative contributions of IPPV, oxygen therapy and CPAP to subsequent lung function status during the first year of life was assessed in 18 infants with IRDS at birth (Stocks and Godfrey, 1976). At discharge from the neonatal unit, most infants had normal lung function. Between 4 and 11 months of age, airway resistance was normal in infants treated with CPAP and/or oxygen, and increased in those given IPPV. However, the latter were of lower birthweight and gestational age than those not given IPPV. Kamper (1978) reported a good long-term prognosis for infants with IRDS treated by mechanical ventilation. When compared some 3–8 years later with controls matched for birthweight, gestation, and socioeconomic characteristics, respiratory illnesses were more common and the likelihood of hospitalization increased. Chest X-rays were 'abnormal' in 21 of 47 IRDS survivors and 9 matched controls. Respiratory rate, lung volumes, oxygen saturation and acid–base status were similar in both groups.

In a prospective clinical and physiological study of 20 infants who received IPPV in the neonatal period and 15 healthy controls matched for birthweight, Wong, Beardsmore and Silverman (1982) reported impairment of lung function (↑ thoracic gas volume, ↓ dynamic compliance and ↓ conductance) during the middle 4 months of the first year. Later in the first year, lung function had returned to normal in the IPPV-treated group, except for those with recurrent respiratory infections. Coates *et al.* (1982) reported respiratory outcome for 2 groups of children who had had IRDS of comparable severity and who received different regimes of oxygen therapy during their illnesses. None had received IPPV. Ten years later, 23 of 102 survivors were recalled for study. Tests of ventilatory function gave similar results in both subgroups. However, analysis of flow–volume curves breathing an oxygen/helium mixture revealed subtle abnormalities in children treated with high concentrations of oxygen in the newborn period. The authors concluded that a high inspired oxygen concentration, in the absence of mechanical ventilation, affected the mechanical properties of the lung of infants with IRDS in the newborn period.

Congenital abnormalities

Congenital diaphragmatic hernia

Herniation of abdominal viscera through the diaphragm may interfere mechanically with the growth of the lung, resulting in a varying degree of hypoplasia on the affected side and reduction in the size and number of airways, alveoli and arteries (Kitagawa *et al.*, 1971). Chatrath, El Hafie and Jones (1971) assessed ventilatory function in 14 children 6–12 years after surgical repair of congenital diaphragmatic hernia in infancy. At operation 5 had 'normal-looking' lungs. At follow-up, 3 children had overinflation of the affected lung on chest X-ray. The FEV_1 and FVC values were significantly reduced in these patients, although lung volumes were within normal limits. Wohl, Griscom and Streider (1977) reported persistent vascular abnormalities in a group of patients 6–18 years following repair of congenital diaphragmatic herniae. Ventilatory function, flow–volume curves breathing air and He/O_2, total respiratory resistance, diffusing capacity and distribution of ventilation using ^{133}Xe were normal in most. However, pulmonary perfusion was reduced on the side of the hernia in 9 patients who were investigated. Lung volumes had become normal with continuing growth of the alveoli, but without a corresponding increase in vascularity.

Tracheo-oesophageal fistula

Respiratory problems are common following repair of oesophageal atresia and tracheo-oesophageal fistulae. Laks, Wilkinson and Schuster (1972) studied 42 such patients 15–25 years following primary repair of these abnormalities and found that 33% had long-term recurrent chest problems. Recurrent aspiration was suggested as the main cause as 15 patients had disordered oesophageal motility on cinefluorographic examination. Dudley and Phelan (1976) reviewed 192 survivors of repaired oesophageal atresia 1–20 years later. About half were studied after 9 years. Persistent cough, recurrent bronchitis and pneumonia were reported in 78% – often necessitating hospitalization. Problems were most common in the first 8 years after operation. Abnormal oesophageal peristalsis was demonstrated in 42 patients. Indirect evidence of milk aspiration was found in 7 children based on examination of tracheal aspirates for fat globules.

Milligan and Levison (1979) found abnormalities of lung function in 23 of 24 patients studied 7–18 years following repair of tracheo-oesophageal fistula. Obstructive airway disease was observed in 13 and restrictive disease in 5. After challenge with methacholine, 15 (63%) had positive responses suggesting an increase in bronchial reactivity. The authors postulated that continuing subclinical aspiration caused lung damage and increased reactivity.

Hydrocarbon ingestion

Gurwitz, Kattan and Levison (1978) studied pulmonary function in 17 asymptomatic children 8–14 years after ingestion of hydrocarbon (petroleum distillate, turpentine, coal oil or cleaning fluid). Mild to severe pneumonia had been present initially. At follow-up, only 1 child had chest X-ray abnormalities persisting from the initial illness. However, 14 (82%) had one or more abnormalities of pulmonary function when compared with matched controls. Taussig *et al.* (1977) studied 3 patients who had swallowed fuel oil or furniture polish more than 7 years later; none showed chest X-ray or pulmonary function abnormalities.

CONCLUSIONS

Socioeconomic status, family factors (size, composition, housing etc.), air pollution and parental smoking may act singly or in combination to effect the occurrence of respiratory symptoms and lung function abnormalities in children. This influence might be direct, or indirect by modifying the prevalence and severity of lower respiratory tract infection. The host factors' atopic predisposition and 'innate' bronchial reactivity may have similar effects. It is difficult to dissociate them from the effect of infection *per se*, but the results of many of the follow-up studies described suggest that infection has an independent effect. There is no proof of a causal link between lower respiratory infection in infancy and diminution of lung function in later childhood and adolescence. Data concerning the transition period between apparent health in adolescence and established respiratory disease in adulthood is likewise inconclusive. Phelan (1984) suggests that functional impairment in asthmatic children continues through adolescence and early adult life to become the forerunner of chronic airflow obstruction in middle age. Confirmation of a particular pathological sequence is still awaited. What cannot be refuted is an association between apparently diverse respiratory illnesses in childhood and subsequent respiratory symptoms, and abnormalities of lung function in older childhood or adulthood. Suboptimal lung growth and bronchial reactivity may be non-specific effects of injury to the lung at a vulnerable time during its development. Genetically determined weakness in host defense mechanisms will almost certainly increase the liability to such injury.

Implications for prevention are clear. Social and environmental determinants of respiratory illness should be minimized by concerted preventive measures. Advances are awaited in the prevention of immaturity at birth, and of methods to ensure that breast-feeding is fully encouraged. There is an urgent need for methods to be introduced which discourage children from starting to smoke cigarettes (Warner and Murt, 1982), as it has proved difficult to influence the smoking habits of adults. In the UK, the limitations of current immunization programmes against pertussis (Robinson, 1981) and measles (Campbell, 1983) must be fully recognized and measures introduced to optimize uptake of these vaccines. Efforts should be intensified to find the means of controlling epidemics of respiratory illness in infants due to RSV (Hall, 1980), and to devise methods of preventing genetically determined lung diseases, such as cystic fibrosis (Weatherall, 1982). The respiratory health of children and adults in the future may well depend on the priority given to developing effective methods for preventing ill-health, and the zeal with which they are applied.

References

AHLSTRÖM, H. (1975) Pulmonary mechanics in infants surviving severe neonatal respiratory insufficiency. *Acta Paediatrica Scandinavica,* **64,** 69–80

BECKERMAN, R. C., TAUSSIG, L. M. and SIEBER, O. F. (1978) Prospective study of lung function in young children. *Pediatric Research,* **12,** 558

BECROFT, D. M. O. (1971) Bronchiolitis obliterans, bronchiotesis and other sequelae of adenovirus type 21 infection in young children. *Journal of Clinical Pathology,* **24,** 72–82

BINDER, L., DUDAS, P., HAIDEKKER, J. and SCHLAFFER, E. (1961) The later fate of children with staphylococcal pneumonia. *Acta Paediatrica Academiae Scientiarum Hungaricae,* **2,** 155–157

BLAND, J. M., BEWLEY, R. B., POLLARD, V. and BANKS, M. H. (1978) Effect of children's and parents' smoking on respiratory symptoms. *Archives of Disease in Childhood,* **53,** 100–105

BLAND, J. M., HOLLAND, W. W. and ELLIOTT, A. (1974) The development of respiratory symptoms in a cohort of Kent schoolchildren. *Bulletin de Physio-pathologie Respiratoire,* **10,** 699–716

BOESEN, I. B. (1953) Asthmatic bronchitis in children. Prognosis for 162 cases, observed 6–11 years. *Acta Paediatrica,* **42,** 87–96

BRITT, E. J., COHEN, B., MENKES, H., BLEECKER, E., PERMUTT, S., ROSENTHAL, R. and NORMAN, P. (1980) Airways reactivity and functional deterioration in relatives of COPD patients. *Chest,* **77,** 260

BURROWS, B., KNUDSON, R. J. and LEBOWITZ, M. D. (1977) The relationship of childhood respiratory illness to adult obstructive airway disease. *American Review of Respiratory Disease,* **115,** 751–760

BURROWS, B. and TAUSSIG, I. M. (1980) 'As the twig is bent, the tree inclines' (perhaps). *American Review of Respiratory Disease,* **122,** 813–816

CAMPBELL, A. G. M. (LA) (1983) Measles immunisation. *Archives of Disease in Childhood,* **58,** 3–5

CERUTI, E., CONTRERAS, J. and NEIRA, M. (1971) Staphylococcal pneumonia in childhood. Long-term follow-up including pulmonary function studies. *American Journal of Diseases of Children,* **122,** 386–392

CHANDRA, R. K. (1979) Prospective studies of the effect of breast feeding on incidence of infection and allergy. *Acta Paediatrica Scandinavica,* **68,** 691–694

CHANY, C., LÉPINE, P., LELONG, M., VINH, L. T., SATGE, P. and VIRAT, J. (1958) Severe and fatal pneumonia in infants and young children associated with adenovirus infections. *American Journal of Hygiene,* **67,** 367–378

CHATRATH, R. L., EL HAFIE, M. and JONES, R. S. (1971) Fate of hypoplastic lungs after repair of congenital diaphragmatic hernia. *Archives of Disease in Childhood,* **46,** 633–635

CLARKE, S. K. R., GARDNER, P. S., POOLE, P. M., SIMPSON, H. and TOBIN, J. O'H. (1978) Respiratory syncytial virus infection – admissions to hospital industrial, urban and rural areas. Report to the Medical Research Council Subcommittee on RSV vaccines. *British Medical Journal,* **2,** 796–798

COATES, A. L., BERGSTEINSSON, H., DESMOND, K., OUTERBRIDGE, E. W. and BEAUDRY, P. H. (1977) Long-term pulmonary sequelae of premature birth with and without idiopathic respiratory distress syndrome. *Journal of Pediatrics,* **90,** 611–616

COATES, A. L., DESMOND, K., WILLIS, D. and NOGRADY, M. B. (1982) Oxygen therapy and long-term pulmonary outcome of respiratory distress syndrome in newborns. *American Journal of Diseases of Children,* **136,** 892–895

COGSWELL, J. J., HALLIDAY, D. F. and ALEXANDER, J. R. (1982) Respiratory infections in the first year of life in children at risk of developing atopy. *British Medical Journal,* **284,** 1011–1013

COLLEY, J. R. T., DOUGLAS, J. W. B. and REID, D. D. (1973) Respiratory disease in young adults: influence of early childhood lower respiratory tract illness, social class, air pollution and smoking. *British Medical Journal,* **3,** 195–198

COLLEY, J. R. T. and HOLLAND, W. W. (1967) Social and environmental factors in respiratory disease. A preliminary report. *Archives of Environmental Health,* **14,** 157–161

COLLEY, J. R. T., HOLLAND, W. W. and CORKHILL, R. T. (1974) Influence of passive smoking and parental phlegm on pneumonia and bronchitis in early childhood. *Lancet,* **ii,** 1031–1034

COLLEY, J. R. T., HOLLAND, W. W., LEEDER, S. R. and CORKHILL, R. T. (1976) Respiratory function of infants in relation to subsequent respiratory disease: an epidemiological study. *Bulletin European de Physio-Pathologie Respiratoire,* **12,** 651–657

COLLEY, J. R. T. and REID, D. D. (1970) Urban and social origins of childhood bronchitis in England and Wales. *British Medical Journal,* **2,** 213–217

COSIO, M., GHEZZO, H., HOGG, J. C. et al. (1978) The relation between structural changes in small airways and pulmonary function tests. *New England Journal of Medicine,* **298,** 1277–1281

COURIEL, J. M., HIBBERT, M., OLINSKY, A. and PHELAN, P. D. (1982) Long-term pulmonary consequences of oesophageal atresia with traceo-oesophageal fistula. *Acta Paediatrica Scandinavica,* **71**(6), 973–978

CUNNINGHAM, A. S. (1979) Morbidity in breast-fed and artificially fed infants 11. *Journal of Pediatrics,* **95,** 685–689

DOUGLAS, J. W. B. and MOGFORD, C. (1953) Health of premature children from birth to four years. *British Medical Journal,* **1,** 748–754

DOUGLAS, J. W. B. and WALLER, R. E. (1966) Air pollution and respiratory function in children. *British Journal of Preventive and Social Medicine,* **20,** 1–8

DOWNHAM, M. A. P. S., SCOTT, R., SIMS, D. G., WEBB, J. K. G. and GARDNER, P. S. (1976) Breast feeding protects against respiratory syncytial virus infections. *British Medical Journal,* **2,** 274–276

DRILLIEN, C. M. (1959) A longitudinal study of the growth and development of prematurely and maturely born children IV. Morbidity. *Archives of Disease in Childhood,* **34,** 210–217

DUDLEY, N. E. and PHELAN, P. D. (1976) Respiratory complications in long term survivors of oesophageal atresia. *Archives of Disease in Childhood,* **51,** 279–282

DUNNILL, M. S. (1962) Post-natal growth of the lung. *Thorax,* **17,** 329

EISEN, A. H. and BACAL, H. L. (1963) The relationship of acute bronchiolitis to bronchial asthma – a 4–14 year follow-up. *Pediatrics,* **31,** 859–861

ELLIS, D. A., THORNLEY, P. E., WIGHTMAN, A. J., WALKER, M., CHALMERS, J. and CROFTON, J. W. (1981) The present outlook in bronchiesctasis: clinical and social study and review of the factors influencing prognosis. *Thorax,* **36**(9), 659–664

EVANS-JONES, G., FIELDING, D. W., TODD, P. J. and TOMLINSON, M. (1978) Breast feeding as protection against respiratory syncytial virus. *British Medical Journal,* **2,** 1434

FALLOT, M. E., BOYD, J. L. III and OSKI, F. A. (1980) Breast feeding reduces incidences of hospital admissions for infection in infants. *Pediatrics,* **65,** 1121–1124

FAWCETT, J. and PARRY, H. E. (1957) Lung changes in pertussis and measles in childhood. A review of 1894 cases with a follow-up study of the pulmonary complications. *British Journal of Radiology,* **30,** 76–82

FERGUSSON, D. M., HORWOOD, L. J. and SHANNON, F. T. (1980) Parental smoking and respiratory illness in infancy. *Archives of Disease in Childhood,* **55,** 358–361

FLETCHER, C., PETO, R., TINKER, C. and SPEIZER, F. E. (1976) *The Natural History of Chronic Bronchitis and Emphysema.* Oxford: Oxford University Press

FOUCARD, T., BERG, T., JOHANSSON, S. G. O. and WAHRAN, B. (1971) Virus serology and serum IgE levels in children with asthmatoid bronchitis. *Acta Paediatrica Scandinavica,* **60,** 621–629

FREEMAN, G. L. and TODD, R. H. (1962) The role of allergy in viral respiratory tract infections. *American Journal of Diseases of Children,* **104,** 44–48

FRICK, O. L., GERMAN, D. F. and MILLS, J. (1979) Development of allergy in children. Associations with virus infections. *Journal of Allergy and Clinical Immunology,* **63,** 228–241

GIVAN, D., SCOTT, P., JEGLUM, E. and EISEN, H. (1981) Lung function and airway reactivity in children 3–10 years after foreign body aspiration. *American Review of Respiratory Disease,* **123,** Suppl: 158 (abstract)

GOLD, R., WILT, J. C., ADHIKARI, P. K. and MACPHERSON, R. I. (1969) Adenoviral pneumonia and its complications in infancy and childhood. *Journal of the Canadian Association of Radiologists,* **20,** 218–224

GURWITZ, D., COREY, M. and LEVISON, H. (1980) Pulmonary function and bronchial reactivity in children after croup. *American Review of Respiratory Disease,* **122,** 95–99

GURWITZ, D., KATTAN, M. and LEVISON, H. (1978) Pulmonary function abnormalities in asymptomatic children after hydrocarbon pneumonitis. *Pediatrics,* **62,** 789–794

GURWITZ, D., MINDORFF, C. and LEVISON, H. (1981) Increased incidence of bronchial reactivity in children with a history of bronchiolitis. *Journal of Pediatrics,* **98,** 551–555

HALL, C. B. (1980) Prevention of infection with respiratory syncytial virus: the hopes and hurdles ahead. *Review of Infectious Diseases,* **2,** 384

HARLAP, S. and DAVIES, A. M. (1974) Infant admission to hospital and maternal smoking. *Lancet,* **i,** 529–532

HARRISON, H. R., TAUSSIG, M. and FULGINITI, V. A. (1982) *Chlamydia trachomatis* and chronic respiratory disease in childhood. *Paediatric Infectious Diseases,* **1,** 29–33

HARROD, J. R., L'HEUREUX, P., WANGENSTEEN, O. D. and HUNT, C. E. (1974) Long-term follow-up of severe respiratory distress syndrome treated with IPPB. *Journal of Pediatrics,* **84,** 277–286

HASSELBLAD, V., HUMBLE, C. G., GRAHAM, M. G. and ANDERSON, H. S. (1981) Indoor environmental determinants of lung function in *American Review of Respiratory Disease,* **123,** 479–485

HENDERSON, F. W., HYDE, W. A., COLLIER, A. M. *et al.* (1979) The etiologic and epidemiological spectrum of bronchiolitis in pediatric practice. *Journal of Pediatrics,* **95,** 183–190

HENRY, R. L., MILNER, A. D., STOKES, G. M., HODGES, I. G. C. and GROGGINS, R. C. (1983) Lung function after acute bronchiolitis. *Archives of Disease in Childhood,* **58,** 60–63

HOGG, J. C., WILLIAMS, J., RICHARDSON, J. B., MACKLEM, P. T. and THURLBECK, W. M. (1970) Age as a factor in the distribution of lower airway conductance and in the pathological anatomy of obstructive lung disease. *New England Journal of Medicine,* **282,** 1283–1287

HOLLAND, W. W. (1982) Beginnings of bronchitis (editorial). *Thorax,* **37,** 401–403

HOLLAND, W. W., BAILEY, P. and BLAND, J. M. (1978) Long-term consequences of respiratory disease in infancy. *Journal of Epidemiology and Community Health,* **32,** 256–259

HOLLAND, W. W., HALIL, T., BENNETT, A. E. and ELLIOTT, A. (1969) Factors influencing the onset of chronic respiratory disease. *British Medical Journal,* **2,** 205–208

HUTCHINSON-SMITH, B. H. (1970) The relationship between the weight of an infant and lower respiratory tract infection. *The Medical Officer,* **123,** 257–262

HUXTABLE, K. A., TUCKER, A. S. and WEDGEWOOD, R. J. (1964) Staphylococcal pneumonia in childhood. *American Journal of Diseases of Children,* **108,** 262–269

HYDE, J. S. and SAED, A. M. (1966) Acute bronchiolitis and the asthmatic child. *Journal of Asthma Research,* **4,** 137–154

INSELMAN, L. S. and MELLINS, R. B. (1981) Growth and development of the lung. *Journal of Pediatrics,* **98,** 1–15

JERNELIUS, H. (1964) Pertussis with pulmonary complications – a follow-up study. *Acta Paediatrica Scandinavica,* **53,** 247–254

JOHNSON, J. D., MALACHOWSKI, N. C., GROBSTEIN, R., WELSH, D., DAILY, W. J. R. and SUNSHINE, P. (1974) Prognosis of children surviving with the aid of mechanical ventilation in the newborn period. *Journal of Pediatrics,* **84,** 272–276

KAMPER, J. (1978) Long-term prognosis of infants with severe idiopathic respiratory distress syndrome. Cardio-pulmonary outcome. *Acta Paediatrica Scandinavica,* **67,** 71–76

KATTAN, M., KEENS, T. G., LAPIERRE, J. G., LEVISON, H., BRYAN, A. C. and REILLY, B. J. (1977) Pulmonary function abnormalities in symptom-free children after bronchiolitis. *Pediatrics,* **59,** 683–688

KATTAN, M., LEVISON, H. and BRYAN, A. C. (1978) Lung mechanics in asymptomatic children after bronchiolitis. *American Review of Respiratory Disease,* **2,** (Suppl.), 357

KIERNAN, K. E., COLLEY, J. R. T., DOUGLAS, J. W. B. and REID, D. D. (1976) Chronic cough in young adults in relation to smoking habits, childhood environment and chest illness. *Respiration,* **33,** 236–244

KITAGAWA, M., HISLOP, A., BOYDEN, E. A. and REID, R. (1971) Lung hypoplasia in congenital diaphragmatic nerma. A quantitative study of airway, artery and alveolar development. *British Journal of Surgery,* **58,** 342–346

KJELLMAN, B. (1968) Lung function in children with pneumonia. *Scandinavian Journal of Respiratory Disease,* **49,** 185–201

LAING, I., RIEDEL, F., YAP, P. L. and SIMPSON, H. (1982) Atopy predisposing to acute bronchiolitis during an epidemic of respiratory syncytial virus. *British Medical Journal,* **284,** 1070–1072

LAKS, H., WILKINSON, R. H. and SCHUSTER, S. R. (1972) Long-term results following correction of esophageal atresia with tracheo-esophageal fistula. A clinical trial and cine flurographic study. *Journal of Paediatric Surgery,* **7,** 591–597

LANNING, P., SIMILA, S. and LINNA, O. (1980) Late pulmonary sequelae after type 7 adenovirus pneumonia. *Annales de Radiologie (Paris),* **23,** 132–136

LAUGHLIN, J. J. and EIGEN, H. (1982) Pulmonary function abnormalities in survivors of near-drowning. *Journal of Pediatrics,* **100,** 26–30

LAUGHLIN, G. M. and TAUSSIG, L. M. (1979) Pulmonary function in children with a history of laryngotracheobronchitis. *Journal of Pediatrics,* **94,** 365–369

LEBOWITZ, M. D. and BURROWS, B. (1976) Respiratory symptoms related to smoking habits of family adults. *Chest,* **69,** 48–50

LEEDER, S. R., CORKHILL, R. T., WYSOCKI, M. J. and HOLLAND, W. W. (1976) Influence of personal and family factors on ventilatory function of children. *British Journal of Preventive and Social Medicine,* **30,** 219–224

LEES, A. W. (1950) Atelectesis and bronchiectasis in pertussis. *British Medical Journal,* **2,** 1138–1144

LEWIS, S. (1968) A follow-up study of the respiratory distress syndrome. *Proceedings of Royal Society of Medicine,* **61,** 771–773

LOURDES, R., LAYAYA-CUASAY, L. R., DE FOREST, A., JUFF, D., LISCHNER, H. and LIUANG, N. N. (1977) Chronic pulmonary complications of early influenza infection in children. *American Review of Respiratory Diseases,* **116,** 617–625

LUNN, J. E., KNOWELDEN, J. and HANDYSIDE, A. J. (1967) Patterns of respiratory illness in Sheffield infant school children. *British Journal of Preventive and Social Medicine,* **21,** 7–16

LUNN, J. E., KNOWELDEN, J. and ROE, J. W. (1970) Patterns of respiratory illness in Sheffield junior school children. A follow-up study. *British Journal of Preventive and Social Medicine,* **24,** 223–228

MACKLEM, P. T. (1973) The pathophysiology of chronic bronchitis and emphysema. *Medical Clinics of North America,* **57,** 669–679

McNICOL, K. N. and WILLIAMS, H. (1973) Spectrum of asthma in children. 1. Clinical and physiological components. *British Medical Journal,* **4,** 7–11

MANSELL, A., BRYAN, C. and LEVISON, H. (1972) Airway closure in children. *Journal of Applied Physiology,* **33,** 711–714

MARTIN, A. J., LANDAU, L. I. and PHELAN, P. D. (1980) Lung function in young adults who had asthma in childhood. *American Review of Respiratory Diseases,* **122,** 609–615

MARTIN, A. J., MCLENNAN, L. A., LANDAU, L. I. and PHELAN, P. D. (1980) The natural history of childhood asthma to adult life. *British Medical Journal,* **1,** 1397–1400

MELLIS, C. M. and LEVISON, H. (1978) Bronchial reactivity in cystic fibrosis. *Pediatrics,* **61,** 446–450

MILLIGAN, D. W. A. and LEVISON, H. (1979) Lung function in children following repair of tracheo-esophageal fistula. *Journal Pediatrics,* **95,** 24–27

MOK, J. Y. Q. and SIMPSON, H. (1982) Outcome of acute lower respiratory tract infection in infants: preliminary report of seven year follow-up study. *British Medical Journal,* **285,** 333–337

MOK, J. Y. Q. and SIMPSON, H. (1984a) Outcome for acute bronchitis, bronchiolitis and pneumonia in infancy. *Archives of Disease in Childhood,* **59,** 306–309

MOK, J. Y. Q. and SIMPSON, H. (1984b) Symptoms, atopy and bronchial reactivity after lower respiratory infection in infancy. *Archives of Disease in Childhood,* **59,** 299–305

MOK, J. Y. Q., WAUGH, P. R. and SIMPSON, H. (1979) *Mycoplasma pneumoniae* infection. A follow-up study of 50 children with respiratory illness. *Archives of Disease in Childhood,* **54,** 506–511

MORSE, J. O. (1978) Alpha-antitrypsin deficiency. *New England Journal of Medicine,* **299,** 1045–1048; 1099–1105

NIEWOEHNER, D. E., KLEINERMAN, J. and RICE, D. B. (1974) Pathological changes in the peripheral airways of young cigarette smokers. *New England Journal of Medicine,* **291,** 755–758

NORMAN-TAYLOR, W. and DICKINSON, V. A. (1972) Danger for children in smoking families. *Community Medicine,* **128,** 32–33

NORTHWAY, W. H., ROSAN, R. C. and PORTER, D. Y. (1967) Pulmonary disease following respiratory therapy of hyaline membrane disease. *New England Journal of Medicine,* **276,** 357–368

OSWALD, N. C., HAROLD, J. T. and MARTIN, W. J. (1953) Clinical patterns of chronic bronchitis. *Lancet,* **ii,** 639–643

OUTERBRIDGE, E. W., NOBRADY, M. B. and BEAUDRY, P. H. (1972) Idiopathic respiratory distress syndrome. Recurrent respiratory illness in survivors. *American Journal of Diseases of Children,* **123,** 99–104

PERRY, K. M. A. and KING, D. S. (1940) Bronchiectasis. A study of prognosis based on follow-up of 1400 patients. *American Review of Tuberculosis,* **41,** 531

PHELAN, P. D. (1984) Does adult chronic obstructive lung disease really begin in childhood. *British Journal of Diseases of the Chest,* **78,** (1), 1–9

PHELAN, P. D., WILLIAMS, H. E. and FREEMAN, M. (1968) The disturbances of ventilation in acute viral bronchiolitis. *Australian Paediatrics Journal,* **4,** 96–104

POLGAR, G. and WENG, T. R. (1979) The functional development of the respiratory system. From the period of gestation to adulthood. *American Review of Respiratory Diseases,* **120,** 625–695

POLMAR, S. H., ROBINSON, L. D. and MINNEFOR, A. R. (1972) Immunoglobulin E in bronchiolitis. *Pediatrics,* **50,** 276–284

PULLAN, C. R. and HEY, E. N. (1982) Wheezing, asthma and pulmonary dysfunction 10 years after infection with respiratory syncytial virus in infancy. *British Medical Journal,* **284,** 1665–1669

REID, D. D. (1969) The beginning of bronchitis. *Proceedings of the Royal Society of Medicine,* **62,** 311–316

REID, L. (1977) The lung: its growth and remodelling in health and disease. *American Journal of Roentgenology,* **129,** 777–788

ROBINSON, R. (LA) (1981) Whooping cough immunisation controversy. *Archives of Disease in Childhood,* **56,** 577–580

RONA, R. J., FLOREY, C. DUV., CLARKE, G. C. and CHINN, S. (1981) Parental smoking at home and height of children. *British Medical Journal,* **283,** 1363

ROONEY, J. C. and WILLIAMS, H. E. (1971) The relationship between proved viral bronchiolitis and subsequent wheezing. *Journal of Pediatrics,* **79,** 744–747

SAMET, J. M., TAGER, I. B. and SPEIZER, F. E. (1983) The relationship between respiratory illness in childhood and chronic air-flow obstruction in adulthood. *American Review of Respiratory Diseases,* **127,** 508–523

SCHILLING, R. S. F., LETAI, A. D., HUI, S. L., BECK, G. J., SCHOENBERG, J. B. and BOUHUYS, A. (1977) Lung function, respiratory disease, and smoking in families. *American Journal of Epidemiology,* **106,** 274–283

SCISLICKI, A., RUDNIK, J., GAWEL, J. and PRYJMA, J. (1978) The risk of bronchial asthma in children with a history of obstructive bronchitis in the first two years of life. *Archivum Immunologiae et Therapiae Experimentalis*, **26**, 723–729

SHARRATT, M. T. and CERNY, F. J. (1979) Pulmonary function and health status of children in two cities of different air quality: a pilot study. *Archives of Environmental Health*, **34**, 114–119

SHEPARD, F. M., JOHNSTON, R. B., KLATTE, E. C., BURKO, H. and STAHLMAN, M. (1968) Residual pulmonary findings in clinical hyaline membrane disease. *New England Journal of Medicine*, **279**, 1063–1071

SIMILA, S., YLIKORKALA, O. and WASZ-HOCKERT, O. (1971) Type 7 adenovirus pneumonia. *Journal of Pediatrics*, **79**, 605–611

SIMON, G. and JORDAN, W. S. JR (1969) Infectious and allergic aspects of bronchiolitis. *Journal of Pediatrics*, **70**, 533–538

SIMS, D. G., DOWNHAM, M. A. P. S., GARDNER, P. S., WEBB, J. K. G. and WEIGHTMAN, D. (1978) Study of 8-year-old children with a history of respiratory syncytial virus bronchiolitis in infancy. *British Medical Journal*, **1**, 11–14

SIMS, D. G., GARDNER, P. S., WIGHTMAN, D., TURNER, M. W. and SOOTHILL, J. F. (1981) Atopy does not predispose to RSV bronchitis or post-bronchiolitic wheezing. *British Medical Journal*, **282**, 2086–2088

SPEIZER, F. E. and TAGER, I. B. (1979) Epidemiology of chronic mucus hypersecretion and obstructive airways disease. *Epidemial Review*, **1**, 124–142

STEBBINGS, J. H. and FOGLEMAN, D. G. (1977) Identifying a susceptible subgroup, effect of the Pittsburgh air pollution episode upon school children. *American Journal of Epidemiology*, **110**, 27–40

STOCKS, J. and GODFREY, S. (1976) The role of artificial ventilation oxygen and CPAP in the pathogenesis of lung damage in neonates: assessment by serial measurements of lung function. *Pediatrics*, 352–362

STOKES, D., SIGLER, A., KHOURI, N. F. and TALAMO, R. C. (Jan. 1978) Unilateral hyperlucent lung (Swyer–James syndrome) after severe mycoplasma pneumoniae infection. *American Review of Respiratory Diseases*, **117**(1), 145–152

STOKES, G. M., MILNER, A. D., HODGES, I. G. C. and GROGGINS, R. C. (1981) Lung function abnormalities after acute bronchiolitis. *Journal of Pediatrics*, **98**, 871–874

STRIEDER, D. J. (1974) Pediatric origins of chronic obstructive lung disease (editorial). *Bull Europeen de Physio-pathologie Respiratoire*, **10**(3), 273–279

TAGER, I. B., WEISS, S. T., MUNOZ, A., ROSNER, B. and SPEIZER, F. E. (1983) Longitudinal study of the effects of maternal smoking on pulmonary function in children. *New England Journal of Medicine*, **309**, 699–703

TAGER, I. B., WEISS, S. T., ROSNER, R. and SPEIZER, F. E. (1979) Effect of parental cigarette smoking on the pulmonary function of children. *American Journal of Epidemiology*, **110**, 15–26

TAUSSIG, L. M., CASTRO, O., LANDAU, L. and BEAUDRY, P. H. (1977) Pulmonary function 8 to 10 years after hydrocarbon pneumonitis. Normal findings in three children carefully studied. *Clinical Pediatrics*, **16**, 57–59

THURLBECK, W. M. (1976) *Chronic Airflow Obstruction in Lung Disease*. Philadelphia: W. B. Saunders Company

THURLBECK, W. M. (1979) Changes in lung structure. In *The Lung in the Transition between Health and Disease*, Eds P. T. Machlem and S. Permutt, pp. 17–41. New York: Marcel Dekker Inc.

TOYAMA, T. (1964) Air pollution and its health effects in Japan. *Archives of Environmental Health*, **8**, 153–173

WAHDAN, M. H. M. E. (1963) Atmospheric pollution and other environmental factors in respiratory disease of children. University of London: PhD thesis

WARNER, K. E. and MURT, H. A. (1982) Impact of the antismoking campaign on smoking prevalence. A cohort analysis. *Journal of Public Health Policy*, **3**(4), 374–390

WATKINS, C. J., LEEDER, S. R. and CORKHILL, R. T. (1979) The relationship between breast and bottle feeding and respiratory illness in the first year of life. *Journal of Epidemiology and Community Health*, **33**, 180–182

WEISS, S. T., TAGER, I. B., SPEIZER, F. E. and ROSNER, B. (1980) Persistent wheeze: its relation to respiratory illness, cigarette smoking, and level of pulmonary function in a population sample of children. *American Review of Respiratory Diseases*, **122**, 697–707

WELLIVER, R. C., KAUL, T. N. and OGRA, P. L. (1979) Cell mediated immune response to respiratory syncytial virus infection: relationship to the development of reactive airway disease. *Journal of Pediatrics*, **94**, 370–375

WETHERALL, D. J. (1982) *The New Genetics and Clinical Practice*. London: The Nuffield Provincial Hospital Trust

WHITE, R., FINBERG, L. and TRAMER, A. (1964) The modern morbidity of pertussis in infants. *Pediatrics*, **33**, 705–710

WILLIAMS, H. and MCNICHOL, K. N. (1969) Prevalence, natural history, and relationship of wheezy bronchitis and asthma in children; an epidemiological study. *British Medical Journal,* **4,** 321–325

WILSON, M. G. and MIKITY, V. G. (1960) A new form of respiratory disease in premature infants. *American Journal of Diseases of Children,* **99,** 489–499

WITTIG, H. J., CRANFORD, N. J. and GLASER, J. (1959) The relationship between bronchiolitis and childhood asthma – a follow-up study of 100 cases of bronchiolitis in infancy. *Journal of Allergy,* **30,** 19–23

WOHL, M. E. B., GRISCOM, J. T. and STREIDER, D. S. (1977) The lung following repair of congenital diaphragmatic hernia. *Journal of Pediatrics,* **90,** 405–414

WOHL, M. E. B., STIGOL, L. C. and MEAD, J. (1969) Resistance of the total respiratory system in healthy infants and infants with bronchiolitis. *Pediatrics,* **43,** 495–509

WONG, Y. C., BEARDSMORE, C. S. and SILVERMAN, M. (1982) Pulmonary sequelae of neonatal respiratory distress in very low birthweight infants: a clinical and physiological study. *Archives of Disease in Childhood,* **57,** 418–424

WOOLCOCK, A., LEEDER, S., PEAT, J. and BLACKBURN, C. (1977) The influence of bronchitis and asthma in infancy and childhood on lung function in schoolchildren. *Chest,* **77** (2 suppl.), 251

YARNELL, J. W. G. and ST LEGER, A. S. (1977) Housing conditions, respiratory illness, and lung function in children in South Wales. *British Journal of Preventive and Social Medicine,* **31,** 183–188

ZAK, M., ERBEN, A. and OLINSKY, A. (1981) Croup, recurrent croup, allergy and airways hyper-reactivity. *Archives of Disease in Childhood,* **56,** 336–341

ZAPLETAL, A., JECH, J. and KASPARJ SAMANEK, M. (1977) Flow–volume curves as a method for detecting airway obstruction in children from an air-polluted area. *Bulletin Europeen de Physiopathologie Respiratoire,* **13,** 803–812

ZAPLETAL, A., JECH, J., PAUL, T. and KASPARJ SAMANEK, M. (1973) Pulmonary function studies in children living in an air polluted area. *American Review of Respiratory Disease,* **107,** 400–409

ZWEIMAN, B., SCHOENWETTER, W. F. and HILDRETH, E. A. (1966) The relationship between bronchiolitis and allergic asthma. A prospective study with allergy evaluation. *Journal of Allergy,* **37,** 48–53

ZWEIMAN, B., SCHOENWETTER, W. F., PAPPANO, J. E. and TEMPEST, B. (1971) Patterns of allergic respiratory disease in children with a past history of bronchiolitis. *Journal of Allergy and Clinical Immunology,* **48,** 283–289

Index